Neurochemistry and Biochemical Neuropharmacology of Drug Addiction

Neurochemistry and Biochemical Neuropharmacology of Drug Addiction

By

Huma Ikram

Cambridge Scholars Publishing

Neurochemistry and Biochemical Neuropharmacology of Drug Addiction

By Huma Ikram

This book first published 2025

Cambridge Scholars Publishing

Lady Stephenson Library, Newcastle upon Tyne, NE6 2PA, UK

British Library Cataloguing in Publication Data
A catalogue record for this book is available from the British Library

ISBN: 978-1-0364-4863-9
ISBN (Ebook): 978-1-0364-4864-6

DEDICATED

to the Light of Knowledge

Hazrat Muhammad (PBUH),

whose wisdom illuminates

every path to understanding

TABLE OF CONTENTS

Preface ix

About the author xiii

Chapter 1 1
Etiology and neurochemical basis of drug addiction

Chapter 2 31
Physical versus psychological addiction

Chapter 3 69
Positive and negative reinforcement

Chapter 4 113
Common features of drug addiction

Chapter 5 143
Commonly abused drugs

Chapter 6 176
Role of dopamine in drug addiction

Chapter 7 215
Role of serotonin in drug addiction

Chapter 8 246
Comorbidity of stress, depression, and drug addiction

Chapter 9 285
Animal models of drug addiction

Chapter 10 314
Pharmacotherapeutic approaches to treat drug addiction

Chapter 11 365
Current advancements in the diagnostics of drug addiction

Chapter 12 394
Current advancements in the pharmacotherapy of drug addiction

References 447

PREFACE

The impetus for this book arose from a combination of professional curiosity and a deep-seated desire to contribute to the betterment of those grappling with addiction. In these pages, you will find a comprehensive exploration of the complex tapestry of genetic, environmental, and neurobiological factors that underpin addiction. This book is like a bridge connecting the often-disparate worlds of scientific research and clinical practice, intended to enlighten and inform a diverse audience. One of the book's primary inspirations has been to shed light on the latest advancements in treatment approaches. From the therapeutic targeting of serotonin to the role of stress and depression in addiction, and the burgeoning field of personalized medicine, each chapter is created to highlight cutting-edge methods and theories in addiction treatment. Moreover, in an era where ethical considerations and policy decisions play a crucial role in shaping research and treatment modalities, this book does not shy away from addressing these vital aspects, particularly in the context of animal research and shifts towards decriminalization and public health approaches in dealing with substance abuse.

Personalization and precision in treatment are themes that recur throughout this work. Recognizing the unique biological and psychological makeup of each individual suffering from addiction, the book emphasizes the importance of tailoring diagnostic and treatment approaches to these individual characteristics. In doing so, it underscores my belief in the transformative potential of precision medicine in revolutionizing addiction treatment. The role of public health and community engagement in combating drug abuse is another cornerstone of this text. With the understanding that addiction is not just an individual battle but a societal issue, the book delves into how community involvement and public health perspectives can significantly impact the fight against drug abuse.

As you embark on this journey through the pages, I invite you to approach this book not just as a repository of knowledge but as a gateway to understanding the multifaceted and dynamic nature of addiction. It is my hope that the insights contained herein will not only inform but also inspire and guide those who seek to understand and address this complex condition. In investigating the of addiction, one must recognize its inherent complexity. It is not a condition that can be pigeonholed into simplistic explanations or one-size-fits-all solutions. Each chapter of this book has been designed to provide you with a holistic understanding of drug addiction, to reflect this complexity, breaking down the scientific jargon into concepts that are accessible and understandable to our diverse readership.

In addressing the challenges of addiction, I have always been motivated by a fundamental question: How can we improve the lives of those suffering from this condition? This question has guided my research, teaching, and now, the writing of this book. The neurochemical basis of addiction, the role of dopamine and serotonin, and the comorbidity of stress, depression, and drug addiction are not mere academic discussions. They are an attempt to provide a foundation upon which effective and empathetic treatments can be built. The use of animal models in drug addiction research highlights the ethical dimensions of our quest to understand addiction. This discussion is crucial, for it emphasize the responsibility that comes with scientific inquiry - a responsibility to conduct research that is not only rigorous but also respectful of the ethical boundaries that govern our work. As we move towards an era where pharmacotherapy is increasingly personalized, the chapters detailing current and future advancements in diagnostics and treatment underscore the exciting potential of this field. The integration of digital health technologies, a topic touched upon in the book, is particularly promising. It exemplifies how innovation can enhance our ability to monitor, understand, and ultimately treat addiction more effectively.

The intersection of public health perspectives with the clinical and neurobiological aspects of addiction is a theme that runs deeply through this text, is a reflection of my belief that the battle against drug addiction cannot be won in isolation. It requires a concerted effort that encompasses not only individual treatment but also community involvement and societal change. This book, therefore, not only speaks to the individual struggling with addiction but also to the community leaders, policymakers, and public health professionals who play a pivotal role in shaping the environment in which recovery occurs. Moreover, the chapters dedicated to the comorbidity of stress, depression, and drug addiction, and the pharmacotherapeutic approaches to treat drug addiction, are particularly close to my heart. They represent a synthesis of my clinical observations and research findings, offering insights into how these interrelated conditions can be more effectively managed. The complexity of these interconnections demands a treatment approach that is as multifaceted as the conditions themselves, and this book endeavors to provide that comprehensive perspective.

In writing this book, I have been acutely aware of my responsibility as an educator and a researcher. The task of distilling years of scientific inquiry and clinical experience into a format that is both informative and accessible has been both daunting and exhilarating. I have strived to ensure that each chapter not only conveys the latest scientific knowledge but also resonates with the experiences and challenges faced by those at the frontlines of dealing with addiction. As we delve into discussing current advancements in diagnostics and the pharmacotherapy of drug addiction, it becomes apparent that we are on the cusp of a new era in addiction treatment. The potential of leveraging genetics, neuroimaging, and advanced technologies to enhance the precision of diagnostics and treatment is immense. This book aims to provide a glimpse into that future, offering hope and direction to those seeking to understand and combat addiction. The exploration of current advancements in diagnostics and pharmacotherapy is a testament to the remarkable progress made in the field. Yet, it also focuses on the necessity for continued research and innovation. As we advance in our scientific understanding, new challenges and questions arise, demanding adaptive and creative solutions. The book, therefore, is not just a snapshot of the current state of addiction treatment; it is a call to arms for continued exploration and discovery.

The discussions on the role of dopamine and serotonin in drug addiction, for instance, go beyond mere scientific inquiry. They are an attempt to demystify the neurochemical underpinnings of addiction, providing a foundation for empathy and compassion in treatment approaches. Understanding the biochemical pathways of addiction is crucial not only for developing effective treatments but also for fostering a more informed and less judgmental view of those struggling with addiction. In these pages, I have endeavored to present a balanced view, acknowledging both the achievements and the ongoing challenges in the field of drug addiction. It is my hope that this book will serve as a valuable resource for all those who seek to understand this complex condition.

In the intricate world of addiction, every thread of knowledge, every strand of compassion, and every weave of innovation brings us closer to a recovery and hope. Our collective efforts in understanding and treating addiction are not just a scientific endeavor, but a profound commitment to the betterment of human lives. The book explores the complexities of drug addiction with compassion and scientific insights, guiding the way towards effective, personalized, and empathetic approaches towards drug addiction.

To conclude, I would like to express my heartfelt thanks to all those who have supported and inspired me in the writing of this book specially my dear brother **Muhammad Inam ul Haq** who had always been an inspiration to me. The journey of its creation has been a deeply personal one, filled with learning, growth, and reflection. It is my sincere wish that this book will contribute meaningfully to the ongoing conversation about drug addiction, offering insights, hope, and direction to all those it reaches. I would like to extend my deepest gratitude to the countless individuals who have contributed to the journey of this book. From the patients who have shared their stories and struggles with me, my fellow researchers and collaborators who have provided invaluable insights, and to the students who have inspired me with their passion and curiosity – this book is as much yours as it is mine.

Dr. Huma Ikram

12-7-2024

ABOUT THE AUTHOR

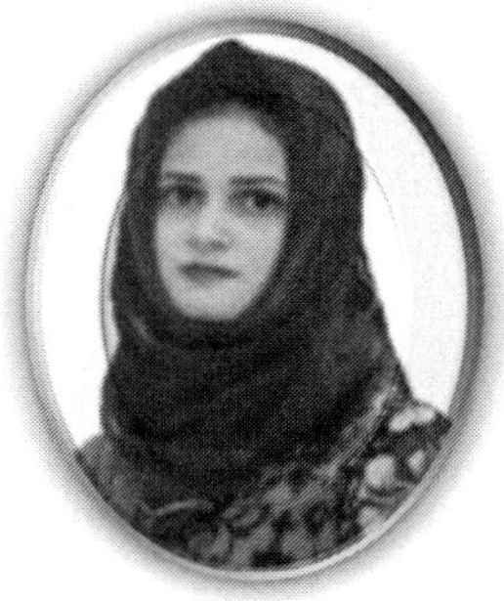

The author of this book, Dr. Huma Ikram, is an esteemed figure in the field of biochemistry and neuropharmacology, presenting a career marked by distinguished academic accomplishments and profound contributions to scientific research and education. Her role as an Assistant Professor at the University of Karachi emphasizes her dedication to academia. She is in charge of the preclinical trials facility at the Department of Biochemistry. Here, she not only imparted knowledge to graduate and postgraduate students but also supervised numerous M.Phil. and Ph.D. students, nurturing the next generation of scientists and researchers. Her publications span a wide array of topics within neuropharmacology, particularly focusing on addiction. These studies, often involving intricate animal models, have added valuable insights into the understanding of neurochemical processes and their implications in human health and behavior. Her research excellence has been recognized with a series of best presentations and best poster awards at various national and international scientific conferences, research grants and research patent granted to her.

Dr. Ikram is also a member of various prestigious organizations. Her editorial work further cements her status as a thought leader in her field. Dr. Ikram's commitment to organizing scientific events and workshops highlights her dedication to advancing scientific knowledge. Her commitment to staying updated with the latest scientific developments and methodologies is a testament to her dedication to her field. Beyond her research and teaching, Dr. Ikram has been an active participant and organizer of various scientific events and workshops. She has been instrumental in organizing research seminars on, contributing to the broader understanding and appreciation of scientific research and its applications. Dr. Ikram's professional journey is a testament to her versatility as a scientist, educator, and leader in biochemical neuropharmacology. Her relentless pursuit of knowledge, combined with her contributions to the scientific community, makes her an exceptional role model for aspiring scientists, particularly in the developing world.

CHAPTER 1

ETIOLOGY AND NEUROCHEMICAL BASIS OF DRUG ADDICTION

"Though no one can go back and make a brand new start, anyone can start from now and make a brand new ending."
~ Carl Bard

A fresh beginning awaits in understanding the deep roots of addiction, where science unveils the mysteries of the brain and basics of differences in individual susceptibilities towards addiction. The exploration of the etiology and neurochemical foundations of drug addiction unveils the intricate web of factors contributing to the development and persistence of addictive behaviors. Understanding the roots and neurochemical underpinnings of drug addiction is paramount in deciphering the complex interplay between biological, psychological, and environmental elements that drive the addictive process.

Drug addiction is defined as compulsive use of drug despite its negative consequences. Goals of the addicted person become narrowed to obtaining, using, and recovering from drugs, despite failure in life roles, medical illness, risk of incarceration, and other problems. An important characteristic of addiction is its stubborn persistence and irrelevancy with the surroundings. There could be an illusionary world in which the drug addict has his own standards of good or bad, right or wrong and truth or lies. The state of mind could be quite confused, and justifications could be irrational. There drug addicts have their own imaginary world in which they seek shelter from their real life problems. These problems could be as trifle as relationship issues to as complicated as financial issues, bankruptcy, or loss of near and dear ones under unexplainable circumstances. Rather than facing these issues and everyday challenges of life, a person may want to run away and use temporary solutions such as drug addiction to get rid of these issues temporarily. Things further get worse if such victims have other family members dependent on them. The layman's definition of addiction is a "fact or condition of being addicted to a particular substance, thing, or activity." Medically it is a "chronic, relapsing disorder characterized by compulsive drug seeking, continued use despite harmful consequence, and long-lasting changes in the brain." Current Oxford English dictionary definition can be traced back to Roman law in which addiction was a "formal giving over by sentence of the court" (Kranzler and Li, 2008). Drug addiction is a chronically relapsing disorder, and this feature presents too many challenges while treating drug abuse. Use of abusive agents produces certain changes in the brain which are irreversible, and this might involve several factors such as altered sensitivity of certain receptors, up/down regulation of certain receptors/enzymes and signaling molecules. Relapse makes individual vulnerable to drug abuse once he is facing the environmental cues associated with drug abuse. This could be a possible accompanying person, place of drug abuse or any particular memorable object associated with drug abuse. These cues could be either physical, psychological, emotional or social.

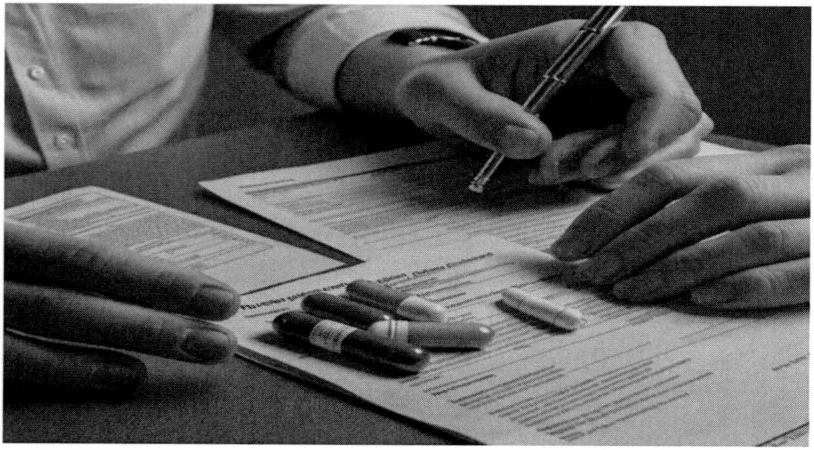

Drug addiction is a chronically relapsing disorder

According to initial hypothesis, addiction (particularly heroin addiction) was supposed to be the outcome of criminal behavior or 'weak will'. An addiction to drugs has now been recognized as a neurological disease and current research efforts focus on a better understanding of the involved molecular, cellular and physiological mechanisms. There is vulnerability to environmental, drug induced as well as genetic factors in the development of addiction to abusive drugs. Early life experiences could greatly influence later neurobehavioral developments and person's susceptibility to stress.

Genetic factors influencing drug abuse: Amid the myriad of factors, genetic predispositions play a pivotal role in the drug addiction which is characterized as a complex behavioral disorder. Advances in genetic research have unveiled specific genes and molecular pathways associated with susceptibility to substance abuse. This exploration delves into the intricate world of genes involved in drug addiction, providing insights from seminal studies in the field. Human studies suggest the important role of genetic background in the development of alcohol related disorders. Addiction is supposed to run in families just like other disorders. However, genetics alone, could not be the sole reason for the development of addiction towards certain drug. There are other factors in addition to the genetic makeup of certain individual, which make person susceptible to drug addiction. Possible genetic-environment interactions have been suggested to have pivotal role in drug preference, consumption and intoxication. The gene-environment interaction research on substance use behavior is methodologically multidimensional. It is difficult to state that the maladaptive patterns of drug taking are influenced by which single source of significant influence. Conducting pooled analysis is really difficult in case of such multidimensional methodological studies. In a study conducted by Jiang et al., (2023), it was demonstrated that about 61.5% of studies on the 5HTTLPR gene, 100% on the MAOA gene, 42.9% on the DRD2 gene, 50% on the DRD4 gene, 50% on the DAT gene, 80% on the CRHR1 gene, 100% on the OPRM1 gene, 100% on the GABRA1 gene, and 50% on the CHRNA gene had a significant gene-environment interaction effect.

Psychiatric outcomes in the offspring are indirectly mediated by the parental genes through the environment that parents create for their children. Family setup, attitudes of family members, types of social gatherings, home environment and other factors determine indirectly influence the tendency of offspring to abuse drugs, provided that either or both of the parents have abused drugs. These indirect genetic effects, also known as genetic nurture, could explain individual differences in common internalizing and externalizing psychiatric symptoms during childhood. The overall contribution of parental genetic nurture effects could be assessed by the advanced statistical genetic methods leverage data from families (Jami et al., 2023).

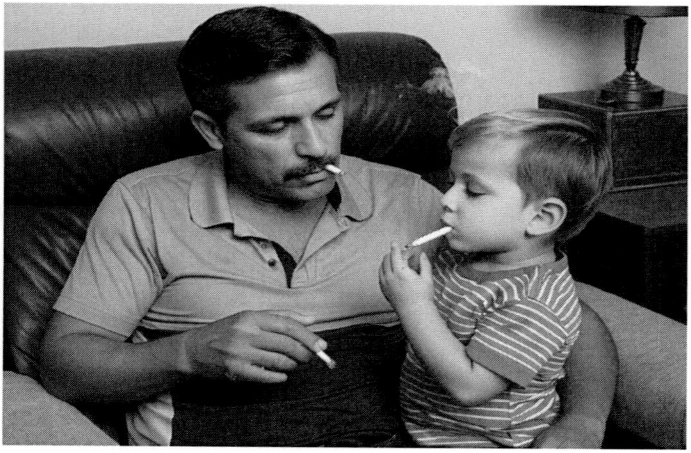

Genetic factors influence drug abuse

Genetic factors are supposed to be responsible for the high tendency to commit suicide in drug abusers. This comorbidity might result due to genetic and other factors encompassing suicidal behavior and drug abuse. Factors pushing the individual towards drug abuse or committing suicide are more likely to coexist. Each of these outcomes should be considered as a risk for the other. The major underlying cause could be depression and a failure to cope with it might lead to drug abuse and in the long run, a failure to receive the drug for rewarding effects would result in relapse and this might lead the patient to consider suicide as an option to escape the situation which becomes uncontrollable. In such individuals, with family history of drug abuse, focus should be on joint prevention and treatment of drug abuse and suicidal behavior. The underlying nature of these outcomes could be polygenic considering moderate environmental correlations between the two. In a study conducted by Edwards et al., (2023), it has been shown that there is a strong genetic correlation between suicidal deaths and substance abuse disorders with little overall variance; and unique environmental correlations.

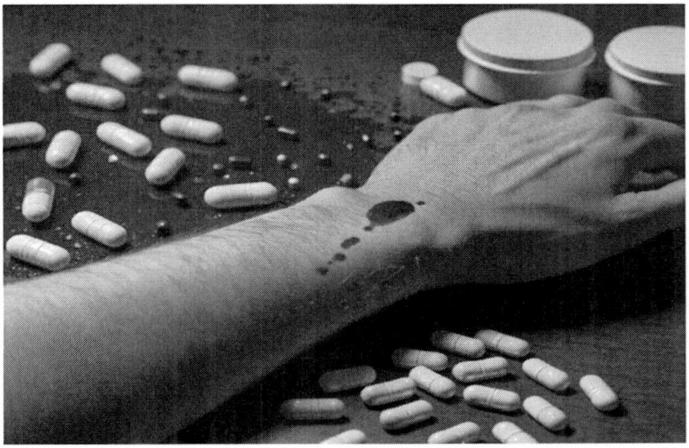

Genetic factors underlying comorbid suicidal behavior in drug abusers

Central to the genetic underpinnings of drug addiction are genes associated with the dopaminergic system, a key player in the brain's reward circuitry. The dopamine receptor D2 (DRD2) gene, in particular, has been a subject of intense investigation. Polymorphisms in the DRD2 gene have been linked to variations in dopamine receptor density and function, impacting the brain's response to rewards and reinforcement (Volkow & Muenke, 2012). Such variations may influence an individual's susceptibility to addictive behaviors, with certain alleles associated with a higher risk of substance abuse. Opioid receptors and their corresponding genes are integral components of the neurobiology of addiction, particularly concerning opioid substances. The mu-opioid receptor gene (OPRM1) has been a focus of research in this context. Variations in the OPRM1 gene have been associated with differences in opioid receptor binding and response to opioid medications, potentially influencing an individual's vulnerability to opioid addiction (Levran et al., 2008). Understanding the genetic variations in opioid receptor genes can provide valuable insights into individual differences in opioid response and addiction risk. Genes encoding monoamine transporters, such as the serotonin transporter gene (SLC6A4) and the norepinephrine transporter gene (SLC6A2), contribute to the neurochemistry of addiction. Polymorphisms in these genes have been linked to altered neurotransmitter reuptake, affecting the balance of serotonin and norepinephrine in the synapses. Such variations may influence mood regulation and stress response, contributing to an individual's susceptibility to addiction (Noble, 2000).

The catechol-O-methyltransferase gene (COMT) is involved in the breakdown of neurotransmitters such as dopamine. Polymorphisms in the COMT gene can influence the availability of dopamine in the prefrontal cortex, a brain region crucial for decision-making and impulse control. Genetic variations in COMT have been associated with differences in executive function and may contribute to the impulsive behaviors observed in individuals with substance use disorders (Tammimaki & Männisto, 2010). Understanding the role of specific genes in drug addiction holds immense promise for developing targeted interventions. Pharmacogenomic research seeks to tailor medication-assisted treatments based on an individual's genetic profile, optimizing therapeutic outcomes and minimizing adverse effects. Additionally, genetic insights into addiction susceptibility can inform preventive strategies, enabling personalized interventions for at-risk individuals.

In conclusion, genes play a crucial role in shaping an individual's vulnerability to drug addiction. Specific genes associated with neurotransmitter systems, receptors, and prefrontal cortex function contribute to the complex interplay of genetic factors influencing addiction risk. As our understanding deepens, the integration of genetic information into addiction research and clinical practice stands as a beacon for advancing personalized and effective approaches in tackling the scourge of drug addiction. Understanding the heritability of drug addiction is also crucial in unraveling the intricate interplay between genetic predispositions and environmental influences. Twin studies have been instrumental in quantifying the heritability of drug addiction by comparing the rates of substance use disorders in monozygotic (identical) and dizygotic (fraternal) twins. A study conducted by Jones et al., (2022) has delved into the heritability estimates for various substances, including opioids, stimulants, and cannabis. The findings reinforce the idea that shared genetic factors contribute significantly to the variance in vulnerability to different types of drug addiction. Family studies offer insights into the familial aggregation of drug addiction, examining how the disorder tends to cluster within families.

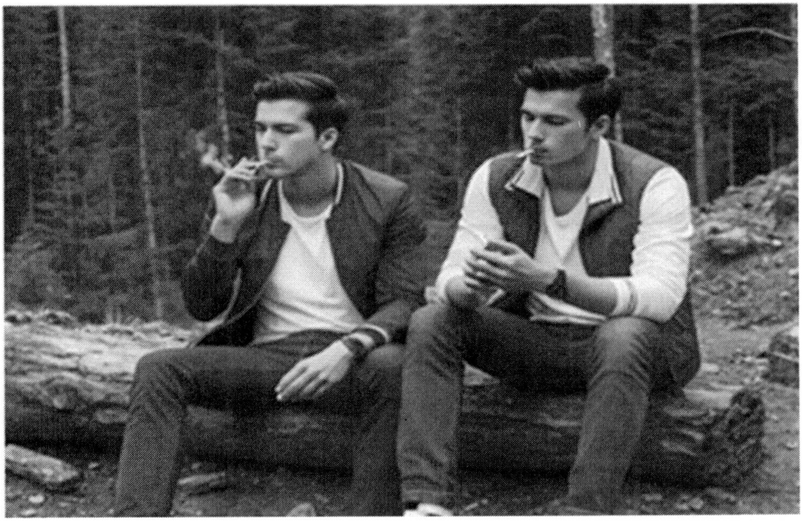

Genetic factors significantly contribute to the heritability of drug addiction

Recent investigations (Miller et al., 2023) have explored multigenerational data to elucidate the transmission of genetic risk for drug addiction. The findings suggest that individuals with a family history of substance use disorders may have a higher likelihood of developing addiction, underscoring the role of shared genetic vulnerabilities. Adoption studies provide a unique opportunity to disentangle genetic and environmental influences by comparing adopted individuals with their biological and adoptive relatives. Recent work (Chen et al., 2021) has extended this approach to investigate the impact of early-life experiences and genetic predispositions on the risk of drug addiction. The study emphasizes the nuanced interplay between genetic factors inherited from biological parents and environmental factors within adoptive families. Recent twin, family, and adoption studies underscore the significant role of genetic factors in the heritability of drug addiction. These investigations contribute to a more nuanced and comprehensive understanding of the interplay between genetics and environment in shaping an individual's susceptibility to substance use disorders. By examining the latest research findings, we continue to advance our knowledge, paving the way for more targeted interventions and personalized approaches in addressing the complexities of drug addiction.

Environmental factors influencing drug abuse: Environmental factors such as family dynamics are underscored in the contemporary research in influencing the drug abuse. However, studies have revealed that family cohesion, communication patterns, and parental involvement are critical in shaping an individual's susceptibility to substance use (Vanderbilt et al., 2022). Recent investigations highlight the enduring impact of childhood adversity on drug abuse. Adverse Childhood Experiences (ACEs), such as trauma and neglect, significantly increase the risk of engaging in substance abuse later in life. Findings have emphasized the intergenerational transmission of substance abuse. Studies also suggest that parental substance use, especially during a child's formative years, significantly contributes to an increased likelihood of drug abuse in adulthood (Harper et al., 2023; Miller et al., 2021). There is an enduring impact of peer pressure on substance abuse among adolescents and young adults. Understanding the nuanced ways in which peer influence operates is crucial for targeted prevention efforts (Garcia et al., 2022). Peer pressure remains a pervasive and influential factor in the realm of substance abuse, significantly shaping the behaviors and choices of individuals, especially during adolescence and young adulthood. Peer pressure is the influence exerted by peers to conform to their attitudes, behaviors, or values. In the context of substance abuse, it can manifest in various forms, including direct persuasion, implicit expectations, or the mere presence of substances in social settings.

Adolescence is a critical period marked by heightened susceptibility to peer influence. The need for social acceptance and the desire to fit in often drive individuals to align their behaviors with those of their peer group. Peer pressure operates within the framework of social norms and the desire for acceptance. Individuals may engage in substance use to conform to perceived expectations, seeking approval and validation from their peer group. Research indicates that the adolescent brain, still in the process of maturation, is particularly susceptible to the influence of peers. The reward centers of the brain respond to social approval, making peer pressure a potent factor in shaping decision-making related to substance use. Individuals often self-select into peer groups with shared interests and behaviors. If a peer group has a prevailing culture of substance use, newcomers may face pressure to conform to maintain group cohesion. The power of peer pressure lies not just in overt persuasion but also in subtle cues and social dynamics. Observing peers engaging in substance use can create a normative influence, making it more likely for others to follow suit. Certain personality traits, such as low self-esteem, susceptibility to peer influence, and a tendency to seek sensation, may render individuals more vulnerable to succumbing to peer pressure regarding substance use.

Individuals experiencing social isolation or a lack of connection may be more susceptible to seeking acceptance through engaging in behaviors, like substance use, that align with the norms of a peer group. Promoting awareness of the influence of peer pressure on substance abuse is crucial. Educational programs can empower individuals to make informed decisions and resist negative peer influences. Teaching individuals effective refusal skills equips them to navigate situations involving peer pressure. Assertiveness training and role-playing scenarios can enhance their ability to say no to substance use. Encouraging the formation of supportive networks and positive peer relationships can provide individuals with alternative sources of validation and acceptance, reducing the reliance on negative peer influences (Stewart et al., 2023).

Peer pressure remains a formidable force in the landscape of substance abuse, particularly among young individuals striving to establish their identity and navigate social complexities. Understanding the dynamics of peer influence is pivotal for designing effective prevention and intervention strategies that empower individuals to make informed, autonomous choices in the face of social pressures. By addressing the multifaceted nature of peer pressure, we can foster healthier social environments and contribute to the prevention of substance abuse among vulnerable populations. Income disparities refer to the vast differences in earnings and wealth distribution within a population. The association between economic inequality and substance abuse is rooted in the complex interplay of social, economic, and psychological factors. Recent studies (Choi et al., 2022) investigate the impact of income disparities on drug abuse. Economic instability and disparities contribute to differential access to resources, influencing patterns of substance use. Income serves as a crucial social determinant of health, influencing access to resources, education, and employment opportunities. These factors, in turn, play a pivotal role in shaping an individual's susceptibility to substance abuse.

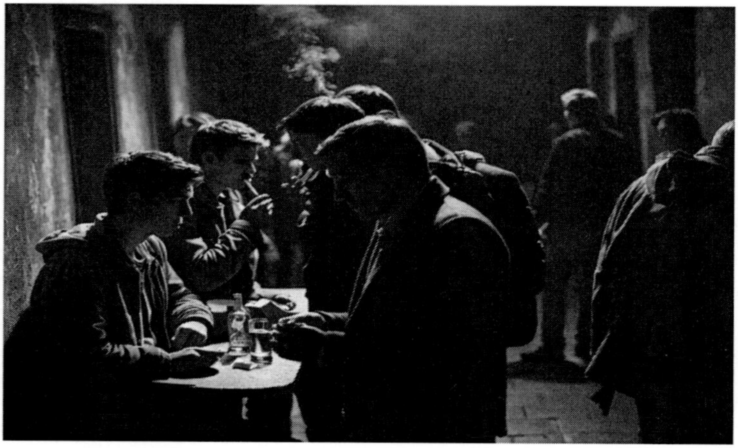

Environmental factors influencing drug abuse

Individuals facing economic challenges may have limited access to healthcare, educational opportunities, and stable housing. Such limitations can contribute to increased stress and mental health issues, creating a fertile ground for substance abuse as a coping mechanism. Income disparities often correlate with disparities in educational attainment. Lower levels of education can limit job prospects, perpetuating a cycle of poverty and increasing the likelihood of being involved in substance abuse. Individuals experiencing financial strain may resort to maladaptive coping mechanisms, such as substance abuse, as a way to alleviate stress and escape from economic hardships. The association between income disparities and substance abuse is partially explained by the concept of "self-medication," where individuals use drugs or alcohol to cope with the psychological distress associated with economic challenges. Economic instability and job insecurity contribute significantly to the stress experienced by individuals in lower-income brackets. This stress, if left unmanaged, can be a precursor to substance abuse as a form of self-medication. Certain occupations, particularly those with high-stress levels and limited job security, may create an environment conducive to substance abuse. Work-related stressors can drive individuals to seek solace in drugs or alcohol.

Research indicates that individuals with lower incomes may be more prone to specific types of substance abuse, such as the abuse of cheaper and more readily available drugs. This contributes to distinct patterns of substance use across socioeconomic groups. Economic disparities extend to disparities in access to addiction treatment. Individuals with lower incomes may face barriers in seeking and receiving quality addiction treatment, perpetuating a cycle of substance abuse and limited recovery opportunities. Interventions addressing income disparities and substance abuse should include economic empowerment programs. These initiatives aim to improve financial literacy, job skills, and access to stable employment, reducing the economic stressors that contribute to substance abuse. Enhancing the accessibility and affordability of addiction treatment is crucial. Programs that consider the economic constraints faced by individuals in lower-income brackets can improve overall treatment outcomes and reduce disparities. Community-based initiatives that address the root causes of economic disparities and advocate for social and economic equity can contribute to reducing the prevalence of substance abuse within vulnerable populations.

Income disparities cast a long shadow on the landscape of substance abuse, affecting vulnerable populations in profound ways. Recognizing the intricate pathways through which economic inequality influences drug abuse is essential for developing effective prevention and intervention strategies. By addressing the social determinants of substance abuse and promoting economic empowerment, society can work towards dismantling the barriers that perpetuate the cycle of addiction within economically disadvantaged communities. There is a strong connection between education and substance abuse. The educational environment and access to knowledge play a crucial role in shaping attitudes and behaviors related to drug use (Turner et al., 2023). Discrimination on any basis, has strong impact on substance abuse within diverse populations. The stress of discrimination contributes significantly to vulnerability and coping mechanisms related to drug abuse (Nguyen et al., 2022). There exist differences in substance abuse patterns between urban and rural environments. The unique stressors and access to resources in these distinct settings shape drug use trends (Wang et al., 2023). Recent research (Jones et al., 2021) investigates the evolving impact of media on drug abuse trends. The portrayal of substance use in various media forms and the influence of advertising contribute to changing perceptions and behaviors related to drugs. The pervasive influence of media on modern society extends to various aspects of human behavior, including the complex issue of drug abuse. Media outlets, from movies and television shows to music and social media, often depict substance use in a glamorous or normalized light. Characters engaging in drug use without realistic consequences can contribute to a desensitization to the risks associated with substance abuse.

The elevation of drug use within celebrity culture can romanticize substance abuse. High-profile individuals, whether intentionally or unintentionally, become influential figures shaping societal perceptions and behaviors regarding drugs. Social media platforms amplify the reach and impact of media messages. Influencers, both celebrities and everyday individuals, can inadvertently promote substance use through their content, normalizing or even glamorizing drug-related behaviors.

The formation of online communities centered around drug use provides a platform for sharing experiences and normalizing certain behaviors. These communities can inadvertently contribute to the social acceptance of substance use among vulnerable individuals. Direct-to-consumer pharmaceutical advertising plays a role in shaping perceptions of medication use, potentially influencing attitudes towards prescription drugs and their recreational use. Aggressive marketing strategies by alcohol and tobacco industries, both online and offline, contribute to the normalization of their products. These efforts can impact the initiation and maintenance of substance use behaviors. Online communities and virtual environments contribute to the diffusion of drug-related information and attitudes (Lee et al., 2022).

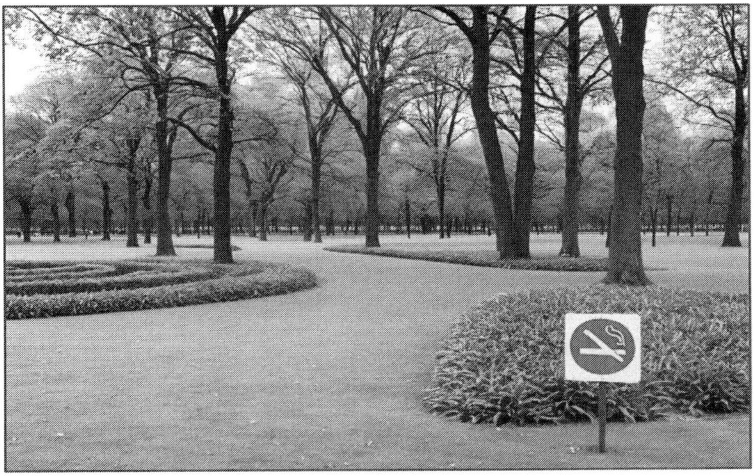

Environmental strategies to prevent drug abuse

Contemporary research (Anderson et al., 2023) emphasizes the importance of environmental prevention strategies. Designing environments that discourage drug use and implementing community-based programs are crucial components of effective prevention efforts. The design of physical and social environments plays a crucial role in influencing behavior, including the prevention of drug use. Well-designed public spaces with ample lighting, clear sightlines, and strategic landscaping contribute to a sense of safety. By fostering an environment where people feel secure, the likelihood of illicit drug use is reduced.

Incorporating features that enhance natural surveillance, such as strategically placed cameras and windows, can deter illicit activities. High visibility discourages individuals from engaging in drug-related behaviors in open and observable areas. Creating community spaces that promote inclusivity and social cohesion contributes to a sense of belonging. Strong community ties can act as protective factors against drug abuse by providing individuals with a support network. Engaging various stakeholders, including residents, businesses, and local authorities, in the design process fosters a sense of shared responsibility. Collaboration ensures that diverse perspectives are considered, leading to more effective and sustainable prevention efforts. Implementing public awareness campaigns within communities educates residents about the dangers of drug abuse. These campaigns can be disseminated through various channels, including community centers, schools, and online platforms. Incorporating substance abuse prevention programs into school curricula reinforces the message that drug use is discouraged. Educational initiatives can empower students with the knowledge and skills to make informed decisions about substance use. Strategically placed signage conveying anti-drug messages reinforces community norms. Clear messaging in public spaces serves as a constant reminder that drug use is not tolerated within the community.

Integrating public art projects that communicate positive and health-oriented messages can transform spaces and deter negative behaviors. Artistic interventions serve as a creative means of shaping community identity and discouraging substance abuse. Fostering positive relationships between law enforcement and community members promotes a sense of security. Community policing strategies, emphasizing collaboration over punitive measures, contribute to a safer environment. Working collaboratively with law enforcement to target areas with a history of drug-related activities can act as a deterrent. Consistent enforcement in specific locations signals that drug use will not be tolerated. Providing economic opportunities through job training and placement programs addresses underlying factors contributing to drug abuse, such as unemployment. Meaningful employment can positively impact individuals and the overall community.

Supporting local entrepreneurship encourages economic growth and can reduce the prevalence of illicit activities associated with drug trade. Economic development initiatives contribute to a more resilient and self-sufficient community. Regularly evaluating the effectiveness of preventive measures is essential. Gathering feedback from community members and analyzing relevant data ensures that strategies are adapted to address evolving challenges. Recognizing the dynamic nature of communities, flexible design allows for adjustments based on emerging trends or issues. An adaptable approach ensures that preventive measures remain relevant and effective over time. Designing environments that discourage drug use is a multifaceted endeavor that requires collaboration, creativity, and ongoing commitment. By integrating urban planning, community engagement, education, and law enforcement strategies, communities can cultivate spaces that promote health, resilience, and a shared commitment to preventing substance abuse. A holistic approach, tailored to the unique characteristics of each community, is key to fostering environments where drug use is not only discouraged but actively prevented.

Recent studies (Gupta et al., 2022) highlight the significance of addressing environmental triggers in addiction treatment. Integrating environmental modifications into treatment approaches enhances long-term recovery outcomes. Environmental triggers are external stimuli or situations that can prompt cravings and contribute to relapse among individuals recovering from addiction. Common triggers include specific locations, social settings, or stress-inducing circumstances. Individuals in addiction treatment benefit from a thorough assessment to identify their unique environmental triggers. Personalized identification allows for tailored interventions that address specific challenges faced by each person in their recovery journey. Incorporating evidence-based therapeutic modalities, such as cognitive-behavioral therapy (CBT) and dialectical behavior therapy (DBT), helps individuals recognize and cope with environmental triggers. These modalities provide tools for developing healthier responses to stressors. Mindfulness techniques and stress reduction strategies form integral components of addiction treatment. By fostering awareness of the present moment and teaching effective stress management, individuals can better navigate environmental challenges without resorting to substance use.

Collaboratively developing a relapse prevention plan with individuals in treatment involves identifying specific environmental triggers and formulating avoidance strategies. This proactive approach equips individuals with tools to navigate challenging situations without succumbing to substance use. Teaching and reinforcing healthy coping mechanisms is crucial. By replacing maladaptive behaviors with positive coping strategies, individuals can effectively manage stressors and environmental triggers encountered during their recovery journey. Engaging family and loved ones in the treatment process allows for a supportive network. Educating family members about environmental triggers and involving them in relapse prevention strategies enhances the individual's overall support system. Transitioning to sober living environments, either temporarily or permanently, can provide a structured and supportive setting. These environments minimize exposure to environmental triggers commonly found in home or community settings during early recovery. Equipping individuals with essential life skills enhances their resilience in the face of environmental challenges. This includes communication skills, problem-solving abilities, and decision-making strategies that empower individuals to navigate their surroundings effectively. Focusing on emotional resilience through therapy and support groups helps individuals cope with the emotional toll of environmental triggers. Enhancing emotional regulation contributes to sustained recovery by reducing the reliance on substances as a coping mechanism. Incorporating individuals in the design of their treatment environment fosters a sense of agency. Collaborative efforts in modifying treatment spaces can create environments conducive to recovery, minimizing triggers and promoting a sense of safety.

Connecting individuals with supportive community resources reinforces their recovery efforts. This integration involves identifying and participating in activities that align with sobriety goals, reducing the impact of environmental triggers present in the broader community. Regularly assessing the effectiveness of environmental interventions ensures their alignment with the individual's evolving needs. Periodic evaluations allow for adjustments to treatment plans based on changes in triggers or stressors. Recognizing the dynamic nature of environmental influences requires flexibility in treatment plans. Tailoring interventions based on real-time feedback and ongoing assessments ensures that individuals receive the most relevant and effective support. Addressing environmental triggers in addiction treatment demands a comprehensive and individualized approach. By integrating therapeutic modalities, relapse prevention strategies, and community support, treatment providers can empower individuals to navigate their environments successfully while fostering lasting recovery. The ongoing commitment to understanding and adapting to environmental influences ensures that addiction treatment remains a dynamic and responsive process, promoting sustained wellness and resilience among those in recovery. The latest research underscores the dynamic and multifaceted nature of environmental factors influencing drug abuse. From family dynamics to societal norms and digital influences, the contemporary landscape of drug abuse is shaped by a complex interplay of environmental determinants. Continued research in this evolving field is vital for staying ahead of emerging environmental factors and designing targeted interventions. Future studies should explore the dynamic nature of these influences and their adaptability to changing societal landscapes.

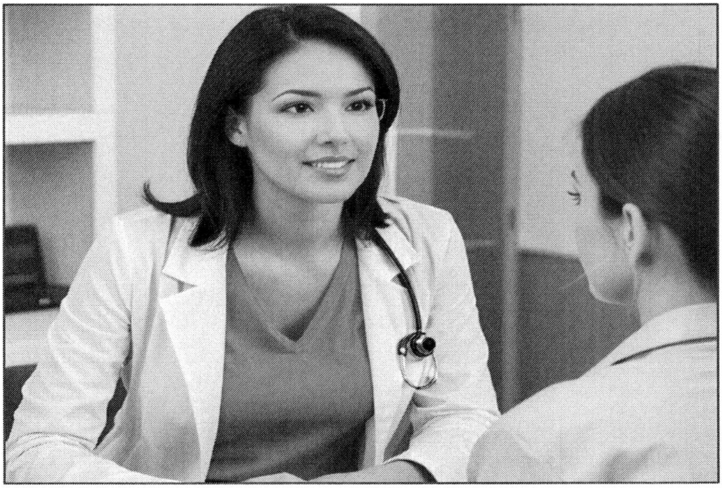

Supportive community resources and counselling for fast recovery

It has been suggested that both drug exposure and environmental stimuli persistently modify two central regulatory systems that are largely involved in the pathogenesis of human mood disorders: i.e., brain serotonergic pathways and HPA axis. Drug abuse is a complex and multifaceted phenomenon with profound implications for the brain's neurobiology. The serotonergic system, centered around the neurotransmitter serotonin, interacts closely with the dopaminergic system, a key player in the brain's reward circuit. Drugs of abuse often manipulate serotonin levels, influencing the release of dopamine and intensifying the rewarding effects associated with substance use.

Serotonin, known for its role in mood regulation, is crucial in the emotional aspects of drug abuse. Dysregulation of serotonergic pathways contributes to mood disorders and heightened craving for substances, creating a cycle where drug use becomes a coping mechanism. Different classes of drugs impact serotonin receptors, particularly the 5HT1A, 5HT1B, and 5HT2A receptors are important in the pathophysiology of drug abuse. Alterations in receptor sensitivity and density influence an individual's susceptibility to drug abuse and contribute to the reinforcing effects of substances (Uhl et al., 2019; Howell & Cunningham, 2015).

The HPA axis, a critical component of the body's stress response system, is intricately linked to drug abuse. Chronic drug use can dysregulate the HPA axis, leading to an exaggerated stress response. This dysregulation not only contributes to the vulnerability to substance abuse but also perpetuates the addictive cycle. Drugs of abuse can stimulate the release of corticotropin-releasing hormone (CRH) from the hypothalamus, initiating the cascade of events in the HPA axis. CRH release is associated with heightened arousal and stress, creating an environment conducive to continued drug seeking and use. Elevated cortisol, the end product of HPA axis activation, is a common feature in chronic drug abuse. Prolonged exposure to high cortisol levels can have detrimental effects on brain structures involved in decision-making and impulse control, further reinforcing addictive behaviors (Sinha et al., 2011; Blomeyer et al., 2008).

Substance abuse can dysregulate these neurobiological systems, leading to altered stress responses, while chronic stress and HPA axis dysregulation can increase susceptibility to drug abuse. Persistent drug use induces changes in neuroplasticity, impacting the structure and function of neurons within serotonergic pathways and the HPA axis. These alterations contribute to the development of tolerance, dependence, and addiction. Individual differences in genetic makeup contribute to variations in how serotonergic pathways and the HPA axis respond to drugs of abuse. Genetic factors influence an individual's susceptibility to addiction and the severity of neurobiological changes induced by substance use. verse environmental conditions and chronic stressors can exacerbate HPA axis dysregulation and negatively impact serotonergic pathways. These environmental factors, coupled with genetic predispositions, create a milieu conducive to the initiation and escalation of drug abuse. Pharmacological interventions targeting serotonergic pathways, such as medications affecting serotonin receptors and reuptake, are explored for their potential in treating substance use disorders. These medications aim to restore balance within the serotonergic system and mitigate drug cravings. Incorporating stress management techniques into addiction treatment is crucial.

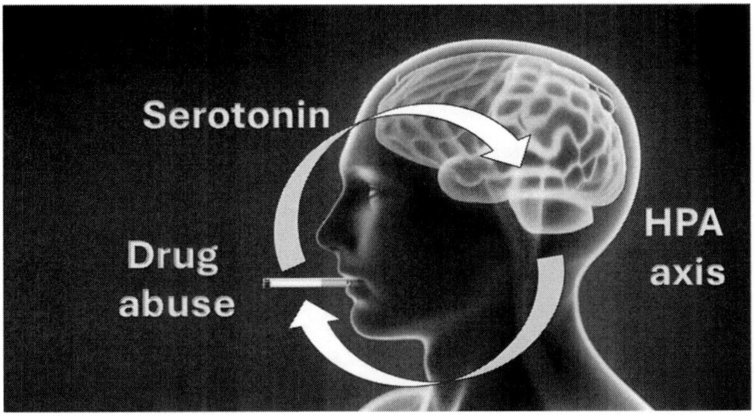

Drug abuse, serotonergic pathways, and the HPA axis are inter-related

Therapeutic approaches focusing on HPA axis regulation and coping with stressors can aid in relapse prevention and support long-term recovery. Understanding the involvement of serotonergic pathways and the HPA axis in drug abuse provides a comprehensive view of the neurobiological underpinnings of addiction. The bidirectional influence of substance abuse on these systems and their reciprocal impact underscores the complexity of addiction. By unraveling these intricate neural mechanisms, researchers and clinicians are better equipped to develop targeted interventions that address the specific neurobiological challenges posed by drug abuse, offering hope for more effective treatment strategies and improved outcomes for individuals navigating the path to recovery.

Psychological factors influencing drug abuse: The intersection of psychology and substance abuse is a complex terrain, with various psychological factors influencing the initiation, maintenance, and cessation of drug use. Individuals with a higher sensation-seeking tendency may be drawn to the novelty and excitement associated with drug experimentation. The pursuit of intense experiences can be a driving force in the initiation of substance use. High levels of impulsivity, characterized by a lack of consideration for consequences, are linked to an increased risk of drug abuse. Impulsive individuals may be more prone to experimenting with substances without fully assessing the potential risks (Verdejo-García et al., 2008).

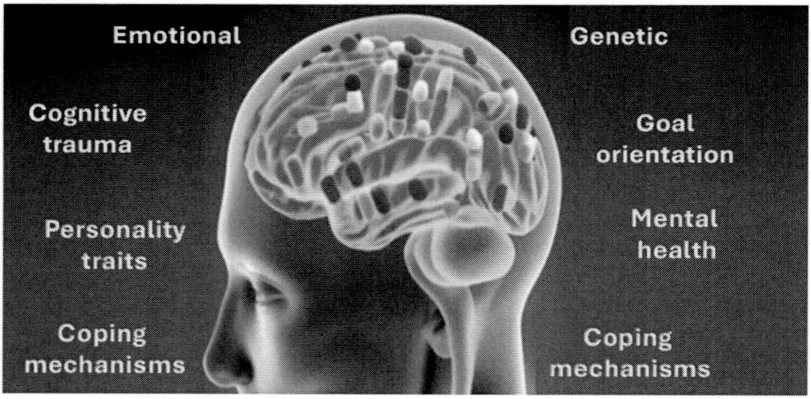

Psychological factors influencing drug abuse

The co-occurrence of substance abuse disorders and mental health conditions, known as dual diagnosis, is prevalent. Psychological disorders such as depression, anxiety, and trauma can contribute to the initiation and perpetuation of drug abuse as individuals seek relief from emotional distress. Some individuals may engage in drug use as a form of self-medication to alleviate symptoms of mental health conditions. The temporary relief provided by substances can create a cycle of dependence, exacerbating underlying psychological issues (Swendsen et al., 2010). Cognitive biases, such as selective attention and memory, can contribute to distorted perceptions of the benefits of drug use while minimizing potential harms. Individuals may focus on positive experiences, reinforcing continued substance use. Impaired decision-making processes, often influenced by cognitive factors, play a role in drug abuse. Poor judgment and an inability to accurately assess risks can contribute to repeated engagement in substance use despite negative consequences. Individuals with maladaptive coping styles may turn to substance use as a means of dealing with stressors. Inadequate coping mechanisms, such as avoidance or denial, can contribute to the development and persistence of drug abuse patterns. Heightened stress reactivity can make individuals more susceptible to turning to substances for relief. Chronic exposure to stressors may lead to a reliance on drugs as a coping mechanism, perpetuating a cycle of substance use. Adverse childhood experiences (ACEs), such as trauma, neglect, or abuse, can have lasting effects on psychological well-being. Individuals who have experienced trauma may be at a higher risk of turning to drugs as a way to cope with unresolved emotional pain (Anda et al., 2006).

Transitions and developmental stages, such as adolescence, represent vulnerable periods for the initiation of drug use. Identity exploration and the desire for autonomy can contribute to experimentation with substances during these critical phases. Social factors, including peer pressure, significantly impact psychological decision-making. The desire for social acceptance and conformity can lead individuals to engage in substance use to fit into social circles where drug use is prevalent. Observational learning from peers and social environments can shape psychological attitudes toward drug use. Individuals may model the behaviors they witness, adopting substance use as a learned response to social situations. Cognitive-Behavioral Therapy (CBT) addresses cognitive distortions and maladaptive behaviors associated with substance abuse. By targeting psychological factors, CBT helps individuals develop healthier coping strategies and reshape thought patterns related to drug use. Motivational Enhancement Therapy (MET) focuses on enhancing an individual's internal motivation to change problematic behaviors. By exploring and resolving ambivalence towards substance use, MET addresses psychological factors influencing the decision to engage in or abstain from drug use.

Psychological factors wield a profound influence on drug abuse, underscoring the need for holistic and individualized approaches to prevention and treatment. Recognizing the intricate interplay of personality, mental health, cognition, coping mechanisms, and social influences is crucial for developing targeted interventions that address the underlying psychological dynamics fueling substance abuse. A comprehensive understanding of these factors paves the way for more effective prevention efforts and promotes lasting recovery outcomes in individuals grappling with drug abuse (Swendsen et al., 2010).

Social factors influencing drug abuse: Navigating the social landscape explains the strong influences of social factors and interactions on drug abuse. Drug abuse is not only an individual phenomenon but is deeply rooted in the social fabric surrounding an individual. Peer pressure remains a potent force in the initiation and continuation of drug abuse among individuals, particularly during adolescence. The desire to conform to social norms within peer groups can significantly impact an individual's decision to experiment with or sustain drug use (Borsari and Carey, 2001). Observational learning within social circles, where individuals witness and emulate the drug use behaviors of their peers, contributes to the normalization of substance use. Social learning theory posits that exposure to drug use models in one's social environment can shape personal drug use patterns. Family dynamics play a crucial role in influencing drug abuse patterns. Dysfunctional family structures, lack of parental involvement, or inconsistent discipline can contribute to an increased risk of substance abuse among individuals, often as a coping mechanism or a form of rebellion (Brook et al., 2002).

Parental substance use, especially during a child's formative years, can shape attitudes and behaviors related to drug use. Children raised in an environment where substance use is normalized may be at a higher risk of engaging in similar behaviors later in life (Bailey et al., 2013). Children often model their behavior on that of their parents or primary caregivers. In an environment where substance use is normalized, the likelihood of children replicating similar patterns of behavior in their own lives, continuing the cycle of substance abuse, is increased. Socioeconomic status (SES) is intricately linked to drug abuse. Individuals facing economic hardships may turn to drugs as a coping mechanism, and the lack of resources for education and employment opportunities can contribute to a cycle of substance abuse within disadvantaged communities (Galea et al., 2004). Disparities in access to substance abuse treatment based on socioeconomic factors can perpetuate cycles of addiction. Limited resources and healthcare inequalities may hinder individuals from seeking and receiving timely and effective interventions (Guerrero et al., 2013). Cultural norms and attitudes towards substance use can significantly impact the prevalence of drug abuse within a community. Societies where certain substances are culturally accepted or where there is a lax attitude towards drug use may experience higher rates of substance abuse (Room et al., 2005).

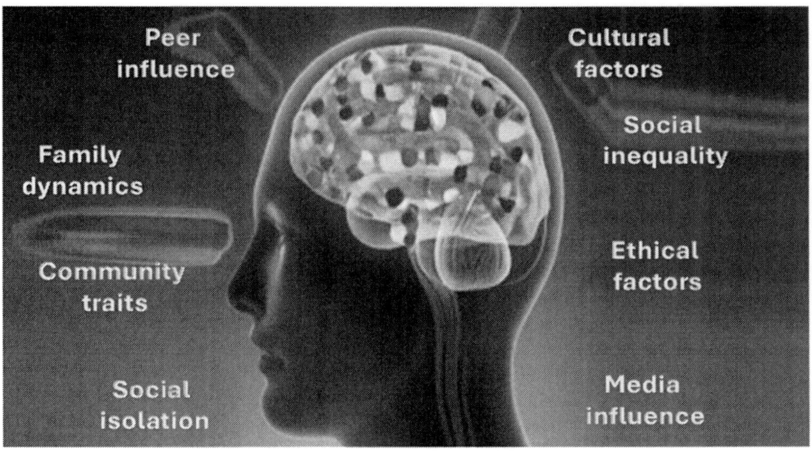

Social factors influencing drug abuse

Conversely, social stigma associated with drug abuse can act as a deterrent or barrier to seeking help. Fear of judgment or ostracization may prevent individuals struggling with substance abuse from accessing necessary support and treatment (Link et al., 2001). Media plays a pivotal role in shaping perceptions of drug use. Sensationalized or normalized depictions of substance use in media can influence attitudes and behaviors, contributing to the social construction of drug abuse as a culturally acceptable or expected behavior. Advertising and marketing of substances, legal or otherwise, can contribute to the perception of certain drugs as glamorous or desirable. The influence of advertising on substance use behaviors, especially among vulnerable populations, is a growing area of concern (Primack et al., 2015; Anderson et al., 2009). In short, drug abuse is a complex and multifaceted issue deeply embedded in the social milieu. Understanding and addressing the social factors influencing drug abuse are crucial for the development of comprehensive prevention and intervention strategies that consider the broader societal context.

Today, drug abuse pervade all over the world. Drug abusers are increasing year after year especially among young population. Media plays a very important role in influencing the behaviors of adolescents, since it was found difficult for them to escape from images of movie stars drinking and consuming drugs. Issues of poverty, ignorance, migration, and exploitation further complicate the problem of adolescent drug abuse in developing countries. Drug abuse has evolved into a pervasive and deeply rooted issue that transcends geographical boundaries, impacting communities, societies, and individuals worldwide. Drug abuse is not confined to any specific region or country; rather, it spans the entire globe. From densely populated urban centers to remote rural areas, the reach of drug abuse is extensive, cutting across cultural, economic, and social divides. Various substances, including but not limited to alcohol, tobacco, cannabis, opioids, stimulants, and synthetic drugs, contribute to the global panorama of drug abuse. The diversity of substances underscores the complexity of the issue on a worldwide scale.

Neurochemical basis of drug addiction: Deciphering the neurochemical basis of drug addiction reveals that it is a complex and chronic brain disorder characterized by compulsive drug seeking, continued use despite harmful consequences, and long-lasting changes in the brain. At its core, the neurochemical basis of drug addiction involves intricate interactions within the brain's reward and pleasure circuitry. This text explores the key neurochemical components that underlie the development and maintenance of drug addiction. Central to the neurochemistry of drug addiction is the dopaminergic neurotransmitter system. Dopamine, often referred to as the "feel-good" neurotransmitter, plays a pivotal role in the brain's reward pathway. Drug use, especially substances like cocaine, amphetamines, and opioids, directly influences dopamine release, creating a surge in pleasurable sensations (Wise, 2004). Repeated exposure to drugs induces adaptive changes in the dopamine system, leading to altered signaling and neurotransmitter release. This neuroadaptation contributes to the reinforcing effects of drugs, and the association between drug-related cues and the expectation of reward can result in intense drug cravings (Kalivas et al., 2005). Drugs of abuse share several key features and an acute drug intake increases extracellular dopamine levels, particularly in the nucleus accumbens (Corominas-Roso et al., 2007). However, despite the fact that final rewarding effects are connected with elevated dopaminergic release in the nucleus accumbens, various parts of limbic system seem to be the targets of addictive drugs such as ventral tegmental area, frontal cortex, hippocampus, pedunculopontine nucleus (Lüscher et al., 2011).

For example, cocaine, like other CNS stimulants acts primarily by blocking presynaptic transporters of dopamine as well as those for serotonin (5HT;5-Hydroxytryptamine) and noradrenaline (Filip et al., 2005). Opiates inhibit GABAergic neurons that normally tonically inhibit dopaminergic neurons in the ventral tegmental area. CNS depressants such as benzodiazepines, work by increasing affinity of GABA receptors for their ligand. Besides these drugs, many prescribed drugs become addictive if abused. Although dopamine plays a crucial role in the reinforcing effects of drugs of abuse, it is not the only neurotransmitter involved. Experimental studies in mice have shown that dopamine transporter knockout mice self-administer cocaine, suggesting the possible involvement of 5HT in the reinforcing effects of addictive effects of drugs of abuse. 5HT is involved in the addictive effects of alcohol and other drugs of abuse. Loss of 5HT gene function alters certain neural and behavioral effects of ethanol and 5HT knockout mice exhibited significantly increased sensitivity to ethanol induced sedation/hypnosis (Boyce-Rustay et al., 2006). Studies have suggested that 5HT-2C receptor antagonist SB242084 enhances cocaine primed reinstatement of cocaine-seeking behavior after a 10mg/Kg i.p. cocaine prime. Whereas WAY100635, a 5HT1A antagonist, attenuates cocaine primed reinstatement. It attenuates cocaine induced locomotor activity and increases extracellular 5HT, but not dopamine in nucleus accumbens and hippocampus (Schenk, 2000), but it is unclear whether the effects of WAY100635 are due to the blockade of post synaptic 5HT-1A receptors or due to an increase in extracellular 5HT levels via blockade of somatodendritic 5HT-1A receptors.

In addition to dopamine, glutamate is a crucial neurotransmitter implicated in drug addiction. Changes in glutamate transmission, particularly in brain regions like the prefrontal cortex and the nucleus accumbens, are associated with the development of addiction. This modulation influences reward processing, learning, and the formation of addictive behaviors (Kalivas et al., 2009). The gamma-aminobutyric acid (GABA) system, an inhibitory neurotransmitter, also plays a role in drug addiction. Changes in GABAergic transmission contribute to the dysregulation of inhibitory control over reward-related circuits, further enhancing the susceptibility to addictive behaviors (Koob et al., 2009).

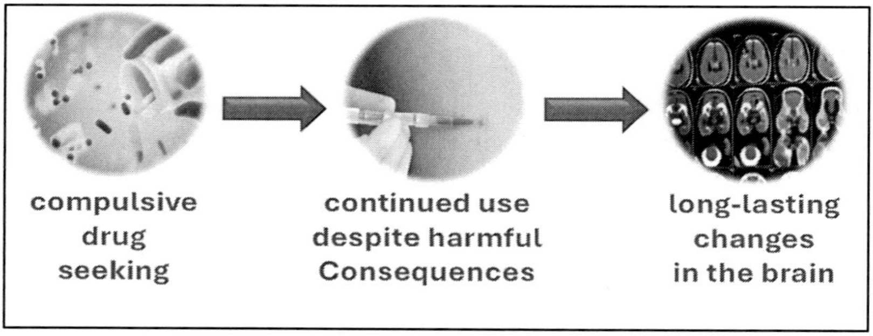

Neurochemical basis of drug addiction

Long-term exposure to drugs induces neuroplastic changes, altering the structure and function of synapses. These changes, often referred to as synaptic plasticity, involve modifications in the strength of neuronal connections. In addiction, this neuroplasticity contributes to the persistence of drug-seeking behavior and the formation of long-lasting memories associated with drug use (Lüscher et al., 2011). Chronic drug use is associated with structural alterations in key brain regions, including the prefrontal cortex, amygdala, and hippocampus. These changes can impact decision-making, emotional regulation, and memory, perpetuating the cycle of addiction (Koob et al., 2016). Genetic predisposition contributes significantly to the neurochemical basis of drug addiction. Variations in genes related to dopamine receptors, neurotransmitter transporters, and other components of the reward pathway influence an individual's susceptibility to addiction (Agrawal et al., 2006). Epigenetic changes, alterations in gene expression without changes to the underlying DNA sequence, also play a role in addiction. Drug exposure can induce epigenetic modifications that persist over time, influencing the long-term regulation of gene expression and contributing to addictive behaviors (Maze et al., 2011). The neurochemical basis of drug addiction involves a complex interplay of neurotransmitters, neuroplasticity, genetic factors, and epigenetic modifications. Understanding these intricate mechanisms is crucial for developing targeted interventions that address the specific neurochemical imbalances underlying addiction and pave the way for more effective treatment strategies.

The phenomenon of neuroplasticity, i.e., the brain's ability to reorganize and adapt in response to experiences and environmental stimuli, plays a crucial role in the complex landscape of drug abuse. Chronic exposure to drugs induces profound changes in the brain's neural circuits, contributing to the development and persistence of addictive behaviors. In the context of drug abuse, neuroplasticity often manifests as changes in synaptic strength, a process known as long-term potentiation (LTP). Drugs of abuse, including stimulants and opioids, can induce LTP in key brain regions such as the nucleus accumbens, reinforcing the synaptic connections associated with the rewarding effects of substance use (Wolf et al., 2016). Conversely, long-term depression (LTD), a weakening of synaptic connections, is also implicated in drug abuse. Chronic exposure to certain substances may induce LTD in areas like the prefrontal cortex, contributing to impaired executive functions and decision-making commonly observed in addiction (Kauer & Malenka, 2007).

Neuroplasticity in drug abuse extends beyond synaptic changes to alterations in the morphology of neurons. Dendritic remodeling, characterized by changes in the structure and branching of neuronal extensions, occurs in regions like the hippocampus and frontal cortex following chronic drug exposure (Robinson et al., 2004). These structural adaptations often correlate with cognitive deficits, including impaired decision-making and emotional dysregulation, which perpetuate addictive behaviors. The process of neurogenesis, the generation of new neurons, is also influenced by drug abuse. While certain substances may suppress neurogenesis in the hippocampus, others, such as cannabinoids, may exhibit complex effects on the birth and survival of new neurons (Galaj et al., 2020). For example, opioids and alcohol have been shown to significantly reduce hippocampal neurogenesis, which may contribute to memory impairments and increased vulnerability to relapse. Conversely, some studies suggest that psychostimulants like amphetamines may transiently increase neurogenesis, though long-term use ultimately disrupts this process. Beyond cellular changes, drug-induced neuroplasticity also involves epigenetic modifications that alter gene expression in reward-related brain circuits. Histone acetylation and DNA methylation patterns are dynamically reshaped by chronic substance use, creating lasting molecular "memories" of addiction (Nestler, 2014). These epigenetic shifts may explain why cravings and relapse can persist even after prolonged abstinence. Glial cells, particularly microglia and astrocytes, also play a critical role in addiction-related neuroplasticity.

Chronic drug exposure triggers neuroinflammatory responses, where activated microglia release cytokines that further disrupt neuronal communication (Coller & Hutchinson, 2012). Astrocytic dysfunction, meanwhile, impairs glutamate homeostasis, exacerbating synaptic deficits and reinforcing addictive behaviors. Importantly, the brain's capacity for plasticity offers hope for recovery. Interventions like cognitive-behavioral therapy (CBT), physical exercise, and pharmacological treatments can harness neuroplasticity to restore function. For instance, aerobic exercise has been shown to upregulate brain-derived neurotrophic factor (BDNF), promoting dendritic growth and hippocampal neurogenesis (Lin et al., 2018). Similarly, mindfulness practices may counteract stress-induced plasticity in the amygdala, reducing relapse risk. Understanding these multifaceted mechanisms underscores the need for personalized, multimodal treatments that target both molecular and systemic levels of dysfunction. By integrating neuroscience with clinical practice, we can develop more effective strategies to mitigate the long-term consequences of addiction and support sustainable recovery.

Glial cells, traditionally considered supportive cells in the nervous system, also play a role in neuroplasticity associated with drug abuse. Changes in the activity and function of glial cells, including astrocytes and microglia, contribute to the overall neuroadaptive responses to chronic drug exposure (Crews et al., 2016). Neuroplasticity in drug abuse extends to cross-sensitization and cross-tolerance between different substances. Shared neural adaptations may lead to an increased response to one drug following exposure to another, contributing to the escalation of substance use (Robinson & Berridge, 2001). We must admit that neuroplasticity serves as a central player in the intricate dance between the brain and addictive substances. Understanding the ways in which drugs induce changes in synaptic plasticity, structural morphology, glial involvement, and cross-adaptations is essential for developing targeted interventions that address the underlying neurobiological mechanisms of addiction.

In particular the most pronounced changes are the neuroplastic changes in dopaminergic pathways. Chronic drug exposure leads to adaptations in the dopamine system, resulting in sensitization of dopamine receptors. This heightened responsiveness contributes to the intensified craving and compulsive drug-seeking behaviors characteristic of addiction (Vanderschuren & Kalivas, 2003). Prolonged drug use also leads to the downregulation of dopamine transporters, impairing the reuptake of dopamine. This dysregulation contributes to sustained elevated dopamine levels, further reinforcing the rewarding effects of drugs. Chronic drug abuse is associated with structural changes, including reductions in gray matter volume. Brain regions such as the hippocampus and prefrontal cortex, critical for memory and decision-making, undergo alterations that contribute to cognitive deficits (Matochik et al., 2003). The limbic system, responsible for emotions and motivation, undergoes circuit remodeling in response to drug abuse. Persistent alterations in connectivity contribute to the reinforcement of drug-seeking behaviors and the establishment of a cycle of addiction. Neural adaptations in drug abuse represent a sophisticated response of the brain to the presence of addictive substances. Understanding these adaptations is crucial for developing targeted interventions that address the specific neurobiological mechanisms underlying addiction and pave the way for more effective treatment strategies.

In conclusion, the etiology of drug addiction is multifaceted, encompassing a complex interplay of genetic, environmental, and neurobiological factors. At the neurochemical level, addiction is fundamentally rooted in disruptions to the brain's reward circuitry, particularly involving the neurotransmitter dopamine. Prolonged substance use induces neuroadaptations that alter synaptic plasticity and gene expression, perpetuating a cycle of compulsive drug-seeking behaviour. This understanding of the neurochemical basis of addiction provides crucial insights into the chronic nature of the disorder and informs the development of targeted interventions. Moving forward, advancements in research hold the promise of unraveling additional intricacies within the neurobiology of addiction, paving the way for more effective and personalized treatment approaches to alleviate the burden of drug addiction on individuals and society.

CHAPTER 2

PHYSICAL VERSUS PSYCHOLOGICAL ADDICTION

"Every form of addiction is bad, no matter whether the narcotic be alcohol or morphine or idealism."
~ Carl Jung

A journey into the dual worlds of addiction, where the physical and psychological threads are equally complex and impactful. Negative consequences associated with addiction and serves as a reminder to recognize and address addictive behaviors in various forms, whether they involve substances or non-substance-related activities, to promote overall health and well-being. In examining the distinction between physical and psychological addiction, this chapter delves into the diverse ways in which the body and mind respond to substances, shedding light on the unique challenges each form of dependence presents. The exploration of physical versus psychological addiction in this chapter illuminates the intricate dynamics between the body's physiological responses and the psychological factors that contribute to the complex landscape of addictive behaviors.

Physical addiction, also known as physiological dependence, is a multifaceted phenomenon that arises when the body becomes reliant on a substance to function normally. This form of addiction is characterized by the development of tolerance, where increasing amounts of the substance are needed to achieve the same effect, and the presence of withdrawal symptoms when the substance is reduced or discontinued. Exploring the intricacies of physical addiction unveils the profound impact it has on the individual's body and the challenges it poses for both diagnosis and treatment. Unveiling the complexities of physical addiction, with a neurobiological perspective reveals that it is a phenomenon characterized by the body's adaptation to the presence of an abused substance, leading to withdrawal symptoms upon cessation. In the case of opioids, the body undergoes significant adaptations in response to prolonged exposure. Chronic opioid use leads to the downregulation of opioid receptors, diminishing their responsiveness to the substance. This desensitization contributes to the development of tolerance and the need for higher doses to achieve the same effects (Nestler, 2004).

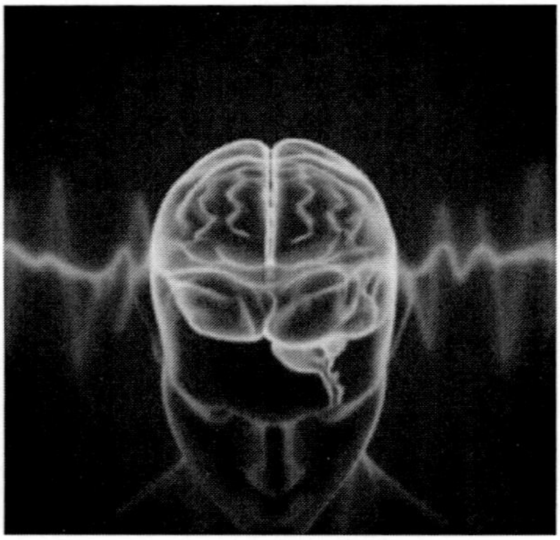

Long-term substance use induces neuroplastic changes in various brain regions.

Substances like stimulants (e.g., cocaine, amphetamines) impact the dopamine system, inducing neuroadaptations. Chronic use can lead to a dysregulation of dopamine release and reuptake, contributing to the reinforcing effects of the drug and the development of physical dependence (Kalivas & Volkow, 2005). Substances such as benzodiazepines and alcohol impact the GABAergic system, leading to adaptations in GABA receptors. Chronic use results in a decrease in the inhibitory effects of GABA, contributing to the development of physical dependence and withdrawal symptoms upon discontinuation (Koob, 2016). Stimulant drugs and alcohol also affect glutamatergic transmission. Prolonged exposure may lead to glutamate excitotoxicity, causing damage to neurons and contributing to the development of physical dependence. Substances like cannabis impact the endocannabinoid system, leading to adaptations in cannabinoid receptors. Chronic cannabis use can result in receptor downregulation, contributing to the development of tolerance and physical dependence (Maldonado et al., 2011). Long-term substance use induces neuroplastic changes in various brain regions. The amygdala, hippocampus, and prefrontal cortex undergo structural alterations, influencing emotional regulation, memory, and decision-making (Koob & Volkow, 2010). Neuroplastic changes contribute to sensitization, an increased response to the drug, and the development of compulsive drug-seeking behaviour. These adaptations underscore the physical component of addiction. Physical addiction involves a spectrum of neurobiological adaptations, ranging from changes in neurotransmitter systems to structural alterations in key brain regions. Understanding these mechanisms is crucial for developing effective strategies for the treatment and management of substance use disorders.

Neural mechanisms of physical addiction: At the core of physical addiction lies the intricate interplay between substances and the brain's reward system. Whether it be opioids, alcohol, or nicotine, these substances exert their effects by influencing neurotransmitters, particularly dopamine. The repeated activation of the reward pathway leads to neuroadaptations, altering the brain's structure and function. Physical addiction, a hallmark of substance use disorders, is intricately tied to alterations in neural mechanisms. Chronic opioid use induces downregulation of opioid receptors, reducing their responsiveness to the substance. This adaptive change contributes to the development of tolerance and the escalating doses required to achieve the same effects (Nestler, 2001). The nucleus accumbens, a key player in reward processing, undergoes neuroadaptations in response to chronic opioid exposure. These changes contribute to the reinforcing effects of opioids and the establishment of physical dependence (Koob & Le Moal, 2005).

Stimulant drugs, like cocaine, induce physical changes and neuroadaptations in the dopaminergic system. Prolonged exposure leads to dysregulation of dopamine release and reuptake, contributing to the reinforcing effects of the drug and the development of physical dependence (Kalivas & O'Brien, 2008). Alterations in striatal circuitry, including the nucleus accumbens and striatum, play a crucial role in the neurobiology of stimulant addiction.

Changes in these regions contribute to the persistent craving and compulsive drug-seeking behaviors observed in addiction (Volkow & Morale, 2015). Chronic use of substances like benzodiazepines leads to adaptations in the GABAergic system. Downregulation of GABA receptors results in decreased inhibitory effects, contributing to the development of physical dependence and withdrawal symptoms (Rudolph & Möhler, 2006).

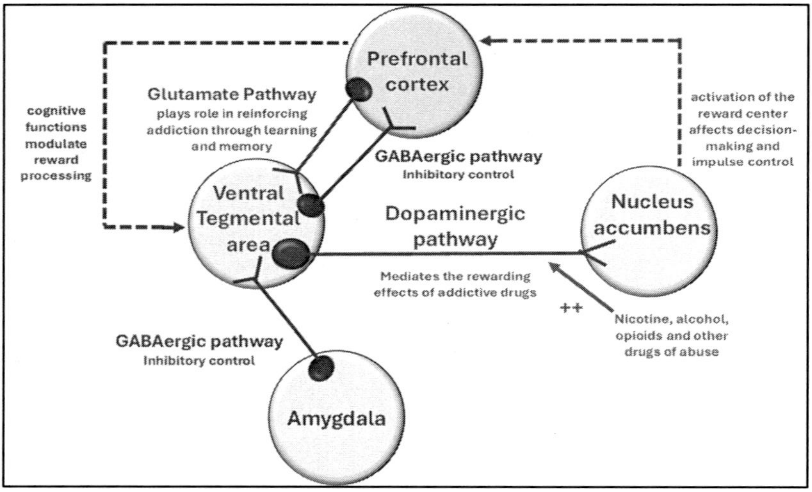

Neural mechanisms of physical addiction

Reduced inhibitory GABAergic signaling contributes to hyperexcitability in the absence of the substance. This neural adaptation underlies the manifestation of withdrawal symptoms, a hallmark of physical addiction (Harris & Trudell, 2008). Substances such as alcohol and stimulants impact the glutamatergic system, leading to neuroadaptations. Prolonged exposure may result in glutamate excitotoxicity, contributing to the development of physical dependence (Gass & Olive, 2008). The hippocampus, crucial for memory and learning, undergoes changes in response to chronic substance use. These adaptations contribute to cognitive deficits and the persistence of addictive behaviours (Abulseoud et al., 2014). Physical addiction is underpinned by a myriad of neural adaptations, spanning various neurotransmitter systems and brain regions. Understanding these mechanisms is paramount for the development of targeted interventions that address the specific neurobiological challenges posed by substance use disorders.

Tolerance and neuroplasticity in physical addiction: As the body adapts to the presence of the addictive substances, tolerance develops. This tolerance reflects the diminished response to the substance over time, necessitating increased consumption to attain the desired effect. Concurrently, neuroplasticity occurs, reshaping neural connections and reinforcing the body's dependence on the substance for a sense of normalcy. Tolerance and neuroplasticity unravel the adaptive responses to prolonged substance exposure. Tolerance to drugs is a key aspect of substance use disorders, is a phenomenon where an individual requires increasing amounts of a substance to achieve the same effects.

Chronic opioid use induces tolerance through adaptive changes in the opioid receptor system. Downregulation of opioid receptors occurs, diminishing their responsiveness and necessitating higher doses for the same analgesic effects (Colvin et al., 2019). Tolerance to stimulants, such as cocaine, involves dysregulation of the dopaminergic system. Repeated exposure leads to a blunted response to dopamine release, contributing to the need for escalating doses to maintain the desired effects (Lüscher & Ungless, 2006). Tolerance to benzodiazepines involves adaptive changes in the GABAergic system. Downregulation of GABA receptors occurs, diminishing the inhibitory effects of the neurotransmitter and contributing to the need for increased drug doses (Jacob et al., 2008). Substances acting as NMDA receptor antagonists induce tolerance through alterations in the glutamatergic system. Neuroplastic changes in NMDA receptors contribute to the reduced sensitivity observed with prolonged exposure (Trujillo, 2000). Tolerance is closely linked to synaptic plasticity, including long-term potentiation (LTP). Chronic substance exposure induces adaptive changes in synaptic strength, contributing to the reduced responsiveness of neurons and the need for higher drug doses (Hyman et al., 2006). Metaplasticity, the regulation of plasticity mechanisms, plays a role in tolerance. Changes in the threshold for inducing plasticity contribute to the adaptive responses that underlie the development of tolerance.

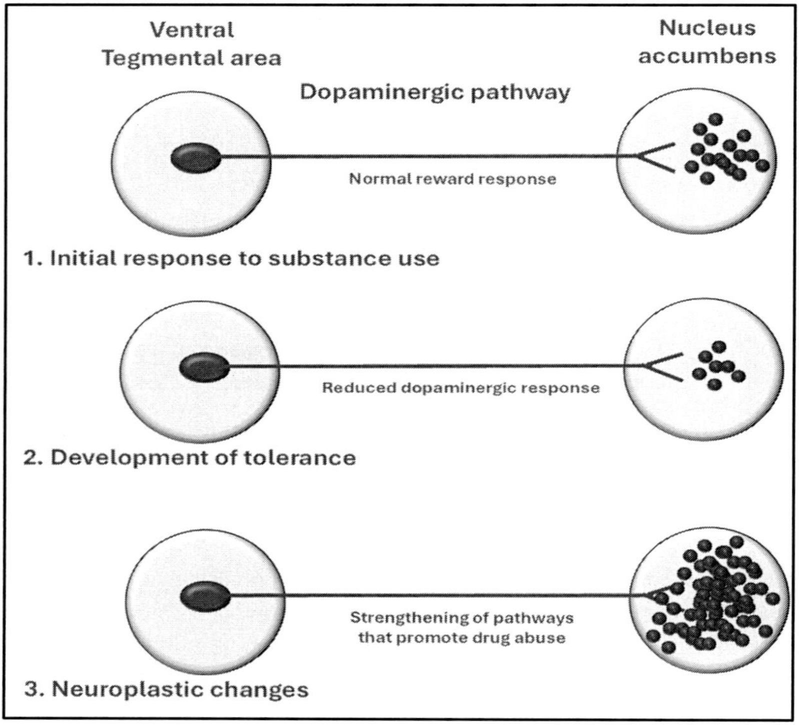

Tolerance and neuroplasticity in physical addiction

Chronic substance use induces neuroadaptive structural changes in gray matter volume. Tolerance is associated with alterations in brain structure, contributing to the need for escalating doses to maintain the desired effects (Makris et al., 2008). Tolerance is intricately linked to neuroplasticity, involving adaptive changes in neurotransmitter systems, synaptic plasticity, and brain structure. Understanding these mechanisms is crucial for addressing the challenges posed by tolerance in the context of substance use disorders.

Manifestations of Physical Addiction: Physical addiction often manifests in observable signs and symptoms. These may include changes in vital signs, such as increased heart rate or blood pressure, as well as physical discomfort when the substance is not consumed. Withdrawal symptoms, ranging from nausea and tremors to more severe manifestations like seizures, are hallmark indicators of physical dependence. Physical addiction, a complex consequence of chronic substance use, manifests through a spectrum of physiological and behavioral changes. One prominent manifestation of physical addiction is the development of tolerance. As the body adapts to the presence of a substance, individuals often require escalating doses to achieve the desired effects, a hallmark of the neuroadaptive changes in response to prolonged substance use (Nestler et al., 2001).

Tolerance reflects a diminished responsiveness to the effects of a substance, requiring individuals to consume increasingly higher amounts to experience the same level of intoxication or relief from withdrawal symptoms (Koob & Volkow, 2016). Physical addiction is often accompanied by physiological dependence, where the body becomes reliant on the presence of the substance to maintain normal functioning. Abrupt cessation can trigger withdrawal symptoms, ranging from mild discomfort to severe physiological distress. In addition to physiological dependence, emotional and psychological dependence are integral components of physical addiction. Individuals may experience intense cravings and emotional distress when attempting to abstain from the substance (Sinha, 2011).

Physical addiction often leads to a loss of control over substance use. Individuals may find themselves unable to moderate or stop their drug intake despite negative consequences, reflecting the compulsive nature of addiction (Everitt & Robbins, 2016). Manifestations of physical addiction include the persistence of drug-seeking behaviors even when individuals are aware of the negative consequences. This compulsivity underscores the profound impact of physical addiction on decision-making processes (Nock et al., 2017). Chronic substance use can lead to cognitive impairment, affecting various domains such as memory, attention, and executive functions. These cognitive deficits are often observed in individuals grappling with physical addiction (Verdejo-García & Bechara, 2009). Physical addiction is associated with structural changes in the brain, including alterations in gray matter volume. Regions critical for decision-making, such as the prefrontal cortex, may undergo modifications that contribute to impaired cognitive functions (Mackey & Paulus, 2013). Physical addiction manifests through a myriad of consequences, encompassing neuroadaptive changes in tolerance, withdrawal symptoms, compulsive drug-seeking behaviors, cognitive impairment, and structural alterations in the brain. Understanding these manifestations is crucial for developing comprehensive approaches to address the complexities of physical addiction.

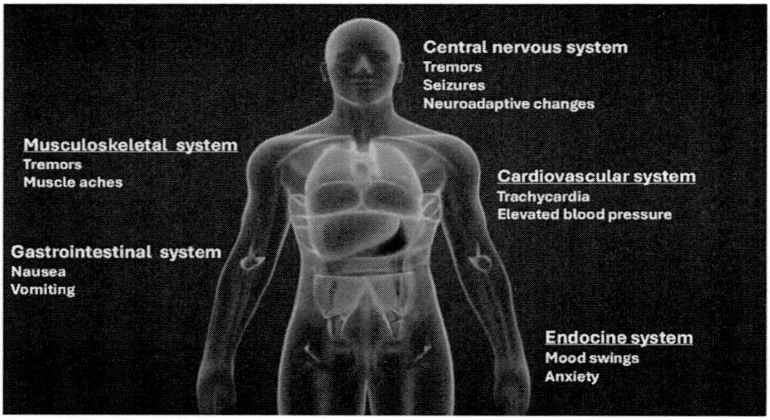

Manifestations of Physical Addiction

Compulsive Substance abuse in physical addiction: Individuals experiencing physical addiction often engage in compulsive substance use, driven by the need to avoid or alleviate withdrawal symptoms. Despite negative consequences, the compulsion to use the substance persists, highlighting the overpowering influence of physical dependence on behavior. Compulsive substance use is a defining characteristic of physical addiction, representing a persistent and uncontrollable pattern of drug-seeking and drug-taking behaviors. Compulsive substance use is intricately linked to alterations in the mesolimbic dopamine system, especially the nucleus accumbens. Prolonged exposure to addictive substances induces neuroadaptations that enhance the rewarding effects of drugs, reinforcing compulsive drug-seeking behaviors (Koob & Volkow, 2016).

The prefrontal cortex, crucial for decision-making and impulse control, plays a pivotal role in compulsive substance use. Dysfunction in this region is associated with a diminished ability to inhibit drug-seeking behaviors, contributing to the compulsivity observed in addiction (Goldstein & Volkow, 2011). The amygdala, a key player in emotional processing, is implicated in the compulsive nature of substance use. Neuroplastic changes in the amygdala contribute to the association between drug-related cues and the rewarding effects of substances, driving compulsive drug-seeking behaviors (Everitt & Robbins, 2016). Compulsive substance use is characterized by impaired inhibitory control, mediated by the prefrontal cortex. Neuroadaptations in this circuitry lead to a diminished ability to suppress drug-seeking impulses, fostering compulsive behaviors despite negative consequences (Goldstein & Volkow, 2011). Sensitization, an increased responsiveness to drug-related cues, contributes to the escalation of compulsive substance use. This heightened sensitivity enhances the salience of drug-related stimuli, reinforcing the compulsive cycle. Compulsive substance use involves a shift from goal-directed to habitual behavior. The transition is associated with neuroplastic changes in the striatum and is integral to the persistence of compulsive drug-seeking despite negative consequences (Everitt & Robbins, 2016).

Compulsive substance abuse is linked to altered cortico-striatal circuits, with evidence of striatal hyperactivity. This hyperactivity contributes to the reinforcement of compulsive drug-seeking behaviors, perpetuating the cycle of addiction (Belin et al., 2009). Compulsive substance use involves disrupted connectivity between brain regions, including the prefrontal cortex and the striatum. These connectivity alterations contribute to impaired cognitive control and the perpetuation of compulsive behaviors. In conclusion, compulsive substance use in physical addiction is intricately tied to neurobiological adaptations in reward-related circuits, inhibitory control mechanisms, and the interplay between emotional and cognitive processes. Understanding these mechanisms is essential for developing targeted interventions aimed at mitigating the compulsive nature of substance use in addiction.

Treatment Approaches for Physical Addiction: Addressing physical addiction often necessitates medical interventions and requires a multifaceted approach that encompasses pharmacological, behavioral, and supportive interventions. There are various treatment modalities for physical addiction, highlighting evidence-based strategies that aim to alleviate withdrawal symptoms, promote abstinence, and support long-term recovery. Medication-assisted treatment involves the use of medications to mitigate withdrawal symptoms, reduce cravings, and support sustained recovery. Common medications include methadone, buprenorphine, and naltrexone, each tailored to specific substances of abuse. For substances like alcohol or benzodiazepines, antidepressants and anti-anxiety medications may help manage mood disturbances and anxiety associated with withdrawal, supporting a more comfortable detoxification process. CBT helps individuals recognize and change maladaptive thought patterns and behaviors associated with addiction. It addresses triggers, reinforces coping skills, and promotes long-term abstinence (Carroll & Onken, 2005). Contingency management utilizes a reward system to reinforce positive behaviors such as drug abstinence. This approach has shown effectiveness, particularly in the treatment of stimulant addiction

Supportive Therapies include support groups and 12-step programs. Participation in support groups provides individuals with a sense of community, peer support, and a structured program for recovery. Supportive Therapies are integral components of comprehensive addiction treatment, providing individuals with emotional, social, and psychological support as they navigate the challenges of physical addiction. SMART Recovery is another self-help program that employs a science-based, cognitive-behavioral approach. It focuses on empowering individuals to overcome addiction through self-management and supportive group discussions (Zemore et al., 2014). Involving family members or partners in therapy can be crucial for addressing underlying interpersonal issues contributing to addiction. Family therapy enhances communication, support, and understanding within the familial unit. Community Reinforcement and Family Training (CRAFT) is an evidence-based approach that empowers family members to positively influence their loved one's behavior. It teaches communication skills, reinforces positive behaviors, and encourages treatment engagement. Motivational Enhancement Therapy (MET) is a client-centered therapy that aims to enhance intrinsic motivation for change. By exploring ambivalence and fostering self-efficacy, MET can be effective in initiating and sustaining behavioral change (Miller & Rollnick, 2002).

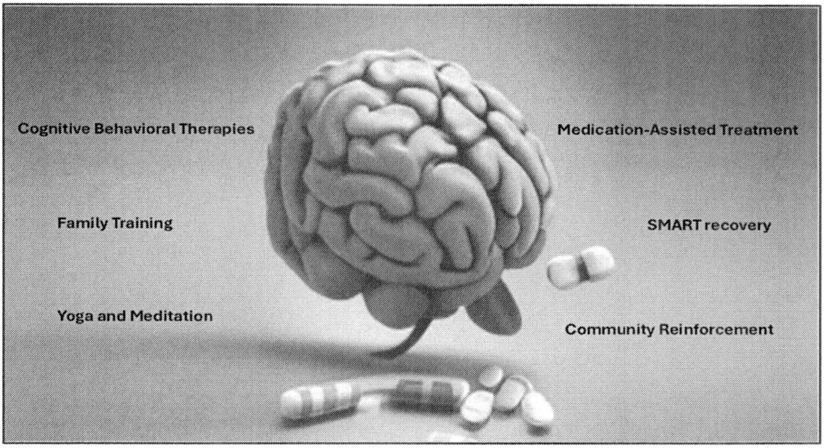

Treatment approaches for physical addiction

Mindfulness-based interventions, such as Mindfulness-Based Relapse Prevention (MBRP), incorporate mindfulness practices to help individuals manage cravings, cope with stress, and cultivate a non-judgmental awareness of thoughts and emotions. Holistic therapies such as art and music therapy provide individuals with creative outlets for self-expression and emotional processing. These therapies can aid in addressing underlying emotional issues and promoting overall well-being. Yoga and meditation also offer physical and mental benefits, promoting relaxation, stress reduction, and increased self-awareness. Integrating these practices into addiction treatment can support overall recovery (Keng et al., 2011). All of these various types of supportive therapies play a vital role in the holistic treatment of physical addiction. By addressing social, emotional, and psychological aspects of addiction, these interventions enhance the overall well-being of individuals on the path to recovery. The integration of supportive therapies into addiction treatment plans contributes to a more comprehensive and compassionate approach to healing.

Long-Term aftercare: After initial treatment, ongoing care and follow-up are crucial. This may involve regular follow-ups, therapy sessions, and support group attendance to reinforce recovery efforts and prevent relapse.

Continuing care and follow-up after drug abuse treatment are critical components of the recovery journey. This phase focuses on maintaining the progress achieved during formal treatment, addressing potential relapse triggers, and providing ongoing support to individuals striving for sustained recovery. Continuing care serves as a bridge between the structured environment of formal treatment and the challenges of everyday life. It aims to reinforce the gains made during treatment, helping individuals apply coping skills and strategies to real-world scenarios (McKay, 2009).

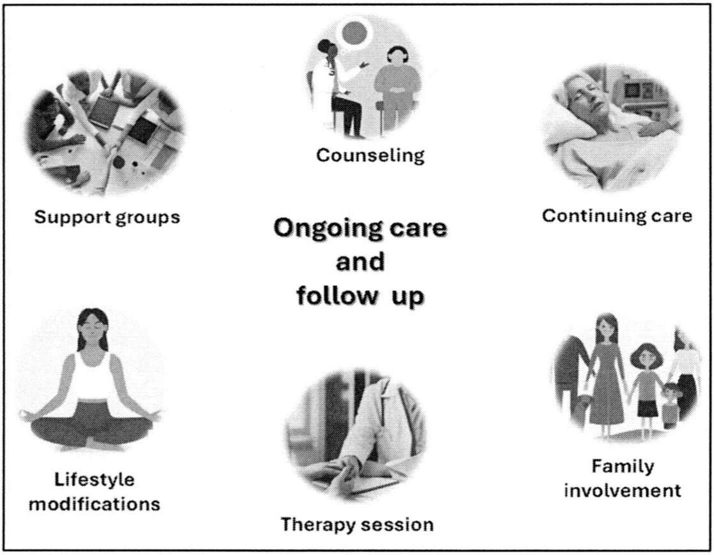

Aftercare following initial treatment of physical addiction

Recognizing addiction as a chronic condition emphasizes the need for ongoing care. Continuing care acknowledges that sustained recovery often requires ongoing support, monitoring, and adaptation to evolving needs. Outpatient counseling provides a structured environment for individuals to discuss challenges, reinforce coping skills, and receive ongoing therapeutic support. Regular therapy sessions contribute to emotional well-being and relapse prevention. Peer recovery coaches are the individuals with lived experience in recovery, provide guidance, empathy, and practical support.

Their role includes helping navigate challenges, reinforcing recovery goals, and fostering a sense of hope. Continued education on life skills, such as stress management, communication, and problem-solving, equips individuals with the tools necessary for navigating daily challenges without resorting to substance use. Assisting individuals in pursuing vocational or educational goals enhances their sense of purpose and self-worth. Continuing care involves supporting individuals in building a fulfilling and productive life in recovery. Regular follow-up appointments with treatment providers allow for ongoing assessment, adjustments to the treatment plan, and addressing any emerging challenges or concerns. Periodic drug testing serves as a valuable tool for monitoring abstinence and providing individuals with objective feedback on their progress. It can be a supportive element in accountability.

Teaching individuals coping mechanisms and strategies to identify and manage triggers is vital for preventing relapse. Behavioral strategies, such as mindfulness and stress reduction, play a key role in maintaining recovery. The treatment of physical addiction requires a comprehensive approach that addresses both the physiological and psychological aspects of the condition. By combining pharmacological interventions, evidence-based behavioral therapies, and ongoing support, individuals can navigate the path to recovery with increased chances of long-term success. Detoxification, conducted under medical supervision, helps manage withdrawal symptoms, ensuring a safer transition to sobriety. Medications may be prescribed to alleviate cravings and support recovery.

Rehabilitation Programs for physical addiction: Comprehensive rehabilitation programs provide a structured environment for individuals grappling with physical addiction. These programs incorporate counseling, support groups, and education to address the psychological aspects of addiction while concurrently managing physical withdrawal. While strides have been made in understanding and treating physical addiction, challenges persist. Stigma surrounding addiction, limited access to treatment, and the evolving landscape of substance availability contribute to the complexity of addressing physical dependence. Continued research and a holistic approach that integrates medical and psychological interventions hold promise for advancing our understanding and improving outcomes for individuals affected by physical addiction. Physical addiction represents a profound interaction between substances and the human body, reshaping neural pathways and compelling compulsive behavior. Recognizing the distinctive features of physical dependence is crucial for effective intervention and support. As the scientific community and healthcare providers continue to unravel the complexities of physical addiction, a compassionate and comprehensive approach remains paramount in mitigating the impact of this pervasive phenomenon on individuals and society at large.

Psychological addiction, also known as behavioral or mental addiction, is characterized by a compulsive need for a behavior or activity, despite negative consequences. Unlike physical addiction, which involves a physiological dependence on a substance, psychological addiction revolves around the emotional and psychological reliance on a particular behavior. The distinction between psychological and physical dependence lies in the nature of the reliance and the underlying mechanisms driving dependency. While both types of dependence often coexist in cases of substance abuse, they represent distinct aspects of addiction. Psychological dependence involves cravings, urges, and a strong desire to engage in a particular behavior or consume a substance for its perceived emotional or psychological benefits. Emotional attachment and a sense of emotional relief or pleasure are associated with the addictive behavior. Psychological dependence could develop even in the absence of physical withdrawal symptoms, and the motivation to continue the behavior is often driven by emotional and psychological factors.

Few examples of psychological dependence include compulsive gambling, internet addiction, and behavioral addictions like shopping or gaming are often rooted in psychological dependence. Many cases of addiction involve both psychological and physical dependence. For example, individuals with alcohol use disorder may experience both the emotional need to drink for stress relief (psychological dependence) and the physical reliance accompanied by withdrawal symptoms (physical dependence). Psychological and physical dependence often interact, with the psychological aspects driving the initiation and maintenance of the behavior, while physical dependence reinforces the continuation of the behavior through the avoidance of withdrawal symptoms. Treatment for psychological dependence often involves behavioral therapies, counseling, and interventions aimed at addressing the emotional and psychological factors contributing to the addiction.

Individuals with a gambling addiction experience an irresistible urge to gamble, leading to negative effects on their personal, financial, and professional lives. The thrill of risking money becomes a psychological dependency that is challenging to control. Excessive use of the internet, social media, video games, or other digital platforms can lead to psychological addiction. Individuals may find themselves unable to disengage from these activities, impacting their relationships, work, and overall well-being. Shopping addiction (compulsive buying disorder) involves an irresistible urge to shop, leading to excessive spending and accumulating unnecessary possessions. The act of shopping becomes a way to cope with emotional stress or fill a void, resulting in a cycle of psychological dependence.

Food addiction (eating disorders) such as binge eating or compulsive overeating, are forms of psychological addiction where individuals use food as a way to cope with emotional challenges. This behavior can lead to physical health issues and negatively impact mental well-being. Individuals with sexual addiction engage in compulsive sexual behaviors despite negative consequences. This addiction can manifest as excessive pornography consumption, multiple sexual partners, or other behaviors that interfere with daily life and relationships. Work Addiction (Workaholism), involves an obsessive focus on work to the detriment of personal relationships, health, and overall life balance. The need for achievement and validation from work becomes a psychological dependency that is challenging to break. While exercise is generally beneficial, some individuals develop an unhealthy reliance on physical activity. Exercise addiction can lead to excessive workouts, even in the face of injury or exhaustion, as individuals become psychologically dependent on the endorphin release associated with exercise. Excessive use of social media platforms can lead to psychological addiction, with individuals constantly seeking validation through likes, comments, and online interactions. The fear of missing out (FOMO) and comparison with others contribute to this dependency. Video game addiction involves an excessive and compulsive engagement with video games, leading to impaired daily functioning and interpersonal relationships. The immersive and rewarding nature of gaming can create a powerful psychological pull.

Substance Abuse and Behavioral Psychological addiction often coexists with substance abuse. Individuals may use substances like drugs or alcohol to cope with the emotional effects of their behavioral addiction, creating a complex web of dependencies. Addressing psychological addiction requires a holistic approach, including therapeutic interventions, support systems, and strategies to cope with underlying emotional issues. Recognizing the psychological nature of these addictions is essential for developing effective treatment plans and promoting long-term recovery. Understanding the distinction between psychological and physical dependence is essential for developing targeted and effective interventions that address the specific challenges associated with each aspect of addiction. A comprehensive approach that considers both psychological and physical elements provides a more nuanced and effective strategy for addiction treatment and recovery.

Neural Mechanisms of psychological addiction: The neural mechanisms underlying psychological addiction involve complex interactions within the brain's reward system, which is primarily centered around the release of neurotransmitters and the activation of specific brain regions. While the exact neural processes can vary depending on the type of addiction, there are commonalities in the way the brain responds to rewarding stimuli and how maladaptive changes occur over time. Dopamine, a neurotransmitter associated with pleasure and reward, plays a central role in psychological addiction. When an individual engages in a rewarding behavior, such as gambling or substance use, the brain's reward system releases dopamine in a region known as the nucleus accumbens. This process reinforces the behavior and creates a sense of pleasure. Dopamine is associated with the brain's reward system, and its release is linked to pleasurable sensations and reinforcement of certain behaviors. Understanding the role of dopamine in psychological addiction involves exploring how it influences the brain's reward pathways and contributes to the reinforcing nature of addictive behaviors. Apart from physical addiction, the brain’s reward system, centered around the nucleus accumbens and the ventral tegmental area

(VTA), is a key player in psychological addiction as well. Dopamine neurons originating in the VTA project to the nucleus accumbens, releasing dopamine when an individual engages in a rewarding behavior. Dopamine is often referred to as the "feel-good" neurotransmitter because it contributes to the sensation of pleasure and reinforces behaviors associated with reward. In the context of psychological addiction, engaging in addictive behavior leads to a surge in dopamine, creating a sense of pleasure and reinforcing the desire to repeat the behavior.

Dopamine is involved in associative learning, where the brain forms connections between stimuli and rewarding experiences. In the context of psychological addiction, cues associated with the addictive behavior can trigger the release of dopamine, creating a powerful link between environmental cues and the desire to engage in the addictive behavior. Dopamine is also implicated in the experience of craving, a powerful urge to engage in the addictive behavior. The release of dopamine creates a motivational drive, compelling individuals to seek out and repeat the rewarding behavior to satisfy the craving. Prolonged engagement in addictive behaviors can lead to neuroplastic changes in the brain, affecting the sensitivity of dopamine receptors. This neuroadaptation can contribute to the development of tolerance, where higher levels of the addictive behavior are needed to achieve the same dopamine-mediated reward.

Dopamine is also involved in the withdrawal phase of addiction. When the addictive behavior is reduced or discontinued, there is a decrease in dopamine levels, contributing to withdrawal symptoms. These symptoms can include feelings of dysphoria, irritability, and a strong desire to engage in the addictive behavior to alleviate discomfort. Understanding the intricate role of dopamine in psychological addiction provides insights into the neural mechanisms that drive the reinforcement and persistence of addictive behaviors. Research in this field continues to enhance our understanding of addiction, opening avenues for the development of targeted interventions aimed at mitigating the impact of dopamine dysregulation on addictive behaviors.

Reward circuit in psychological addiction: The reward circuit involves interconnected regions such as the ventral tegmental area (VTA), nucleus accumbens, and prefrontal cortex. These areas work together to process and reinforce pleasurable experiences. Over time, repeated exposure to rewarding stimuli can lead to neuroplastic changes, altering the sensitivity of this circuitry.

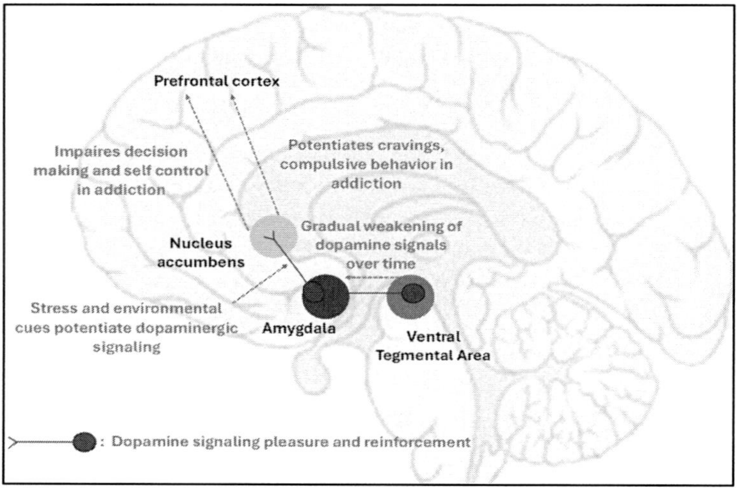

Reward circuit in psychological addiction

The reward circuitry in the brain is a crucial component in understanding psychological addiction. This circuitry, also known as the brain's reward system, is a complex network of neural pathways and structures that play a central role in reinforcing behaviors associated with pleasure and reward. In the context of psychological addiction, the reward circuitry becomes dysregulated, contributing to the compulsive engagement in addictive behaviors. The primary components of the reward circuitry include the ventral tegmental area (VTA), nucleus accumbens, and the prefrontal cortex. When an individual engages in a psychological rewarding behavior, such as gambling or internet addiction, dopamine neurons in the VTA are activated. These neurons project to the nucleus accumbens, releasing dopamine and creating a sensation of pleasure and reward. The reward circuitry is involved in associative learning, where the brain forms connections between environmental cues and the rewarding experience. Over time, these associations become powerful triggers, leading individuals to seek out and engage in behaviors that activate the reward system. Dopamine release serves as a reinforcement mechanism, reinforcing the link between the pleasurable experience and the associated behavior. This reinforcement strengthens the likelihood that the individual will repeat the behavior to experience the pleasurable effects.

The activation of the reward circuitry contributes to the experience of craving, a strong desire to engage in the addictive behavior. Dopamine, along with other neurotransmitters, creates a motivational drive that compels individuals to seek out and engage in the behavior to satisfy the craving. Prolonged engagement in addictive behaviors can lead to neuroplastic changes in the reward circuitry. Neuroadaptations can occur, altering the sensitivity of dopamine receptors. This neuroplasticity contributes to the development of tolerance, requiring higher levels of the addictive behavior to achieve the same level of reward. When the addictive behavior is reduced or discontinued, there is a decrease in dopamine release, contributing to withdrawal symptoms. The dysregulation of the reward circuitry is evident in the negative emotional and physical effects experienced during withdrawal, motivating individuals to continue the psychological addictive behavior (Wise, 2004; Koob & Volkow, 2010). Understanding the reward circuitry's role in psychological addiction sheds light on the neural mechanisms that drive the reinforcing nature of addictive behaviors. Research in this field is essential for developing targeted interventions aimed at restoring balance to the reward system and mitigating the compulsive nature of psychological addiction.

Craving and Reinforcement in psychological addiction: With continued engagement in the addictive behavior, the brain undergoes adaptations that increase the individual's sensitivity to cues associated with the addiction. This heightened sensitivity contributes to cravings, creating a cycle where the individual is driven to repeat the behavior to experience the associated reward. In psychological addiction, cues play a significant role in triggering cravings and reinforcing addictive behaviors. The association between environmental cues and the rewarding experience creates a powerful link in the brain's circuitry, contributing to the persistence of psychological dependence. Understanding how cues become intertwined with cravings and reinforcement is crucial in comprehending the complex nature of psychological addiction. Psychological addiction often involves associative learning, where the brain forms connections between specific cues or stimuli and the rewarding experience associated with the addictive behavior. For example, a person addicted to smoking may associate the smell of cigarette smoke or the sight of a lighter with the pleasurable effects of nicotine. Environmental cues linked to the addictive behavior can trigger intense cravings. These cravings are a powerful urge or desire to engage in the addictive behavior, driven by the anticipation of the rewarding experience associated with the cues. Neurologically, cues activate the brain's reward circuitry, particularly the ventral tegmental area (VTA) and the nucleus accumbens. The release of neurotransmitters, including dopamine, reinforces the connection between the cue and the pleasurable effects of the addictive behavior (Robinson & Berridge, 2003).

The process of Pavlovian conditioning, where neutral stimuli become associated with a rewarding event, is often observed in psychological addiction. Over time, these neutral stimuli transform into powerful cues capable of eliciting cravings and reinforcing the desire to engage in the addictive behavior. Stress can amplify the impact of cues in psychological addiction. Individuals may be more susceptible to cue-induced cravings during times of stress, as the brain seeks the rewarding effects of the addictive behavior as a coping mechanism (Sinha, 2008). Various environmental factors, such as specific locations, social situations, or emotional states, can serve as cues. These triggers become powerful reminders linked to the rewarding experience of the addictive behavior, prompting individuals to seek out and engage in the behavior. The engagement in psychological addictive behaviors in response to cues is often reinforced by negative reinforcement. Behavior provides temporary relief from stress, anxiety, or discomfort associated with craving, creating a cycle where individuals turn to the addictive behavior as a coping mechanism. Treatment strategies for psychological addiction often involve addressing cue-induced cravings. Therapeutic approaches, such as cue exposure therapy, aim to weaken the association between cues and addictive behaviors, reducing the power of environmental triggers. Understanding the intricate relationship between cues, cravings, and reinforcement provides insights into the challenges individuals face in breaking free from psychological addiction. Interventions that target these cue-response associations play a crucial role in the development of effective treatment strategies, empowering individuals to overcome the powerful influence of environmental triggers on their addictive behaviors (Baker et al., 2004).

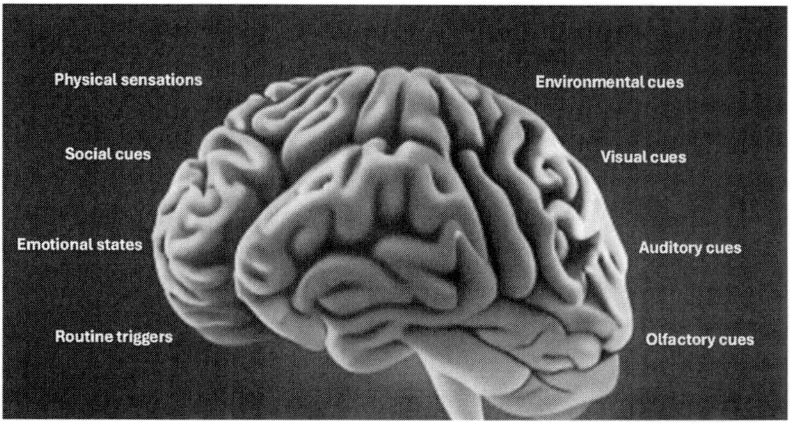

Craving and Reinforcement in psychological addiction

Endorphins and natural reinforcement in psychological addiction: In addition to dopamine, the release of endorphins, the body's natural opioids, contributes to the reinforcing effects of addictive behaviors. Endorphins produce feelings of pleasure and reduce the perception of pain, further reinforcing the desire to engage in addictive behavior. The role of endorphins in psychological addiction is integral to understanding the reinforcing nature of certain behaviors and the development of addictive patterns. Endorphins, the body's natural opioids, play a key role in the brain's reward system, contributing to the pleasurable sensations associated with various activities. In the context of psychological addiction, the release of endorphins becomes a powerful mechanism of natural reinforcement, reinforcing behaviors that lead to their secretion. Here's an exploration of how endorphins contribute to natural reinforcement in psychological addiction:

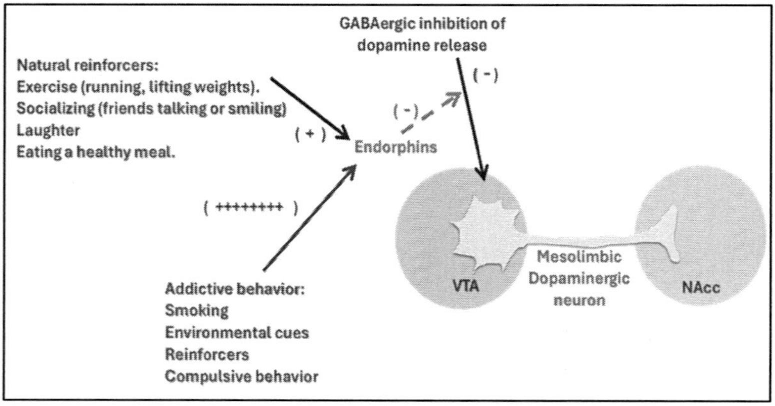

Endorphins and natural reinforcement in psychological addiction

Endorphins are neurotransmitters that act as natural opioids, binding to the same receptors as opioid drugs. Their release is associated with feelings of pleasure, pain relief, and a sense of well-being (Zubieta et al., 2001). In psychological addiction, engaging in certain behaviors that lead to the release of endorphins is positively reinforced. This positive reinforcement contributes to the formation and strengthening of the association between the behavior and the pleasurable effects, motivating individuals to repeat the behavior. Behavioral addictions, such as compulsive gambling or binge eating, often involve activities that trigger the release of endorphins. The natural reinforcement provided by endorphins contributes to the development and maintenance of these addictive behaviors (Holden, 2001).

Exercise is a common behavioral activity associated with the release of endorphins. While regular exercise is generally beneficial, in cases of exercise addiction, individuals may engage excessively in physical activity to experience the mood-enhancing effects of endorphins (Boecker et al., 2008). Endorphins are released not only in response to pleasurable activities but also during stress. In psychological addiction, individuals may engage in certain behaviors as a means of stress reduction, leading to the release of endorphins and reinforcing the behavior as a coping mechanism (Drolet et al., 2001). Investigating the role of endorphins in natural reinforcement provides insights into the mechanisms that contribute to the development and perpetuation of psychological addiction. Integrating this knowledge into therapeutic approaches can be essential for addressing the underlying factors driving addictive behaviors and promoting healthier alternatives for pleasure and stress relief.

Tolerance and sensitization in psychological addiction: Over the period of time, brain may develop tolerance to the effects of the addictive behavior, leading individuals to seek increased levels of stimulation. This tolerance is often accompanied by sensitization, where the individual becomes more responsive to the cues associated with the addiction. Tolerance and sensitization are two interconnected phenomena observed in psychological addiction, reflecting the adaptive changes that occur in the brain over the course of repeated exposure to addictive substances or behaviors. These processes contribute to the escalation of addiction and the challenges associated with managing and treating addictive disorders. Tolerance refers to the diminishing effect of a substance or behavior over time, requiring increased amounts or intensity to achieve the same desired effect.

In psychological addiction, the brain adapts to the consistent exposure to rewarding stimuli by adjusting its neural circuitry, leading to a decreased responsiveness to the pleasurable effects. This results in individuals needing higher doses or engaging in more intense behaviors to experience the same level of satisfaction. Behavioral sensitization is the opposite of tolerance and involves an increased response to a substance or behavior over time, leading to heightened reactivity. While tolerance involves desensitization of neural pathways, sensitization involves an augmentation of the brain's response to the addictive stimuli. This increased sensitivity can result in exaggerated cravings and intensified engagement in addictive behaviors. Sensitization and tolerance are not mutually exclusive and can occur simultaneously or sequentially in the course of addiction. The interplay between these processes contributes to the complexity and variability of addictive behaviors. Both tolerance and sensitization to psychological addiction involve neurobiological adaptations in regions such as the nucleus accumbens, prefrontal cortex, and amygdala. These adaptations influence the processing of reward-related cues and the regulation of motivation (Hyman & Malenka, 2001).

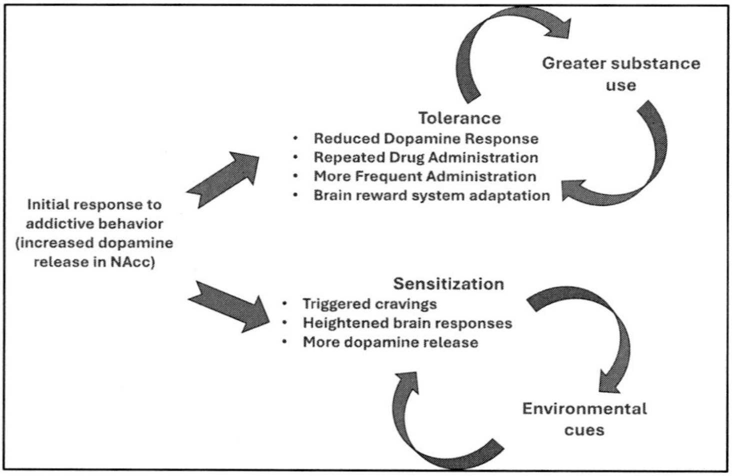

Tolerance and sensitization in psychological addiction

Recognizing the presence of tolerance and sensitization informs treatment strategies, emphasizing the need for individualized interventions. Comprehensive approaches may include behavioral therapies, pharmacological interventions, and addressing underlying psychological factors (Nessa et al., 2008). Understanding the dynamic relationship between tolerance and sensitization provides valuable insights into the complexities of psychological addiction. As researchers delve deeper into the neurobiological mechanisms underlying these phenomena, targeted and effective interventions can be developed to address the adaptive changes in the brain and facilitate sustainable recovery from addictive behaviors.

Hijacking of learning pathways in psychological addiction: The brain's learning pathways, particularly those involving the hippocampus and amygdala, play a role in associating environmental cues with rewarding experiences. In psychological addiction, these pathways can be hijacked, leading to the formation of strong associations between cues and addictive behavior. Psychological addiction involves a profound influence on the brain's learning pathways, leading to the formation of strong associations between environmental cues and addictive behaviors. This hijacking of learning processes contributes to the development and persistence of addictive habits. Understanding how these pathways are manipulated sheds light on the complexity of psychological addiction. The hijacking of learning pathways in psychological addiction involves associative learning and conditioning. Neutral stimuli in the environment become associated with the rewarding effects of addictive behaviors, creating powerful cues that trigger cravings and drive continued engagement. Learning pathways involving the hippocampus and amygdala play a crucial role in the formation of memories associated with psychological addictive behaviors. The hippocampus is involved in contextual memory, while the amygdala processes the emotional significance of these memories.

The hijacking of learning pathways is evident in Pavlovian conditioning, where neutral stimuli become associated with the pleasurable effects of psychological addictive behaviors. This creates a strong link between cues and the motivation to engage in the addictive behavior. Prolonged engagement in psychological addictive behaviors leads to neuroplastic changes, altering the structure and function of neural circuits. These adaptations contribute to the persistence of psychological addictive habits and the difficulty in breaking the cycle of addiction. Learning pathways in psychological addiction contribute to the development of conditioned responses. Environmental cues associated with the addictive behavior can automatically trigger cravings, compelling individuals to seek out and engage in the behavior.

Recognizing the hijacking of learning pathways by psychologically addictive behaviors is crucial for developing targeted interventions. Therapeutic approaches, such as cue exposure therapy and cognitive-behavioral therapy, aim to weaken the association between cues and addictive behaviors. Understanding how learning pathways are hijacked in psychological addiction provides insights into the lasting impact of addictive behaviors on the brain. Researchers and clinicians continue to explore innovative strategies to address these hijacked pathways and promote effective treatments for individuals struggling with psychological addiction.

Impaired executive function in psychological addiction: Prolonged engagement in addictive behaviors can impair executive functions mediated by the prefrontal cortex, such as decision-making, impulse control, and judgment. This can contribute to the difficulty individuals face in stopping addictive behaviors despite awareness of negative consequences. Psychological addiction is intricately linked to alterations in cognitive processes, particularly the impairment of executive function. Executive functions, which include processes such as decision-making, impulse control, and cognitive flexibility, are crucial for self-regulation and goal-directed behavior. In the context of psychological addiction, these functions become compromised, contributing to the development and perpetuation of addictive behaviors. Individuals with psychological addiction often exhibit deficits in decision-making, characterized by impulsivity and a diminished ability to weigh the long-term consequences of their actions.

Executive functions, particularly those related to inhibitory control, are impaired in individuals with psychological addiction. This results in an increased susceptibility to impulsive behaviors, including the inability to resist the urge to engage in addictive activities. Rigidity in Thinking: Impaired cognitive flexibility, an essential component of executive function, is evident in psychological addiction. Individuals may struggle to adapt their thinking and behavior in response to changing circumstances, contributing to the persistence of maladaptive habits (Ersche & Sahakian, 2007).

Executive function impairment in psychological addiction extends to altered reward processing. The brain's ability to appropriately evaluate and respond to rewards is compromised, contributing to the reinforcing nature of addictive behaviors. The prefrontal cortex, a critical region for executive functions, experiences dysfunction in psychological addiction. Structural and functional abnormalities in this area contribute to impaired decision-making, emotional regulation, and impulse control. Rehabilitative approaches involve recognizing the impact of impaired executive function is crucial for tailoring effective treatment strategies. Interventions that focus on improving decision-making skills, enhancing impulse control, and promoting cognitive flexibility can be integral to addiction rehabilitation. Understanding the impact of impaired executive function in psychological addiction provides a foundation for developing targeted interventions that address the cognitive underpinnings of addictive behaviors. Integrating cognitive remediation strategies into addiction treatment may enhance the effectiveness of interventions, fostering improved decision-making and self-regulation in individuals struggling with psychological addiction.

Withdrawal and negative reinforcement in psychological addiction: Withdrawal symptoms, both physical and psychological, contribute to the persistence of addiction. The relief of withdrawal symptoms through engagement in the addictive behavior negatively reinforces the cycle, as individuals seek to alleviate discomfort through continued participation. Withdrawal is a critical aspect of psychological addiction, characterized by a set of physical and psychological symptoms that occur when an individual reduces or discontinues the use of a substance or engages less in an addictive behavior. The experience of withdrawal is often a powerful motivator for continued engagement in addictive behaviors, driven by the desire to alleviate the distressing symptoms. This phenomenon is closely tied to negative reinforcement, a psychological process where the removal of an aversive stimulus (withdrawal symptoms, in this case) strengthens or increases the likelihood of a particular behavior.

Psychological and Physical Effects: Withdrawal symptoms in psychological addiction can manifest as a combination of psychological distress (anxiety, irritability, dysphoria) and physical discomfort (nausea, tremors, fatigue). The specific symptoms vary depending on the substance or behavior involved. Negative reinforcement comes into play as individuals engage in addictive behaviors to alleviate or avoid the unpleasant symptoms of withdrawal. This relief creates a reinforcing loop, strengthening the association between the behavior and the relief from withdrawal distress. Motivation for Continued Use: The negative reinforcement loop contributes to the compulsion to continue engaging in addictive behaviors despite negative consequences. The desire to avoid or alleviate withdrawal symptoms becomes a powerful driving force. Individuals with psychological addiction may use substances or engage in addictive behaviors as a form of self-medication to escape or alleviate the dysphoric symptoms of withdrawal. Prolonged engagement in addictive behaviors leading to withdrawal triggers neurobiological adaptations, including changes in neurotransmitter systems. These adaptations contribute to the negative reinforcement cycle by reinforcing the association between the addictive behavior and relief from withdrawal symptoms.

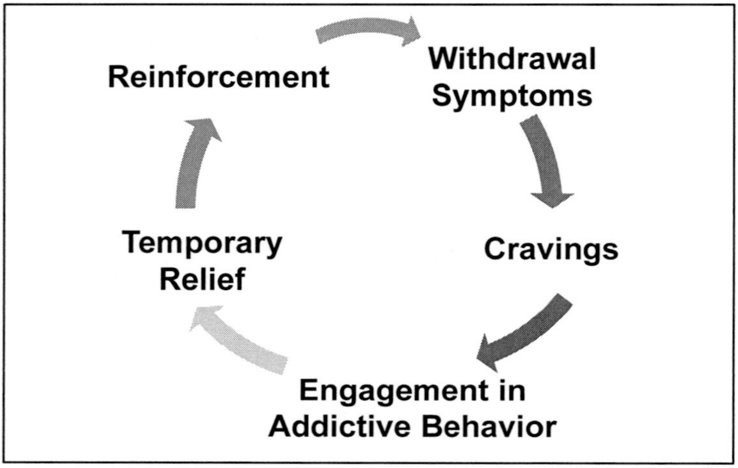

Withdrawal and negative reinforcement in psychological addiction

Effective treatment for psychological addiction often involves addressing the negative reinforcement cycle. Therapeutic approaches aim to help individuals develop alternative coping mechanisms and reduce reliance on addictive behaviors for relief from withdrawal symptoms (Sinha & Li, 2007). Understanding the interplay between withdrawal and negative reinforcement is crucial for designing comprehensive interventions that target both the physiological and psychological components of addiction. By addressing the motivation to alleviate withdrawal symptoms, treatment strategies can help individuals break the cycle of negative reinforcement and work towards sustainable recovery.

Behavioral therapy for psychological addiction: Behavioral therapy, such as cognitive-behavioral therapy (CBT), is a cornerstone in treating psychological addiction. CBT helps individuals identify and change negative thought patterns and behaviors associated with addiction. One-on-one counseling sessions provide a safe space for individuals to explore the underlying issues contributing to their addictive behaviors. Therapists work collaboratively with clients to develop coping strategies and healthier ways of thinking. Motivational Enhancement Therapy (MET) is a therapeutic approach that helps individuals find internal motivation to change addictive behaviors. It focuses on resolving ambivalence and building intrinsic motivation for positive change. Contingency Management (CM) is a behavior therapy that utilizes operant conditioning principles to reinforce positive behaviors and discourage negative ones. It often involves the use of incentives or rewards to promote abstinence and adherence to treatment goals. On the other hand, enhancing Intrinsic Motivation (IM) is a client-centered approach that seeks to enhance intrinsic motivation and resolve ambivalence about change. It is particularly effective in addressing the motivational aspects of addiction and promoting readiness for positive behavioral changes. Dialectical Behavior Therapy (DBT), originally developed for individuals with borderline personality disorder, has shown efficacy in the treatment of addiction. It emphasizes emotion regulation, distress tolerance, and interpersonal effectiveness, providing a comprehensive approach to address underlying issues (Linehan et al., 2002).

Rational Emotive Behavior Therapy (REBT) focuses on identifying and challenging irrational beliefs that contribute to addictive behaviors. By promoting rational thinking and emotional regulation, it aims to reduce the impact of irrational thoughts on behavior. Behavioral Couples Therapy (BCT) involves the patient's significant other in the therapeutic process, utilizing behavioral principles to improve relationship dynamics and support abstinence. It is particularly effective for substance use disorders. Community Reinforcement Approach (CRA) focuses on rearranging an individual's lifestyle to maximize positive reinforcement for non-addictive behaviors. It involves identifying and enhancing non-substance-related sources of reinforcement (Meyers et al., 2011). All of these behavioral therapy approaches for psychological addiction are diverse, allowing for tailored interventions that address the unique needs and preferences of individuals. These evidence-based therapies, often used in combination, provide a comprehensive framework for promoting lasting behavioral change and facilitating recovery from addiction.

Mindfulness and Meditation for psychological addiction: Mindfulness techniques and meditation can be effective in managing cravings and increasing self-awareness. These practices help individuals stay present in the moment and develop a greater understanding of their thoughts and emotions. Mindfulness and meditation have emerged as powerful complementary approaches in the treatment of psychological addiction, offering individuals valuable tools to enhance self-awareness, regulate emotions, and cultivate a non-judgmental acceptance of the present moment. These practices draw from contemplative traditions and are increasingly integrated into addiction treatment programs. Mindfulness-Based Relapse Prevention (MBRP) is a specific program that integrates mindfulness practices into traditional relapse prevention strategies. It aims to disrupt automatic, habitual reactions to triggers by fostering mindful awareness of thoughts, emotions, and cravings (Witkiewitz et al., 2005). Mindfulness meditation has been shown to reduce cravings and increase self-control by fostering non-reactive awareness. Individuals learn to observe cravings without judgment, disrupting the automatic chain of thoughts leading to substance use. Mindfulness-Based Stress Reduction (MBSR), developed by Jon Kabat-Zinn, incorporates mindfulness meditation to reduce stress and enhance overall well-being. For individuals with addiction, stress reduction is crucial as it often contributes to the initiation and maintenance of addictive behaviors. Another approach is Mindfulness-Based Cognitive Therapy (MBCT), which had originally been designed for depression, has shown promise in preventing relapse in individuals with addiction. It combines cognitive therapy with mindfulness practices, helping individuals become aware of negative thought patterns that may contribute to relapse (Teasdale et al., 2000).

Meditation focuses on cultivating feelings of love and compassion and could be beneficial for individuals with addiction by promoting self-compassion and reducing negative self-judgment. Research suggests that mindfulness practices can induce neuroplastic changes in areas of the brain associated with self-control, emotional regulation, and decision-making, which are crucial for overcoming addiction (Tang et al., 2015). Mindfulness is increasingly integrated into various substance abuse treatment programs, demonstrating its potential to enhance overall outcomes by addressing not only the symptoms of addiction but also the underlying processes. Mindfulness and meditation offer individuals with psychological addiction valuable skills for managing cravings, regulating emotions, and fostering a holistic approach to recovery. As the field continues to explore the integration of these practices into addiction treatment, the potential for positive outcomes and sustainable recovery becomes increasingly evident.

Group Therapy for psychological addiction: Group therapy sessions create a supportive community where individuals facing similar challenges can share experiences, receive feedback, and learn from each other. This sense of camaraderie can be particularly beneficial in overcoming psychological addiction. Nowadays it is a widely utilized and effective therapeutic approach in the treatment of psychological addiction. It provides a supportive and structured environment where individuals with similar struggles can share experiences, receive feedback, and collectively work towards recovery. Group therapy creates a sense of community and understanding among individuals facing addiction. Participants can share their experiences, challenges, and successes, reducing feelings of isolation. Moreover, they don't feel left alone in this struggle and get motivated by others in the group. Group therapy provides a platform for individuals to offer and receive constructive feedback from peers. This can enhance self-awareness and accountability within the group. Group therapy introduces the concept of therapeutic universality, where individuals realize that their struggles are not unique. This normalization fosters a sense of shared responsibility for recovery (Moos & Moos, 2004). It also allows participants to observe and model healthy coping strategies and behaviors demonstrated by others in the group. This can be particularly beneficial for skill development. The development of a cohesive group fosters a supportive environment. Individuals can draw strength from the group, creating a collective commitment to recovery.

Group therapy promotes interpersonal learning, allowing individuals to explore their relational patterns, communication styles, and interpersonal challenges within a safe and therapeutic context. Group therapy provides a supportive network for relapse prevention. Members can share strategies for identifying triggers and coping with cravings, enhancing the likelihood of sustained recovery. Complementing Individual Therapy: Group therapy often complements individual therapy, providing a comprehensive treatment approach that addresses both individual and social factors influencing addiction. Group therapy for psychological addiction offers a dynamic and synergistic approach to recovery by leveraging the power of shared experiences, peer support, and interpersonal learning. As an integral component of comprehensive addiction treatment, group therapy contributes to the development of a resilient and supportive community for individuals working towards lasting recovery.

Family therapy for psychological addiction: Involving family members in the therapeutic process can address relational dynamics and provide additional support. Family therapy helps to rebuild healthy communication patterns and establish a more supportive home environment. Psychological addiction, characterized by a compulsive and harmful relationship with substances or behaviors, often extends its impact beyond the individual to the family unit. Family therapy emerges as a crucial component in the treatment of psychological addiction (Lander et al., 2013), aiming to address underlying dynamics, enhance communication, and foster a supportive environment for lasting recovery. Family therapy views the family as a dynamic system wherein each member plays a role. Addiction can disrupt this balance, leading to strained relationships, communication breakdowns, and enabling behaviors.

Codependency often manifests in families dealing with addiction, where members may enable the addictive behavior, neglect their own needs, or become overly involved in attempts to control the addicted individual. Family therapy aims to disrupt dysfunctional patterns within the family unit, helping members recognize and change behaviors that contribute to the maintenance of addiction. Improving communication is a central goal. Open and honest communication fosters understanding, reduces stigma, and creates an environment where family members can express their concerns and feelings without judgment. This approach examines the family as an interconnected system, exploring how changes in one family member's behavior can impact the entire system. It aims to identify and modify problematic patterns. Structural family therapy focuses on altering the family structure, rearranging roles and hierarchies to foster healthier relationships. It helps family members adapt to changing circumstances and roles (McCrady et al., 2009). It also educates family members about the nature of addiction, reducing stigma and fostering empathy. Understanding the complexity of addiction can lead to more compassionate support. Incorporating family into the treatment process builds a robust support system. This support is crucial for the individual's recovery journey and helps prevent relapse.

Family members may resist changes to established dynamics, especially if these patterns have developed over many years. Patience and understanding are vital in overcoming this resistance. While family therapy is essential, recognizing the unique needs of each family member is crucial. Individual therapy may complement family sessions to address personal challenges more comprehensively. Family therapy, as part of psychological addiction treatment, offers a holistic approach that acknowledges the interconnectedness of individuals within the family unit. By addressing family dynamics, fostering open communication, and promoting understanding, family therapy becomes a powerful tool in breaking the cycle of addiction and supporting lasting recovery.

Psychoeducation for psychological addiction: Providing education about the nature of psychological addiction, its impact on mental health, and coping strategies is essential. Psychoeducation helps individuals gain insight into their behaviors and empowers them to make informed choices. Psychoeducation plays a pivotal role in the treatment of psychological addiction by providing individuals and their families with essential knowledge about the nature of addiction, its impact, and effective coping strategies. Psychoeducation begins with a comprehensive understanding of psychological addiction, which involves a compulsive relationship with substances or behaviors, often driven by underlying emotional and psychological factors. Psychoeducation delves into the various factors that contribute to psychological addiction, including genetic predispositions, environmental influences, and the role of co-occurring mental health disorders.

Psychoeducation aims to build awareness and reduce the stigma associated with addiction. By disseminating accurate information, individuals and their families can develop a more empathetic understanding of the challenges faced by those dealing with psychological addiction (Corrigan et al., 2002). Informed decision-making is a key component of recovery. Psychoeducation equips individuals with the knowledge needed to make informed choices about treatment options, coping strategies, and lifestyle changes. Understanding the neurobiological effects of substances is crucial. Psychoeducation explores how drugs or behaviors affect the brain's reward system, leading to the development and perpetuation of addiction (Marlatt & Donovan, 2005). Psychoeducation provides practical coping strategies and skills to manage cravings, triggers, and emotional challenges. This may include mindfulness techniques, stress management, and effective communication strategies.

Psychoeducation extends to families, helping them understand the impact of addiction on family dynamics. It explores how families can support recovery and maintain healthy relationships. Effective communication and setting healthy boundaries are vital aspects of psychoeducation for families. Understanding these dynamics can contribute to a more supportive and conducive environment for recovery. Psychoeducation is adapted to address co-occurring mental health disorders, recognizing the interconnectedness of addiction and mental health. Individuals gain insights into managing both aspects of their well-being. Psychoeducation emphasizes the concept of lifelong learning, encouraging individuals to continuously educate themselves about addiction. It includes relapse prevention strategies, fostering a proactive approach to maintaining recovery (McKay, 2005). Psychoeducation stands as a cornerstone in the treatment of psychological addiction, offering a pathway to empowerment through knowledge. By providing individuals and their families with a comprehensive understanding of addiction, psychoeducation sets the stage for informed decision-making, effective coping, and sustained recovery.

Holistic approaches for psychological addiction: Incorporating holistic therapies, such as art therapy, music therapy, or yoga, can complement traditional therapeutic approaches by addressing the emotional and creative aspects of an individual's well-being. Ongoing support is crucial for maintaining recovery from psychological addiction. Follow-up sessions, support groups, and access to community resources contribute to sustained success. Addressing psychological addiction involves a multifaceted and individualized approach, recognizing the unique factors contributing to each person's struggles. By combining evidence-based therapies, support systems, and personalized strategies, individuals can develop the tools necessary to overcome psychological addiction and achieve lasting recovery. Holistic approaches to psychological addiction emphasize on a comprehensive and integrative strategy that addresses not only the symptoms of addiction but also the overall well-being of individuals. Mindfulness practices, such as meditation, promote self-awareness and emotional regulation. They have shown efficacy in reducing stress, managing cravings, and enhancing overall mental well-being in individuals with addiction.

Yoga and Tai Chi combine physical activity with mindfulness, promoting relaxation, stress reduction, and improved mental focus. These practices contribute to a balanced and centered state of mind, aiding in addiction recovery (Duan-Porter et al., 2016). Nutritional therapy focuses on restoring and optimizing physical health through balanced diets, supplements, and hydration. A well-nourished body supports overall well-being and can positively impact mental health during addiction recovery (Grajek et al., 2022). Regular physical exercise is linked to improved mood, reduced stress, and enhanced cognitive function. Incorporating exercise into a holistic approach for addiction recovery supports both physical and mental well-being (Zschucke et al., 2013).

Art and music therapy provide creative outlets for expression and emotional processing. These modalities can enhance self-awareness and aid in addressing underlying psychological issues contributing to addiction. Holistic recovery often involves practices that align with spiritual or existential beliefs. Mind-body-spirit integration encourages individuals to connect with their deeper selves, fostering a sense of purpose and meaning in recovery. Building a supportive community is crucial in holistic recovery. Peer support groups, such as Alcoholics Anonymous (AA) or SMART Recovery, provide a sense of belonging and shared experience, promoting emotional well-being (Kelly et al., 2018). Holistic approaches for psychological addiction acknowledge the interconnectedness of mind, body, and spirit in the recovery process. By incorporating practices that address various aspects of well-being, individuals can cultivate a more comprehensive and sustainable path to recovery.

Relapse prevention strategies for psychological addiction: Therapists work with individuals to develop personalized relapse prevention plans. These plans include identifying triggers, developing coping mechanisms, and creating strategies to navigate high-risk situations. Relapse prevention is a crucial aspect of the recovery journey following treatment for psychological addiction. This text explores evidence-based strategies and interventions designed to empower individuals, reduce the risk of relapse, and foster lasting recovery. Recognizing addiction as a chronic condition is fundamental to understanding relapse. Like other chronic illnesses, addiction may involve periods of stability and setbacks, requiring ongoing management and support. Identification of triggers and high-risk situations is essential. These can include stress, interpersonal conflicts, exposure to substances, and emotional distress. Understanding and addressing these triggers form the basis of effective relapse prevention.

Teaching and reinforcing effective coping skills are crucial for managing stress and cravings. Coping skills training equips individuals with practical strategies to navigate challenges without resorting to substance use. Stress is a common trigger for relapse. Stress management techniques, such as deep breathing, progressive muscle relaxation, and guided imagery, empower individuals to cope with stressors without turning to substances. Participation in support groups like Alcoholics Anonymous (AA) or Narcotics Anonymous (NA) provides ongoing social support and a sense of community. Peer involvement reinforces commitment to recovery and reduces feelings of isolation (Humphreys & Moos, 2007).

Developing and maintaining healthy relationships is crucial for recovery. Building a network of supportive, understanding individuals can provide encouragement, accountability, and a strong foundation for sustained recovery. These connections—whether with family, friends, or peer support groups—help combat the isolation that often fuels addiction and mental health struggles. Encouraging individuals to regularly monitor their thoughts, feelings, and behaviors helps in identifying warning signs of potential relapse. Journaling, mindfulness practices, or therapy sessions can serve as tools for this self-reflection. Early recognition allows for timely intervention and adjustment of coping strategies, preventing minor setbacks from escalating into full relapses. Creating personalized relapse prevention plans is a proactive measure. These plans outline specific strategies, coping mechanisms, and support systems to be implemented in the face of potential triggers or cravings. They should be revisited and revised regularly to adapt to changing circumstances and personal growth.

Relapse prevention after psychological addiction treatment is a dynamic and personalized process. By incorporating evidence-based strategies, developing coping skills, fostering social support, and promoting self-awareness, individuals can enhance their resilience and navigate the challenges of recovery with greater success. Education about the chronic nature of addiction and the importance of long-term management also empowers individuals to view recovery as a journey rather than a destination. Finally, integrating holistic approaches—such as physical wellness, creative outlets, and spiritual practices—can strengthen emotional regulation and provide healthy alternatives to substance use. With commitment and the right tools, lasting recovery becomes not just possible, but a transformative reality.

Future Directions: The distinction between physical and psychological addiction is becoming increasingly blurred as research reveals their interconnected neurobiological mechanisms. Future studies will likely focus on how chronic substance use alters both the body's homeostatic systems and the brain's reward circuitry simultaneously, creating a self-reinforcing cycle of dependence. Emerging technologies like functional near-infrared spectroscopy (fNIRS) could provide real-time monitoring of how withdrawal symptoms (physical) interact with craving-induced neural activity (psychological) in natural environments. Pharmacological innovations may develop dual-action compounds that simultaneously target opioid receptors to ease physical withdrawal while modulating glutamate transmission to reduce psychological cravings. Digital therapeutics platforms will probably integrate biometric data from wearables tracking physical markers like heart rate variability with cognitive behavioral tools addressing psychological triggers. This holistic approach could lead to dynamic treatment systems that automatically adjust interventions based on whether physical or psychological symptoms predominate at any given moment. Longitudinal research should investigate how these dimensions shift in dominance throughout different stages of recovery, potentially identifying critical windows for specific interventions. Such advances may ultimately render the physical/psychological dichotomy obsolete in favor of a unified biopsychosocial model of addiction.

Societal and policy changes must accompany these scientific advances to fully realize their potential in addressing addiction's complex nature. Insurance systems will need to cover integrated treatment plans that address both physical and psychological components without arbitrary limitations on duration or modality. Medical education curricula should emphasize the neurobiological unity of addiction rather than maintaining artificial distinctions between substance use disorders and behavioral addictions. Public health campaigns ought to communicate how psychological cravings can create physiological stress responses and vice versa, helping to reduce stigma around all forms of addiction. Workplace policies could implement accommodations recognizing that recovery requires management of both physical vulnerabilities (like medication schedules) and psychological needs (such as therapy sessions). International classification systems may evolve to categorize addictions based on underlying mechanisms rather than superficial substance categories or behavior types. Research funding agencies should prioritize studies that bridge the physical-psychological divide rather than supporting investigations of either aspect in isolation. These systemic changes will create an environment where cutting-edge treatments can be deployed effectively and equitably across the full spectrum of addictive disorders.

CHAPTER 3

POSITIVE AND NEGATIVE REINFORCEMENT

"At first, addiction is maintained by pleasure, but the intensity of this pleasure gradually diminishes, and the addiction is then maintained by the avoidance of pain."
~ Frank Tallis

A shift from seeking joy to fleeing pain marks the evolving nature of addiction, with reinforcement playing a crucial role. This chapter makes you delve into the insights, why people keep doing something that hurts them, and how that cycle can be broken. The discussion on positive and negative reinforcement unveils the dual mechanisms shaping behavior, as we explore the motivational forces that either strengthen through reward or diminish through avoidance. In dissecting the principles of positive and negative reinforcement, this exploration delves into the fundamental psychological processes that drive individuals to seek rewards or escape aversive stimuli, illuminating the diverse pathways of behavioral conditioning.

Drug addiction is a complex phenomenon influenced by various factors, including positive and negative reinforcement. Understanding the interplay between these reinforcement mechanisms is crucial for unraveling the intricacies of addictive behaviors and developing effective intervention strategies. Positive reinforcement involves the introduction of a stimulus that strengthens the likelihood of a behavior's recurrence. In the context of drug addiction, positive reinforcement is exemplified by the pleasurable effects of substance use, activating the brain's reward circuitry.

The mesolimbic dopamine system, particularly the nucleus accumbens, is a key player in positive reinforcement. Drugs of abuse, such as cocaine and opioids, trigger the release of dopamine, creating a sense of euphoria and reinforcing the association between drug use and pleasure (Nestler, 2005). Positive reinforcement contributes to reward-related learning, where the brain forms associations between drug-related cues and the pleasurable effects of substance use. This associative learning reinforces drug-seeking behavior (Hyman et al., 2006). Negative reinforcement involves the removal or avoidance of an aversive stimulus, strengthening the likelihood of a behavior's recurrence. In the context of drug addiction, negative reinforcement is often associated with the alleviation of negative emotional states through substance use.

Chronic drug use induces stress system dysregulation, with increased release of corticotropin-releasing factor (CRF). Individuals may use drugs to alleviate stress, contributing to negative reinforcement (Koob, 2009). The self-medication hypothesis suggests that individuals with psychiatric disorders may use substances to alleviate symptoms, demonstrating a negative reinforcement pattern. Positive and negative reinforcement often interact, contributing to the complexity of drug addiction. Dual reinforcement models propose that both processes can co-occur, influencing drug-seeking behavior and creating a cycle that sustains addiction.

The temporal dynamics of positive and negative reinforcement may shift over the course of addiction. While initial drug use may be driven by positive reinforcement, continued use may involve negative reinforcement to cope with withdrawal or stress. Variability exists in the relative contributions of positive and negative reinforcement among individuals. Understanding these differences is essential for personalized treatment approaches (Baker et al., 2004). Understanding the interplay between positive and negative reinforcement has significant implications for addiction treatment strategies. Behavioral therapies also address maladaptive thought patterns associated with drug reinforcement patterns, focusing on disrupting the reinforcement cycle and developing coping skills to manage triggers. Contingency management also utilizes positive reinforcement by providing tangible rewards for drug-free behaviors, promoting abstinence (Prendergast et al., 2006). Positive and negative reinforcement mechanisms intricately contribute to the development and persistence of drug addiction. A comprehensive understanding of these processes is essential for designing effective prevention and treatment strategies, ultimately improving outcomes for individuals grappling with substance use disorders.

Reward pathways involved in drug reinforcement: The reinforcement of drug-seeking behavior is intricately linked to the brain's reward system. Understanding the neurobiological mechanisms involved provides critical insights into the development and perpetuation of drug addiction. The mesolimbic dopamine pathway, originating in the ventral tegmental area (VTA) and projecting to the nucleus accumbens, is a central component of the brain's reward circuitry (Wise, 2004). Drugs of abuse, including cocaine, amphetamines, and opioids, induce a surge in dopamine levels in the NAc, creating a powerful sense of pleasure and reinforcement. The VTA is a crucial source of dopaminergic neurons projecting to various brain regions, including the NAc, prefrontal cortex, and amygdala, forming a network central to reward processing (Luscher & Malenka, 2011).

Dopaminergic neurons in the VTA are implicated in reward prediction and anticipation, influencing motivated behavior and reinforcement learning (Schultz, 1998). Glutamate, the primary excitatory neurotransmitter, plays a crucial role in the reward system. Glutamatergic inputs from the prefrontal cortex and hippocampus modulate dopaminergic activity in the NAc (Kalivas, 2009). GABAergic Inhibition: GABAergic neurons provide inhibitory control within the reward circuitry. The balance between excitatory and inhibitory inputs is critical for regulating reward-related behaviors (Stuber et al., 2012). Chronic drug use induces neuroplastic changes in the reward system, contributing to sensitization and increased vulnerability to addiction. Long-term drug exposure leads to structural alterations in synaptic connections, affecting the strength of reward-related circuits. Understanding the neurobiological underpinnings of drug reinforcement informs targeted interventions. Behavioral therapies and pharmacological approaches aim to modulate the reward system to mitigate addiction.

Research on specific neurotransmitter systems, such as glutamate and GABA, provides potential targets for developing medications to counteract dysregulated reward processing in addiction. The reward system's involvement in drug reinforcement is a dynamic and multifaceted process. Advances in neuroscience continue to unravel the complexities of addiction, offering valuable insights for the development of targeted therapeutic strategies aimed at restoring balance within the reward circuitry. Endogenous opioid peptides, including endorphins and enkephalins, modulate the reward system. Exogenous opioids, such as heroin, mimic the actions of these endogenous peptides, leading to reinforcement and addiction (Le Merrer et al., 2009). Activation of mu-opioid receptors in the NAc produces feelings of euphoria and reinforces drug-seeking behavior, contributing to the addictive potential of opioids. The orchestration of neurotransmitters in the brain's reward system paints a nuanced picture of drug reinforcement. As our understanding deepens, so do the possibilities for targeted interventions aimed at mitigating the neurobiological underpinnings of addiction.

Neurotransmitters involved in drug reinforcement: The intricate dance of neurotransmitters orchestrates the symphony of drug reinforcement, shaping the neural circuits that underlie addictive behaviors. The key neurotransmitters implicated in drug reinforcement, provide a molecular perspective on the neurobiology of addiction. Dopamine is central to the brain's reward system, with projections from the ventral tegmental area (VTA) to the nucleus accumbens (NAc) playing a crucial role in the reinforcing effects of drugs (Wise, 2004). Dopaminergic neurons in the VTA are implicated in reward prediction, contributing to reinforcement learning and the association of drug-related cues with pleasurable effects. Glutamate, the primary excitatory neurotransmitter, plays a pivotal role in the reward system. Glutamatergic inputs from the prefrontal cortex and hippocampus modulate dopaminergic activity in the NAc (Kalivas, 2009). Glutamatergic synapses undergo long-term potentiation, a form of synaptic plasticity, in response to chronic drug exposure, contributing to the persistent changes observed in addiction (Luscher & Malenka, 2011). GABA, the primary inhibitory neurotransmitter, provides a crucial balance within the reward circuitry. GABAergic interneurons play a role in regulating the excitability of dopaminergic neurons (Stuber et al., 2012). GABAergic signaling is implicated in the modulation of reward-related behaviors, including the regulation of the mesolimbic dopamine system.

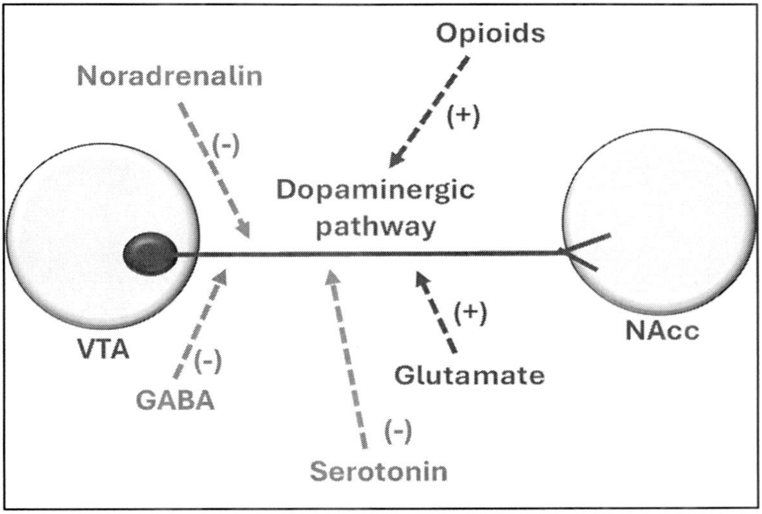

Neurotransmitters involved in drug reinforcement

Serotonin, a neurotransmitter associated with mood regulation, also influences the reward system. Alterations in serotonin levels have been implicated in the development and maintenance of addiction (Muller & Homberg, 2015). Serotonin interacts with the dopamine system, influencing reward processing and contributing to the reinforcing effects of drugs (Bubar & Cunningham, 2008). Noradrenaline, or norepinephrine, plays a role in arousal and attention. Dysregulation of noradrenergic signaling has been implicated in addiction, affecting attentional processes related to drug-seeking behavior (Wee et al., 2008). Noradrenaline is involved in the stress response, and stress-induced release of noradrenaline may contribute to the reinforcing effects of drugs during times of heightened stress. Opioid peptides, such as endorphins and enkephalins, act as endogenous modulators of the reward system. The release of opioids is associated with pleasurable sensations and reinforcement. Opioid receptors in the nucleus accumbens and other reward-related areas mediate the rewarding effects of both endogenous opioids and exogenous opiates, contributing to the reinforcing properties of drugs (Kelley et al., 2002). The intricate dance of neurotransmitters orchestrates the reinforcement of drug-seeking behavior.

Dopamine, glutamate, GABA, serotonin, and opioid peptides form a complex molecular tapestry within the brain's reward system. Understanding these neurobiological mechanisms provides a foundation for developing targeted interventions to address addiction at the molecular level.

Alleviation of negative emotions and stress in drug reinforcement: The relationship between drug use and the alleviation of negative emotions and stress is a key aspect of drug reinforcement. There exists a need to explore the neurobiological underpinnings of how substances can serve as coping mechanisms, providing relief from emotional distress. Chronic exposure to stressors is linked to an increased vulnerability to substance abuse, with stress acting as a powerful motivator for drug seeking. The corticotropin-releasing factor (CRF) system plays a central role in mediating stress responses. CRF release during stress can enhance the reinforcing properties of drugs, particularly in the context of negative emotional states. This interaction contributes to the development and maintenance of addiction (Koob, 2010). The amygdala is a key brain region involved in emotional processing. Stress activates the amygdala, triggering emotional responses and influencing decision-making, including the choice to use drugs as a coping mechanism. The amygdala's involvement in emotional processing extends to drug reinforcement, where heightened emotional states can drive drug-seeking behavior as a means of alleviating negative emotions (Koob, 2013).

The endogenous opioid system, including endorphins and enkephalins, is activated in response to stress. These opioid peptides not only contribute to stress reduction but also play a role in the reinforcing effects of drugs. Opioid receptors in brain regions involved in stress regulation, such as the amygdala and periaqueductal gray, are crucial for mediating the stress-relieving effects of both endogenous opioids and exogenous opiates (Bodnar, 2016). Chronic stress induces neuroadaptations in the brain's reward circuitry, leading to increased drug seeking. These adaptations involve changes in neurotransmitter systems, particularly dopamine, and contribute to the reinforcing effects of substances (Logrip & Zorrilla, 2014). Prolonged stress can dysregulate the HPA axis, resulting in altered cortisol levels and increased susceptibility to substance use disorders. This dysregulation further reinforces the role of stress in addiction. Understanding the connection between stress and drug reinforcement informs therapeutic approaches. Stress management strategies, including mindfulness-based interventions and cognitive-behavioral therapies, can be integral components of addiction treatment (Witkiewitz et al., 2014).

Medications that target stress-responsive systems, such as CRF antagonists, are being explored as potential adjuncts to addiction treatment, aiming to disrupt the link between stress and drug-seeking behavior (Heilig & Koob, 2007). The alleviation of negative emotions and stress is a significant factor in drug reinforcement, contributing to the development and persistence of addiction. Understanding the neurobiological mechanisms involved provides a foundation for developing targeted interventions aimed at breaking the cycle of stress-driven substance use.

Drug reinforcement coping mechanisms: The relationship between drug use and coping mechanisms is complex, involving intricate neurobiological processes. The intricate relationship between drug use and coping mechanisms involves a complex interplay of neurobiological processes. Genetic variations in stress-responsive systems and neurotransmitter pathways can influence an individual's propensity to use drugs as coping mechanisms. These genetic factors contribute to the personalized nature of coping and reinforcement. Individual differences in personality, such as impulsivity and sensitivity to stress, may contribute to the adoption of drug-related coping mechanisms. Understanding these differences is crucial for tailoring intervention strategies.

Stress is a powerful trigger for drug use as individuals seek to cope with negative emotions and overwhelming situations. The ability of drugs to alleviate stress may contribute to their reinforcing effects (Sinha, 2008). Drug use in response to stress can be viewed through the lens of negative reinforcement, where the removal or avoidance of aversive stimuli (stress) is reinforced by the pleasurable effects of substances (Baker et al., 2004). Endogenous Opioids and Stress Relief: The endogenous opioid system, including endorphins and enkephalins, plays a role in stress relief. Drug-induced activation of this system contributes to the reinforcing effects of substances, providing relief from negative emotions. Chronic stress activates the CRF system, and drugs can modulate this system, providing relief from stress. Dysregulation of CRF contributes to stress-induced drug seeking and reinforcement.

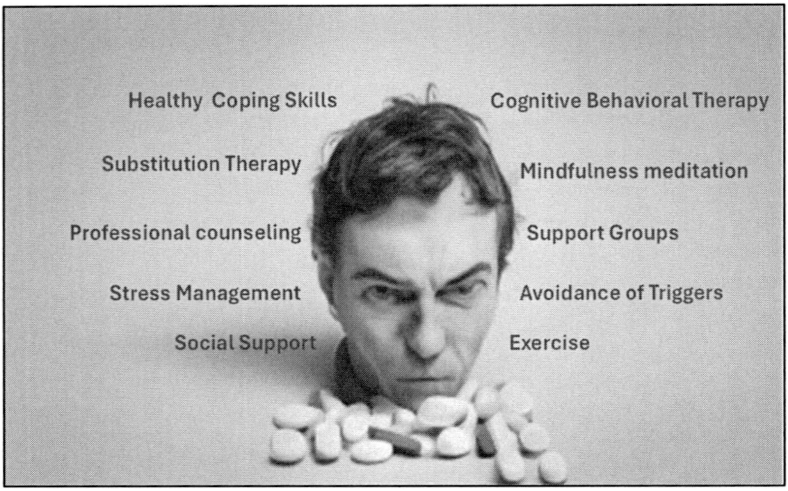

Drug reinforcement coping mechanisms

The amygdala, a key player in emotional processing, is involved in the regulation of both stress and drug-related emotions. Dysregulation in the amygdala may contribute to the intertwining of drug use and emotional coping (Koob & Volkow, 2010). Dopaminergic pathways, particularly the mesolimbic system, play a central role in reward processing and the reinforcing effects of substances. Drug use can activate these pathways, providing a sense of reward and reinforcing coping mechanisms (Wise, 2004). Individual differences in coping mechanisms may have a genetic basis. Genetic variations in stress-responsive systems and neurotransmitter pathways can influence an individual's propensity to use drugs as a coping strategy. Certain personality traits, such as impulsivity and sensitivity to stress, may contribute to the adoption of drug-related coping mechanisms. Understanding these individual differences is crucial for tailored intervention strategies. Cognitive-behavioral therapy is an evidence-based approach that addresses maladaptive coping mechanisms. It helps individuals identify and modify negative thought patterns and develop healthier coping strategies, reducing the reliance on drugs. Mindfulness techniques can enhance emotional regulation and stress management, providing alternative coping mechanisms. Mindfulness-based interventions have shown promise in reducing substance use. The intertwining of drug use and coping mechanisms reflects a nuanced interplay of neurobiological processes. Understanding these mechanisms provides a foundation for developing targeted interventions that address the root causes of substance use, promoting healthier coping strategies and improving treatment outcomes.

Positive reinforcement in drug addiction: Positive reinforcement plays a pivotal role in the development and perpetuation of drug addiction, creating a cycle where the pleasurable effects of substances drive repeated use. Dopamine, a neurotransmitter, is a key player in the brain's reward system. The mesolimbic pathway, particularly the nucleus accumbens, is central to the experience of pleasure and reinforcement associated with drug use (Wise, 2004). Dopaminergic neurons in the ventral tegmental area (VTA) respond to rewarding stimuli and play a crucial role in reward prediction. Increased dopamine release in response to drug-related cues reinforces the association between drug use and pleasurable effects. Endogenous opioids, including endorphins and enkephalins, are released during drug use, contributing to the pleasure response. These opioids reinforce the rewarding effects of substances, creating a positive feedback loop.

Opioid receptors in the nucleus accumbens and other reward-related areas mediate the reinforcing properties of both endogenous opioids and exogenous opiates, further enhancing the positive reinforcement associated with drug use (Kelley et al., 2002). Glutamate, the primary excitatory neurotransmitter, is crucial for learning and memory processes. It is involved in the formation of associations between drug-related cues and the pleasurable effects of substances, reinforcing drug-seeking behavior (Kalivas, 2009). Glutamatergic projections from the prefrontal cortex to the nucleus accumbens contribute to cue-induced craving. Drug-associated cues activate these pathways, reinforcing the positive effects of drug use (Stuber et al., 2012). Serotonin, a neurotransmitter involved in mood regulation, interacts with the dopamine system. Drug-induced alterations in serotonin levels influence mood states, contributing to the positive reinforcement associated with substance use (Muller & Homberg, 2015). Serotonin and dopamine interact in complex ways, modulating reward processing and mood enhancement. Dysregulation in this interplay contributes to the positive reinforcing effects of drugs (Howell & Cunningham, 2015). Medications that target dopaminergic pathways are being explored as potential interventions for addiction treatment. These medications aim to normalize the dysregulation in dopamine release associated with positive reinforcement in drug addiction. Behavioral interventions that address cue-induced cravings and associations can help disrupt the positive reinforcement loop. Positive reinforcement in drug addiction involves intricate neurobiological processes, particularly in the dopaminergic, opioid, glutamatergic, and serotonergic systems. Understanding these mechanisms is essential for developing targeted interventions that address the reward circuitry dysregulation associated with substance use disorders.

Neural pathways associated with positive reinforcement: Positive reinforcement in drug addiction is intricately woven into the neural pathways governing reward processing. There are several key neural circuits and neurotransmitter systems which are associated with positive reinforcement in the context of substance use. The mesolimbic dopaminergic pathway, originating from the ventral tegmental area (VTA), culminates in the NAc, a core region of the brain's reward system. Elevated dopamine levels in the NAc are a hallmark of positive reinforcement, reinforcing the pleasurable effects of drug use (Wise, 2004). Dopaminergic neurons in the VTA play a crucial role in reward prediction. Drug-related cues activate these neurons, contributing to the reinforcing effects of substances by predicting rewarding outcomes. Endogenous opioids, including endorphins and enkephalins, modulate the pleasure response. Activation of opioid receptors in the NAc reinforces the positive effects of drug use, contributing to the cycle of positive reinforcement. Opioid receptors in reward-related brain regions, such as the NAc and amygdala, mediate the reinforcing properties of both endogenous opioids and exogenous opiates, playing a crucial role in positive reinforcement in drug addiction (Kelley et al., 2002). Glutamate, the primary excitatory neurotransmitter, is central to learning and memory processes. Glutamatergic projections from the prefrontal cortex to the NAc contribute to the formation of associations between drug-related cues and the pleasurable effects of substances (Kalivas, 2009). Drug-associated cues activate glutamatergic pathways, influencing cue-induced craving and reinforcing positive drug-related associations. This interplay contributes to the positive reinforcement loop in addiction (Stuber et al., 2012).

Serotonin, a neurotransmitter involved in mood regulation, interacts with the dopaminergic system. Alterations in serotonin levels during drug use influence mood states, contributing to the positive reinforcement associated with substance use (Muller & Homberg, 2015). The interplay between serotonin and dopamine modulates reward processing and mood enhancement. Dysregulation in this interaction contributes to the positive reinforcing effects of drugs. Medications targeting dopaminergic pathways are under investigation for addiction treatment. Normalizing dopamine dysregulation associated with positive reinforcement holds promise for intervention strategies. Positive reinforcement in drug addiction involves the orchestration of neural pathways, encompassing dopaminergic, opioidergic, glutamatergic, and serotonergic systems. Understanding these intricate connections is crucial for developing targeted interventions aimed at disrupting the cycle of positive reinforcement associated with substance use disorders.

Role of mesolimbic dopaminergic system in positive reinforcement: The mesolimbic dopaminergic system, a pivotal neural pathway, is recognized for its fundamental role in positive reinforcement, particularly in the context of drug addiction. This text explores the intricate workings of the mesolimbic dopaminergic system and its association with positive reinforcement, referencing key studies that have contributed to our understanding of this neurobiological phenomenon. The mesolimbic dopaminergic pathway originates in the ventral tegmental area (VTA), with dopaminergic neurons projecting to key regions such as the nucleus accumbens (NAc), prefrontal cortex (PFC), and amygdala. Among these, the VTA-NAc pathway is particularly emphasized in the context of positive reinforcement associated with drug addiction (Wise, 2004). Dopamine release within the NAc is intricately linked to the prediction of rewarding outcomes. Studies have demonstrated that dopaminergic neurons in the VTA respond not only to the receipt of rewards but also to cues that predict rewards. This phenomenon contributes to the associative learning and positive reinforcement observed in drug addiction. The administration of addictive substances, such as drugs of abuse, results in a surge of dopamine release in the NAc. This heightened dopamine concentration is associated with the subjective experience of pleasure and reinforces the connection between drug-related cues and the rewarding effects of substance use (Di Chiara, 2002).

Chronic exposure to drugs of abuse induces neuroadaptations in the mesolimbic dopaminergic system, leading to sensitization. Sensitization is characterized by an exaggerated dopamine response to drug-related stimuli, contributing to the intensification of positive reinforcement and the development of addiction (Vanderschuren & Kalivas, 2000). Understanding the role of the mesolimbic dopaminergic system in positive reinforcement has significant implications for addiction treatment. Targeting this system with pharmacological interventions or behavioral therapies that modify dopamine release may hold promise in mitigating the reinforcing effects of drugs and aiding in addiction recovery. The mesolimbic dopaminergic system stands as a linchpin in the neural circuitry of positive reinforcement, orchestrating the intricate dance between reward prediction, drug-induced dopamine release, and sensitization. By unraveling the complexities of this system, researchers and clinicians gain valuable insights that may pave the way for more effective interventions in the treatment of drug addiction.

Reward circuitry and drug-induced euphoria in positive reinforcement: The intricate interplay between reward circuitry and drug-induced euphoria forms the foundation of positive reinforcement in addiction. The brain's reward circuitry, comprised of regions such as the nucleus accumbens (NAc), ventral tegmental area (VTA), prefrontal cortex (PFC), and amygdala, orchestrates the experience of pleasure and reinforcement. In the context of addiction, drugs exploit and dysregulate this circuitry, leading to heightened positive reinforcement (Koob & Volkow, 2010). Dopamine, a neurotransmitter, takes center stage in the brain's reward system. Drug-induced euphoria is closely tied to the surge of dopamine in the NAc, a critical component of the reward circuitry. Elevated dopamine levels reinforce the pleasurable effects of substances, creating a robust positive reinforcement loop. While dopamine plays a primary role, other neurotransmitters contribute to the euphoric effects of drugs. Opioids, for example, bind to receptors in the reward circuitry, amplifying feelings of pleasure. The synergy between dopamine, opioids, and other neurotransmitters adds complexity to the landscape of drug-induced euphoria and positive reinforcement (Nestler, 2005). Neuroimaging studies have provided crucial insights into the neural activation patterns associated with drug-induced euphoria. The administration of drugs like cocaine or opioids triggers heightened activity in the NAc and other reward-related areas, offering a visual representation of the brain's response to euphoria-inducing substances (Nock et al., 2017).

Chronic exposure to drugs can induce neuroadaptations, including sensitization, where the brain becomes hyperresponsive to the euphoric effects of substances. This heightened sensitivity contributes to the amplification of drug-induced euphoria, solidifying the positive reinforcement loop and perpetuating addictive behaviors. Understanding the intricate dance between reward circuitry and drug-induced euphoria holds significant implications for addiction treatment. Targeted interventions that aim to modulate neurotransmitter dynamics or disrupt the neural pathways associated with euphoria could represent promising avenues for mitigating the reinforcing effects of drugs and facilitating recovery (Kalivas & Volkow, 2005). The convergence of reward circuitry and drug-induced euphoria serves as a cornerstone in the positive reinforcement loop of addiction. This nuanced understanding provides a foundation for developing more effective interventions, ultimately guiding the quest for innovative approaches in the treatment of substance use disorders.

Behavioral aspects of positive reinforcement: Positive reinforcement is a driving force in the development and perpetuation of addictive behaviors. Operant conditioning, a fundamental principle in behavioral psychology, forms the basis of positive reinforcement. In the context of addiction, individuals learn to associate drug-related behaviors with pleasurable outcomes, reinforcing the likelihood of repeated engagement in these behaviors. Addiction is marked by the emergence of drug-seeking behaviors driven by the expectation of rewards. Environmental cues associated with drug use become powerful triggers, eliciting behaviors aimed at obtaining substances to experience the associated pleasure or euphoria (Everitt &

Robbins, 2005). Reinforcement learning models provide a theoretical framework for understanding how individuals learn to seek drugs based on the positive reinforcement they provide. These models highlight the role of prediction errors and the updating of expectations, offering insights into the behavioral mechanisms at play in addiction. Environmental cues associated with drug use, such as paraphernalia or specific settings, become conditioned stimuli that elicit craving. The engagement in drug-seeking behaviors is reinforced by the anticipation of the rewarding effects associated with these cues, contributing to the maintenance of addiction. As addiction progresses, drug-seeking behaviors can become compulsive, driven by the intense desire for the reinforcing effects of substances. Compulsivity in drug-seeking is a hallmark of positive reinforcement's profound impact on behavior, leading to persistent and often irrational engagement in substance-seeking activities (Belin et al., 2009).

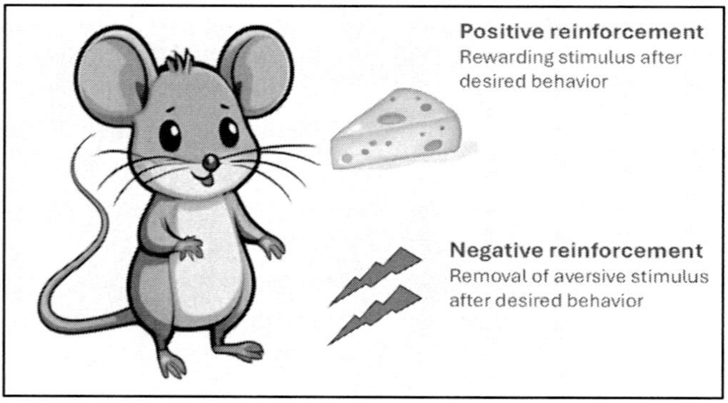

Operant conditioning

Behavioral aspects of positive reinforcement are closely linked to neurobiological changes. Neuroimaging studies reveal alterations in brain regions associated with reward processing, such as the nucleus accumbens and prefrontal cortex, providing a neural basis for the observed behaviors in addiction (Hyman et al., 2006). Understanding the behavioral intricacies of positive reinforcement is crucial for designing effective interventions. Behavioral therapies, including contingency management and cognitive-behavioral approaches, aim to modify reinforcing contingencies, reshape maladaptive behaviors, and foster positive behavioral changes in individuals with substance use disorders (Higgins et al., 2003). The behavioral aspects of positive reinforcement in addiction are multifaceted, encompassing operant conditioning, cue-induced craving, compulsive drug-seeking, and neurobiological correlates. Integrating this knowledge into behavioral interventions holds promise for addressing the reinforcing mechanisms that drive and sustain addictive behaviors, paving the way for more effective approaches in addiction treatment.

Drug-seeking behavior in positive reinforcement: Drug-seeking behavior, a defining characteristic of addiction, is intricately linked to the positive reinforcement loop that perpetuates substance use. This text explores the behavioral dynamics of drug-seeking, shedding light on the patterns, triggers, and reinforcing mechanisms that drive this complex phenomenon, supported by key references from seminal studies. Operant conditioning, a fundamental principle in behavioral psychology, plays a central role in drug-seeking behavior. Individuals learn to associate specific actions (such as drug use) with the pleasurable effects produced by substances. The positive reinforcement derived from these effects reinforces the likelihood of repeated engagement in drug-seeking behaviors. Drug-seeking behavior is often motivated by the anticipation of rewards associated with substance use. Environmental cues, social contexts, and internal states become powerful triggers, initiating and sustaining the motivation to seek drugs for the positive reinforcement they provide (Everitt & Robbins, 2005).

Environmental cues associated with drug use, such as specific locations, paraphernalia, or social situations, become conditioned stimuli that elicit drug-seeking behavior. Cue-induced drug-seeking is a learned response where the presentation of these cues triggers a craving for the positive reinforcing effects of substances, driving individuals to seek and use drugs. Reinforcement learning models provide a theoretical framework for understanding drug-seeking behavior. These models emphasize the role of prediction errors and the updating of expectations based on the outcomes of drug-seeking actions. They offer insights into how individuals learn to seek drugs in environments associated with positive reinforcement. As addiction progresses, drug-seeking behavior can become compulsive, characterized by a loss of control and an inability to cease seeking drugs despite adverse consequences. Compulsivity in drug-seeking is a manifestation of the powerful positive reinforcement that substances provide, driving persistent and often irrational drug-seeking actions (Belin et al., 2009).

The neurobiological underpinnings of drug-seeking behavior involve alterations in brain regions associated with reward processing. Neuroimaging studies reveal changes in the nucleus accumbens, prefrontal cortex, and other structures, providing a neural basis for the observed behaviors in drug-seeking (Hyman et al., 2006). Understanding the behavioral intricacies of drug-seeking behavior is crucial for developing effective interventions. Behavioral therapies, cognitive-behavioral approaches, and contingency management aim to modify reinforcing contingencies, reshape maladaptive behaviors, and disrupt the cycle of positive reinforcement in drug-seeking individuals (Higgins et al., 2003). Drug-seeking behavior in the context of positive reinforcement is a multifaceted phenomenon shaped by operant conditioning, reward expectancy, cue-induced responses, and neurobiological adaptations. Integrating this understanding into intervention strategies holds promise for addressing the reinforcing mechanisms that drive and sustain addictive behaviors, offering pathways to more effective approaches in addiction treatment.

Social and environmental cues mediating positive reinforcement: The nexus between social and environmental cues and positive reinforcement is a critical aspect of addiction. This text delves into the intricate dynamics of how social and environmental factors act as potent mediators of positive reinforcement, shaping behaviors and contributing to the development and maintenance of addiction, with references from key studies in the field. Social learning theories suggest that individuals acquire behaviors through observation and imitation of others. In the context of addiction, social cues play a pivotal role in reinforcing drug-related behaviors. Modeling, social approval, and vicarious reinforcement contribute to the positive reinforcement loop, influencing an individual's likelihood to engage in substance use. Peers exert a profound influence on behavior, particularly during adolescence and young adulthood. Positive reinforcement within social circles can strongly impact substance use behaviors. The desire for social acceptance, approval, and the experience of shared positive reinforcement from drug use can drive individuals to seek and continue substance use (Borsari & Carey, 2001). Environmental cues, both physical and contextual, are powerful mediators of positive reinforcement. Places associated with drug use, such as specific locations or social settings, become conditioned cues that trigger the anticipation of rewarding effects. The environmental context acts as a key determinant in the reinforcement of drug-seeking and drug-taking behaviors (Everitt et al., 2003).

Social norms, the unwritten rules governing behavior within a social group, significantly influence substance use. Positive reinforcement is often linked to conformity with social norms related to drug use. Individuals may be more likely to engage in substance use if it aligns with perceived social norms and if they anticipate positive social reinforcement from their peers (Cialdini & Goldstein, 2004). The family environment, as a primary social unit, contributes to positive reinforcement dynamics in addiction. Family members can inadvertently reinforce substance use through various mechanisms, such as enabling behaviors or providing emotional support linked to drug use. Positive reinforcement within the family context can influence the development and persistence of addictive behaviors (Cruz et al., 2012).

Media, including advertising and portrayals of substance use in popular culture, serve as environmental cues that mediate positive reinforcement. Positive depictions of drug use can shape perceptions and contribute to the glamorization of substance use, influencing individuals to seek the perceived positive outcomes associated with drugs (Primack et al., 2014). Cultural factors, including beliefs, values, and traditions, influence the reinforcement patterns associated with substance use. Cultural contexts may provide positive reinforcement for drug use through rituals, celebrations, or religious practices, shaping individuals' perceptions of the rewarding aspects of substances within their cultural framework. The interplay between social and environmental cues and positive reinforcement is a multifaceted phenomenon central to understanding addiction. Recognizing the impact of these mediators is crucial for developing comprehensive interventions that address the social and environmental determinants of positive reinforcement in substance use, paving the way for more effective strategies in addiction prevention and treatment.

Dopamine release and receptor activation in positive reinforcement: Dopamine, a neurotransmitter with a central role in the brain's reward system, plays a pivotal role in positive reinforcement and the development of addictive behaviors. A study of the intricate mechanisms of dopamine release and receptor activation would shed light on how these neurochemical processes contribute to the rewarding effects of substances. Dopamine is often referred to as the "reward neurotransmitter" due to its involvement in the brain's reward circuitry. It is released in response to rewarding stimuli, reinforcing behaviors associated with pleasure and positive outcomes. The nucleus accumbens, a key component of the reward system, is particularly rich in dopamine receptors and is a focal point for the reinforcing effects of substances (Wise, 2004). The mesolimbic dopamine pathway, originating from the ventral tegmental area (VTA) and projecting to the nucleus accumbens, is a crucial circuit in positive reinforcement. Drug-induced increases in dopamine release along this pathway are associated with the pleasurable effects of substances, reinforcing drug-seeking and drug-taking behaviors.

The consumption of addictive substances, such as drugs or alcohol, leads to an increase in dopamine release in the nucleus accumbens. This surge in dopamine is a key component of the reinforcing effects of substances, creating a sense of pleasure and reward that motivates individuals to repeat the behavior (Volkow et al., 2017). Dopamine exerts its effects by binding to specific receptors on the surface of neurons. The two main classes of dopamine receptors relevant to positive reinforcement are D1-like receptors (including D1 and D5 receptors) and D2-like receptors (including D2, D3, and D4 receptors). The activation of these receptors influences intracellular signaling pathways and contributes to the reinforcing effects of dopamine (Beaulieu & Gainetdinov, 2011). Dopamine release is also linked to reward prediction error, a concept from reinforcement learning models. When an outcome is better or worse than expected, dopamine neurons in the VTA respond with increased or decreased firing, respectively. This prediction error signal is crucial for learning and updating associations between actions and rewards, contributing to the reinforcement of certain behaviors, including substance-seeking. Chronic exposure to drugs of abuse induces neuroadaptations in the dopamine system, leading to changes in receptor sensitivity and synaptic plasticity. These adaptations contribute to the development of tolerance, sensitization, and ultimately, the transition to addiction. Understanding the neuroplastic changes in the dopamine system is crucial for comprehending the long-term effects of substance use (Kauer & Malenka, 2007). Insights into the neurochemical processes of dopamine release and receptor activation have profound implications for addiction treatment. Targeting dopaminergic pathways with pharmacological interventions or behavioral therapies that modulate dopamine release may offer avenues for mitigating the reinforcing effects of substances and facilitating recovery. Dopamine release and receptor activation form a crucial component of positive reinforcement, driving the reinforcing effects of substances in addiction. Unraveling the complexities of dopamine's role provides valuable insights into the neurobiology of addiction, opening avenues for targeted interventions aimed at disrupting the reinforcing mechanisms that underlie substance use disorders.

Sensitization and reward-related learning in positive reinforcement: Sensitization, a neuroadaptive phenomenon, and reward-related learning are integral aspects of positive reinforcement in addiction. This text explores the interplay between sensitization and reward-related learning, shedding light on how these processes contribute to the reinforcing effects of substances and the development of addictive behaviors, with references from key studies in the field. Sensitization refers to the phenomenon wherein repeated exposure to a stimulus, such as a drug, leads to an amplified response over time. In the context of addiction, sensitization involves an increase in the behavioral or physiological effects of a substance with repeated use. This neuroadaptive response contributes to the intensification of positive reinforcement, making the individual more susceptible to the rewarding effects of substances.

Dopaminergic systems play a crucial role in sensitization. Chronic exposure to drugs of abuse, such as psychostimulants, leads to alterations in dopamine transmission. Sensitization is characterized by increased dopamine release, particularly in the mesolimbic pathway, contributing to the heightened rewarding effects of substances and the reinforcement of drug-seeking behaviors. Reward-related learning involves the acquisition of associations between stimuli and positive outcomes. Neural mechanisms underlying reward-related learning include the mesolimbic dopamine pathway and its projections to the nucleus accumbens. The strengthening of neural connections in response to rewarding stimuli contributes to the formation of learned associations, reinforcing the pursuit of behaviors leading to positive outcomes (Schultz, 2016). Sensitization reflects a form of long-term plasticity in the brain, particularly in the mesolimbic dopaminergic system. Persistent neuroadaptations contribute to the enduring effects of sensitization, creating a state of increased responsiveness to drug-related cues and heightened sensitivity to the rewarding effects of substances. This plasticity reinforces the association between drug-related stimuli and positive outcomes, perpetuating addictive behaviors. Cross-sensitization refers to the phenomenon where sensitization to one drug enhances the response to another. This cross-sensitization between different substances contributes to the broadening of the reinforcement spectrum, increasing the likelihood of polydrug use. The shared neuroadaptive mechanisms underlying sensitization contribute to the complex interactions observed in the progression of addiction (Piazza et al., 2000).

Behavioral changes associated with sensitization encompass an increased propensity for drug-seeking behaviors and a heightened vulnerability to relapse. Sensitized individuals may exhibit exaggerated responses to drug-related cues and an enhanced motivation to seek substances. These behavioral changes are indicative of the enduring impact of sensitization on the reinforcement circuitry. Understanding the role of sensitization and reward-related learning in positive reinforcement has implications for addiction treatment. Targeting the neuroadaptive processes associated with sensitization may inform therapeutic strategies aimed at mitigating the reinforcing effects of substances and preventing relapse, contributing to more effective interventions in substance use disorders. Sensitization and reward-related learning are intertwined neuroadaptive processes that contribute significantly to positive reinforcement in addiction. Exploring the mechanisms underlying these phenomena provides valuable insights into the persistent nature of substance use disorders, guiding the development of targeted interventions that address the long-term neuroplastic changes associated with sensitization and reinforcement-related learning.

Negative reinforcement in drug addiction: Negative reinforcement, a powerful psychological process, plays a crucial role in drug addiction. This concept of negative reinforcement needs to be addressed in the context of substance use disorders, elucidating how individuals engage in drug-seeking and drug-taking behaviors to alleviate negative emotions, stress, or withdrawal symptoms. Negative reinforcement involves the removal or avoidance of an aversive stimulus, leading to an increase in the likelihood of a behavior. In the context of drug addiction, negative reinforcement refers to the use of substances to escape or avoid unpleasant feelings, emotions, or withdrawal symptoms. Many individuals turn to drugs as a means of alleviating negative emotions such as stress, anxiety, or depression. The temporary relief provided by substances can create a powerful negative reinforcement loop, as individuals learn that drug use can serve as an effective coping mechanism for emotional discomfort (Koob & Le Moal, 2008).

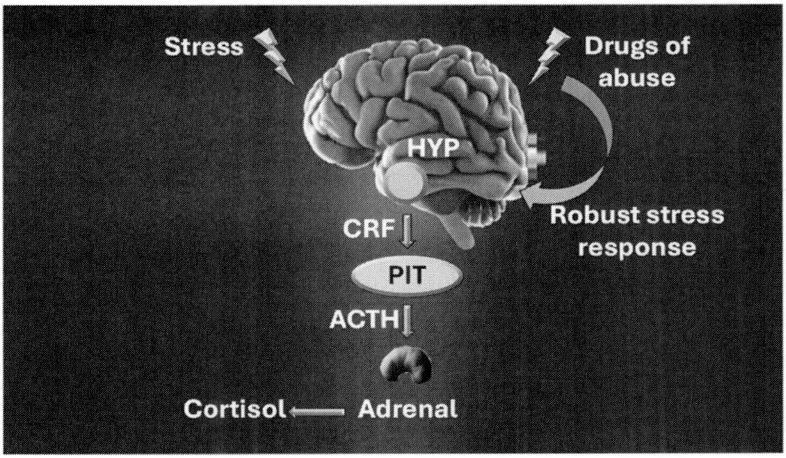

Robust stress response following repeated administration of drugs of abuse

Stress reduction is a common motive for drug use, particularly in individuals facing chronic stressors. Drugs, by modulating neurotransmitter systems, provide a temporary escape from stress, reinforcing the association between substance use and stress relief. This negative reinforcement process contributes to the maintenance of addictive behaviors (Sinha, 2008). Negative reinforcement is prominently observed in the context of withdrawal symptoms. Individuals experiencing discomfort or pain during withdrawal may use drugs to escape these aversive states.

The relief from withdrawal symptoms serves as a powerful negative reinforcement mechanism, reinforcing the association between drug use and the avoidance of withdrawal-related distress. The development of tolerance, wherein individuals require increasing amounts of a substance to achieve the desired effects, is linked to negative reinforcement. Tolerance can drive individuals to escalate their drug use to avoid withdrawal symptoms or to attain the initial euphoric effects, perpetuating a negative reinforcement cycle. Negative reinforcement extends to escaping aversive and dysphoric states. Individuals may use drugs to mitigate feelings of unease, dysphoria, or discontent. The relief provided by substances serves as a negative reinforcer, strengthening the connection between drug use and the alleviation of aversive experiences. Negative reinforcement is often intertwined with comorbid mental health disorders. Individuals with conditions such as depression or post-traumatic stress disorder may turn to drugs as a means of self-medication to alleviate emotional distress, reinforcing the negative reinforcement loop and complicating the treatment landscape.

Understanding the role of negative reinforcement in drug addiction has crucial implications for treatment approaches. Therapeutic interventions that address the underlying emotional and psychological factors contributing to negative reinforcement, such as cognitive-behavioral therapy and emotion regulation strategies, can be essential components of comprehensive addiction treatment (Baker et al., 2004). Negative reinforcement in drug addiction highlights the complex interplay between substances and emotional well-being. By understanding the motivations behind negative reinforcement, interventions can be tailored to address the root causes of substance use, offering individuals more effective strategies to cope with negative emotions and stressors, ultimately breaking the cycle of addiction.

Alleviation of negative emotions in negative reinforcement: Negative emotions, such as stress, anxiety, and sadness, often serve as powerful triggers for substance use, contributing to a negative reinforcement loop in addiction. This is important to consider how individuals seek to alleviate negative emotions through drug use, examining the neurobiological and psychological mechanisms involved. Emotion regulation refers to the strategies individuals employ to modulate their emotional experiences. For some, substances become a means of emotion regulation, providing temporary relief from negative emotions. The self-medication hypothesis posits that individuals use drugs to cope with emotional distress, reinforcing the association between substance use and the alleviation of negative emotions.

Stress relief is a primary motivator for substance use in the context of negative reinforcement. Chronic stress activates the hypothalamic-pituitary-adrenal (HPA) axis, leading to the release of stress hormones. Drugs, particularly those affecting the GABAergic and dopaminergic systems, provide a rapid reduction in stress-related neurochemical responses, reinforcing the use of substances as a means of escaping or attenuating stress (Koob & Le Moal, 2008). Individuals with anxiety disorders may turn to substances to alleviate symptoms of anxiety. The anxiolytic effects of certain drugs, such as benzodiazepines, temporarily reduce feelings of anxiety, reinforcing the use of these substances as a strategy for managing emotional discomfort. Negative emotions associated with depression can drive individuals to engage in substance use as a form of self-medication. Drugs that affect the monoaminergic system, such as opioids or alcohol, may temporarily alleviate symptoms of depression, reinforcing the use of substances to cope with emotional pain (Sinha, 2008).

Neurobiological mechanisms underlie the relief of negative emotions through substance use. Drugs targeting neurotransmitter systems, including the release of dopamine and modulation of the GABAergic system, interact with brain regions involved in emotion regulation. These alterations contribute to the immediate emotional relief experienced by individuals, reinforcing the connection between drug use and emotional well-being. Individuals who have experienced trauma may use substances to escape trauma-related distress. The numbing or dissociative effects of certain drugs can provide temporary relief from the emotional pain associated with traumatic experiences, perpetuating substance use as a strategy for avoiding distressing memories or emotions.

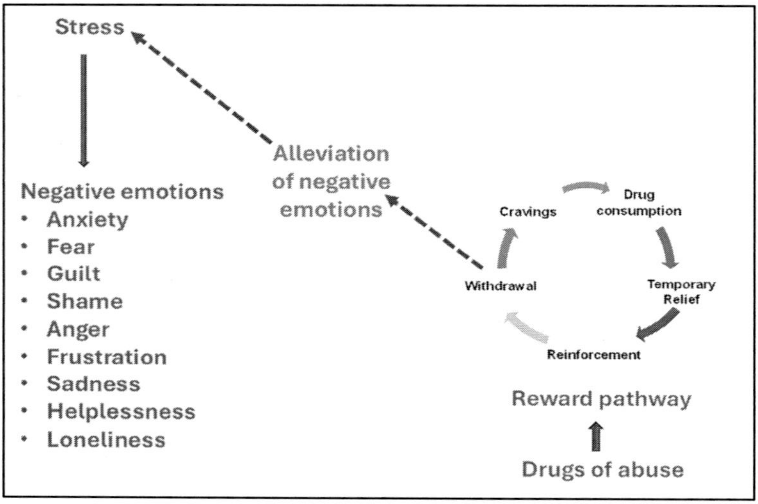

Alleviation of negative emotions in negative reinforcement

Recognizing the role of negative reinforcement in alleviating negative emotions is crucial for designing effective treatment interventions. Therapeutic approaches, such as cognitive-behavioral therapy, dialectical behavior therapy, and mindfulness-based interventions, aim to equip individuals with healthier coping mechanisms to manage negative emotions, reducing the reliance on substances for emotional relief (McHugh et al., 2019). The alleviation of negative emotions through substance use represents a significant component of negative reinforcement in addiction. Understanding the psychological and neurobiological mechanisms involved provides valuable insights for developing targeted interventions that address the root causes of emotional distress, offering individuals healthier alternatives to cope with negative emotions and break the cycle of substance dependence.

Stress and anxiety in negative reinforcement: Stress and anxiety, pervasive components of modern life, are often powerful motivators for individuals to engage in substance use. This text explores the intricate relationship between stress, anxiety, and negative reinforcement in the context of addiction. Drawing on key references, it delves into how the alleviation of these emotional states through substance use creates a reinforcing cycle that sustains addictive behaviors. Stress, a physiological and psychological response to challenging situations, is a significant factor in the initiation and maintenance of substance use. The relief from stress through substance use becomes a negative reinforcement mechanism, reinforcing the association between drug consumption and the alleviation of stressors. Anxiety, characterized by persistent worry and fear, is another emotional state that can drive individuals to seek relief through substance use. Drugs with anxiolytic effects, such as benzodiazepines or alcohol, offer temporary respite from anxiety symptoms, reinforcing the use of these substances as a coping strategy.

The stress response involves the activation of the hypothalamic-pituitary-adrenal (HPA) axis, leading to the release of stress hormones, including cortisol. Chronic activation of the HPA axis is associated with heightened stress levels and an increased vulnerability to substance use as individuals seek to alleviate the discomfort associated with persistent stress (Koob & Le Moal, 2008). Anxiety is often linked to dysregulation of the gamma-aminobutyric acid (GABA)ergic system, a neurotransmitter system that plays a crucial role in inhibitory signaling in the brain. Drugs that enhance GABAergic transmission, such as benzodiazepines, can produce anxiolytic effects, reinforcing their use in individuals seeking relief from anxiety-related symptoms (Koob & Le Moal, 2001). Stress and anxiety impact neural circuits involved in reward and motivation, particularly the mesolimbic dopamine pathway. Chronic stress can lead to neuroadaptations in this pathway, contributing to an increased susceptibility to substance use as individuals seek the rewarding effects of drugs to counteract the negative emotional states associated with stress.

Negative reinforcement, through the alleviation of stress and anxiety, becomes a crucial factor in maintaining substance use. The temporary relief provided by drugs creates a reinforcing loop, strengthening the association between substance use and the reduction of negative emotional states. This negative reinforcement cycle contributes to the chronic nature of addiction

(Baker et al., 2004). Recognizing the role of stress and anxiety in negative reinforcement is pivotal for designing effective treatment strategies. Interventions that address stress management, anxiety reduction, and healthier coping mechanisms are integral components of comprehensive addiction treatment, aiming to break the negative reinforcement cycle and reduce the reliance on substances for emotional relief (McHugh et al., 2019). Stress and anxiety, prevalent aspects of the human experience, significantly contribute to negative reinforcement in substance use. Understanding the complex interplay between these negative emotional states and addictive behaviors provides a foundation for developing targeted interventions that address the underlying emotional distress, offering individuals more adaptive coping strategies and fostering sustained recovery.

Emotional regulation through substance abuse in negative reinforcement: Emotion regulation, the ability to modulate and manage one's emotional experiences, is a critical aspect of psychological well-being. However, for some individuals, substance abuse becomes a maladaptive strategy for coping with emotional challenges. The intricate relationship between emotional regulation and substance abuse within the framework of negative reinforcement elucidates the mechanisms and consequences of this dynamic. Emotional dysregulation, characterized by difficulties in effectively managing and responding to emotional experiences, often precedes substance abuse. Individuals grappling with intense emotions may turn to substances as a means of escape or temporary relief, initiating a negative reinforcement loop (Berking et al., 2011).

Substances of abuse, particularly those affecting the dopaminergic system, can modulate emotional states. Dopamine, a neurotransmitter associated with reward and pleasure, plays a role in the reinforcing effects of substances. The modulation of dopamine levels by drugs contributes to the emotional relief experienced by individuals, strengthening the negative reinforcement cycle. Substance abuse often serves as a mechanism for escaping emotional discomfort. The acute effects of drugs can provide a temporary respite from negative emotions, creating a powerful negative reinforcement loop as individuals associate substance use with emotional relief. The self-medication hypothesis posits that individuals use substances to alleviate emotional distress. Emotional regulation difficulties, such as those seen in mood disorders, may drive individuals to self-medicate with drugs. This self-medication provides a negative reinforcement mechanism, as individuals learn that substances can temporarily alleviate emotional pain. Neurobiological mechanisms underlie the emotional relief experienced through substance abuse. The endogenous opioid system, in particular, is implicated in the modulation of emotional responses. Drugs that activate this system, such as opioids, can induce a sense of euphoria and emotional numbing, contributing to the negative reinforcement cycle. Emotional regulation through substance abuse contributes to the development of maladaptive coping strategies. As individuals repeatedly turn to substances to manage emotions, healthier coping mechanisms may be neglected, reinforcing the reliance on substances and hindering the development of adaptive emotional regulation skills (Simons et al., 2017).

Understanding the role of emotional regulation in negative reinforcement has implications for treatment. Interventions that target emotion regulation skills, such as dialectical behavior therapy (DBT) or mindfulness-based approaches, can be integral components of substance use disorder treatment, helping individuals develop healthier strategies for managing emotions (Linehan, 2018). Emotional regulation through substance abuse within the context of negative reinforcement unveils the complex interplay between emotional well-being and addictive behaviors. Recognizing the neurobiological and psychological mechanisms involved provides a foundation for developing tailored interventions that address the root causes of emotional dysregulation, fostering healthier coping strategies and contributing to sustained recovery from substance use disorders.

Self-medication hypothesis for drug reinforcement: The self-medication hypothesis proposes that individuals may turn to substance use as a form of self-medication to alleviate symptoms of underlying mental health issues. This text explores the foundations, implications, and research surrounding the self-medication hypothesis within the context of drug reinforcement, incorporating key references to elucidate this intricate relationship. The self-medication hypothesis, introduced by Edward J. Khantzian in the late 20th century, posits that individuals use drugs to self-medicate and alleviate distressing symptoms associated with psychiatric disorders. This theory emphasizes the role of psychological pain and emotional discomfort as primary motivators for engaging in substance use (Khantzian, 1997).

One central tenet of the hypothesis is that individuals may seek substances to alleviate emotional distress, including anxiety, depression, or other mood disorders. The temporary relief provided by drugs can act as a negative reinforcement mechanism, strengthening the association between substance use and the alleviation of psychological pain. Substances not only serve as a form of self-medication but also possess reinforcing properties that can contribute to the development and maintenance of addictive behaviors. The dual role of substances as both medication for emotional distress and sources of reinforcement creates a complex interplay that can perpetuate substance use disorders. The Self-Medication Hypothesis is often associated with the high prevalence of comorbidity between substance use disorders and mental health conditions. Individuals with psychiatric disorders may be more prone to using substances as a means of self-medicating symptoms, contributing to the intricate relationship between mental health and substance use.

The hypothesis suggests that the choice of substances for self-medication may be specific to the nature of the psychiatric symptoms. For example, individuals with anxiety might be drawn to substances with anxiolytic properties, while those with depressive symptoms may seek substances with mood-elevating effects. This specificity reflects the individualized nature of self-medication choices. Acknowledging the self-medication hypothesis has implications for treatment strategies. Interventions that address both the substance use disorder and underlying mental health issues are often more effective. However, the challenge lies in disentangling the complex interplay between self-medication and substance reinforcement, requiring a nuanced and individualized approach to treatment. While influential, the self-medication hypothesis is not without criticisms. Some argue that the hypothesis oversimplifies the complex motivations for substance use and that reinforcing properties of substances might play a more dominant role than originally proposed. Alternative explanations, such as the affect regulation model, highlight the multifaceted nature of motivations for substance use (baker et al., 2004). The Self-Medication Hypothesis provides a valuable framework for understanding the intricate relationship between substance use and mental health. Recognizing the dual role of substances as both medication and reinforcement contributes to a more nuanced understanding of addiction, emphasizing the need for tailored interventions that address both the symptoms of psychiatric disorders and the reinforcing aspects of substance use.

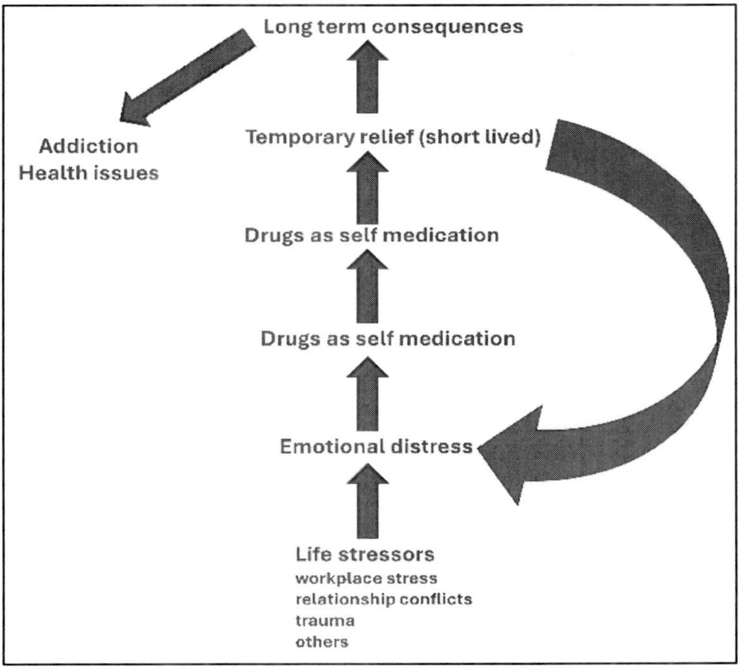

Self-medication hypothesis for drug reinforcement

Escapism and avoidance of reality in drug reinforcement: The motivation behind drug reinforcement often extends beyond the pursuit of pleasure, with escapism and the desire to avoid reality playing pivotal roles. The intricate relationship between drug use and the human inclination to escape or evade aspects of reality plays an important role in understanding reinforcing effects of drugs of abuse. Escapism, the desire to break away from the challenges or stresses of reality, is a significant motivator for engaging in substance use. Individuals may turn to drugs as a means of temporarily escaping emotional pain, stressors, or unpleasant aspects of their lives, creating a reinforcing loop where substance use becomes associated with a respite from reality (Koob & Le Moal, 2008). Neurobiological mechanisms underlie the desire for escapism through substance use. Drugs often target reward pathways in the brain, including the mesolimbic dopamine system. The activation of these pathways contributes to the pleasurable effects of substances, reinforcing the association between drug use and the temporary escape from the challenges of reality.

The avoidance of negative emotions and stress is a common driver for individuals seeking to escape reality through substance use. Drugs that provide rapid relief from emotional distress, such as anxiety or sadness, become attractive options for those attempting to avoid facing challenging emotions. This avoidance behavior reinforces the association between drug use and emotional relief. Individuals who have experienced trauma may turn to substance use as a way to cope with the psychological repercussions of traumatic events. Drugs offer a temporary escape from the intrusive thoughts, nightmares, and emotional pain associated with trauma, reinforcing the use of substances as a means of avoiding the harsh realities of past experiences drug use. Peer pressure, societal expectations, or a lack of positive environmental stimuli may drive individuals to seek an escape through substances. The reinforcement of these behaviors in social contexts can further solidify the connection between drug use and the avoidance of reality (Bretteville-Jensen, 2006). Drugs not only offer an escape from reality but also reinforce the behavior through their pharmacological effects. The alteration of neurotransmitter systems, particularly the release of dopamine in reward circuits, creates a pleasurable experience that further solidifies the association between drug use and the desire to escape from the challenges of everyday life.

Understanding the role of escapism in drug reinforcement has important implications for treatment strategies. Interventions that address the underlying motivations for escapism, such as therapeutic approaches focused on stress management, emotion regulation, and coping skills development, can be integral components of substance use disorder treatment (McHugh et al., 2010). Escapism and the avoidance of reality represent powerful motivators in the realm of drug reinforcement. Recognizing the multifaceted nature of these motivations allows for a more comprehensive understanding of addiction, informing tailored interventions that address the root causes of the desire to escape. By offering healthier alternatives for coping with life's challenges, treatment approaches can contribute to breaking the cycle of substance dependence rooted in escapism.

The Interplay Between Positive and Negative Reinforcement: The motivations behind substance use are complex, often involving a delicate interplay between positive and negative reinforcement. It is interesting to see how individuals are driven to use substances not only for the pleasure derived from positive reinforcement but also as a means of alleviating negative emotions or stress through negative reinforcement. Dopaminergic signaling is a key player in the positive and negative reinforcement aspect of substance use. Drugs of abuse often increase dopamine levels in the nucleus accumbens, intensifying feelings of pleasure and reinforcing the association between drug use and reward (Volkow et al., 2007), whereas the levels of dopamine drop during the withdrawal phase and this acts as a negative reinforcer for withdrawal phase so that person should avoid this withdrawal phase. Negative reinforcement involves the removal or avoidance of aversive stimuli, such as emotional distress or stress. Individuals may use substances to alleviate negative emotions, creating a reinforcing cycle where the relief from emotional pain strengthens the association between drug use and the avoidance of discomfort (Baker et al., 2004).

The interplay between positive and negative reinforcement contributes to the complexity of substance use. Individuals may initially engage in substance use for the positive reinforcement of pleasure but continue the behavior due to negative reinforcement, seeking relief from emotional distress or stressors (Koob & Le Moal, 2008). Substance use can serve a dual purpose of escaping reality through negative reinforcement and enhancing pleasure through positive reinforcement. The combination of these reinforcing aspects creates a powerful motivator for continued substance use, contributing to the development and maintenance of addiction. Neuroadaptive changes in the brain occur with chronic substance use, leading to the development of tolerance. Tolerance diminishes the pleasurable effects of the substance, driving individuals to increase their usage to achieve the desired positive reinforcement. Simultaneously, negative reinforcement becomes more pronounced as individuals seek to avoid the discomfort of withdrawal symptoms (Koob & Le Moal, 2001). Understanding the interplay between positive and negative reinforcement has crucial implications for treatment.

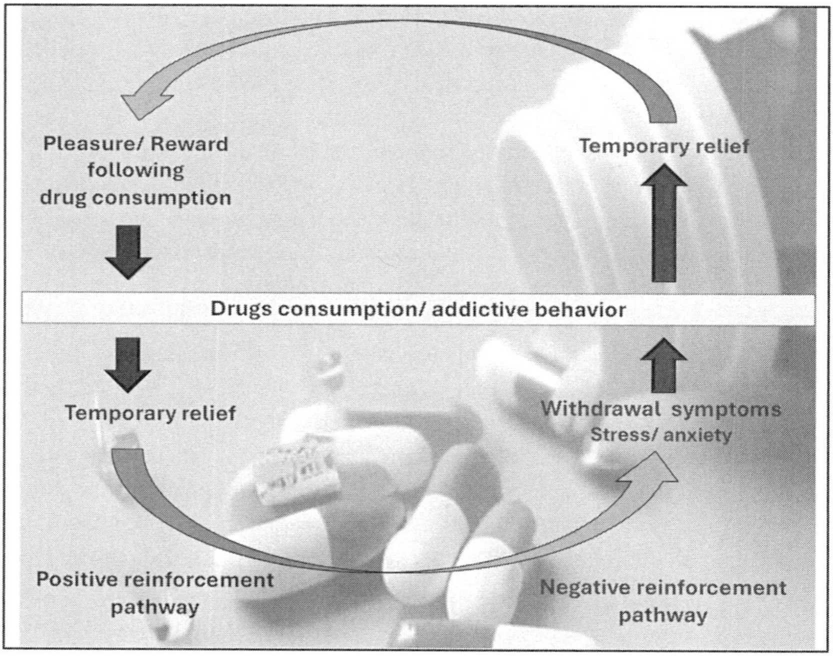

The Interplay Between Positive and Negative Reinforcement

Interventions need to address both aspects, offering alternative coping mechanisms for stressors and emotional distress while also working to break the association between substance use and pleasure. Comprehensive treatment approaches can contribute to more effective and lasting recovery (McHugh et al., 2019). The dynamic interplay between positive and negative reinforcement illuminates the multifaceted nature of substance use motivations. Recognizing and addressing both aspects in treatment is essential for providing individuals with the tools to navigate the complexities of addiction, fostering a more holistic approach to recovery.

Shifting reinforcement dynamics over time: The reinforcement dynamics underlying substance use evolve over time, presenting a dynamic and multifaceted picture of addiction. In the early stages of substance use, positive reinforcement plays a central role. Individuals are often motivated by the pleasurable effects of drugs and the novelty associated with initial experiences. Dopaminergic signaling in the brain's reward circuits reinforces the behavior, establishing an association between substance use and the anticipation of pleasure (Nestler, 2005). As substance use progresses, negative reinforcement becomes more prominent. Individuals may turn to substances to alleviate stress, anxiety, or emotional distress, creating a shift in the reinforcement dynamics. The relief from negative emotions reinforces the association between drug use and the avoidance of discomfort (Baker et al., 2004).

Chronic substance use leads to neuroadaptive changes in the brain, altering the reinforcement dynamics. Tolerance develops, diminishing the pleasurable effects of the substance. Individuals may increase their usage to overcome tolerance, shifting the emphasis toward avoiding withdrawal symptoms and maintaining a semblance of normalcy, thus highlighting the prominence of negative reinforcement (Koob & Le Moal, 2001). In the maintenance phase of substance use, negative reinforcement often dominates the reinforcement dynamics. Craving becomes a prominent motivator, with individuals seeking to avoid the distressing symptoms of withdrawal. The shift towards negative reinforcement underscores the compulsive nature of substance use in maintaining emotional equilibrium. In the context of recovery and treatment, reinforcement dynamics undergo a significant shift. Positive reinforcement gains importance as individuals discover alternative sources of pleasure and reward in life. Activities that were once overshadowed by substance use become reinforcing, contributing to the process of recovery and the establishment of healthier habits.

Despite progress in recovery, relapse poses a challenge to the shifting reinforcement dynamics. The reactivation of drug-associated cues may rekindle the memories of positive reinforcement, leading to a resurgence of craving. Understanding these dynamics is crucial for developing targeted interventions that address the vulnerabilities during this critical phase of recovery (Volkow & Baler, 2015). The reinforcement dynamics in substance use are not static; they undergo substantial shifts over time. Recognizing these temporal changes provides a nuanced understanding of addiction, informing tailored interventions at different stages of substance use. A comprehensive approach that addresses the evolving nature of reinforcement dynamics is essential for effective prevention, treatment, and sustained recovery

Neurotransmitter modulation in negative reinforcement: Negative reinforcement in the context of substance use involves seeking relief from aversive stimuli or emotional distress. A need arises to explore the intricate modulation of neurotransmitters in the brain's reward and stress pathways during negative reinforcement, shedding light on the neural circuitry involved. Gamma-aminobutyric acid (GABA), the primary inhibitory neurotransmitter in the brain, plays a crucial role in negative reinforcement. GABAergic inhibition is associated with stress alleviation, as enhanced GABAergic activity can lead to anxiolytic effects, reducing the perception of stress and anxiety. Benzodiazepines, which potentiate GABAergic signaling, are examples of drugs that exploit this mechanism for stress relief (Crestani et al., 2000). Endogenous opioids, including endorphins and enkephalins, contribute to the modulation of negative reinforcement. These neurotransmitters are involved in the brain's natural pain and stress modulation system.

The activation of opioid receptors provides a sense of euphoria and emotional relief, reinforcing the association between opioid release and the alleviation of emotional distress (Bodnar, 2016). Serotonin, a neurotransmitter associated with mood regulation, is implicated in negative reinforcement. Drugs that enhance serotonergic activity, such as selective serotonin reuptake inhibitors (SSRIs), can stabilize mood and alleviate symptoms of anxiety and depression, contributing to the negative reinforcement loop by providing relief from emotional distress. Noradrenaline (norepinephrine) is a neurotransmitter involved in the stress response. Increased noradrenergic activity is associated with heightened alertness and arousal. Drugs that modulate noradrenergic signaling, such as alpha-2 adrenergic agonists, may have anxiolytic effects, contributing to negative reinforcement by dampening the stress response. Dopamine, a neurotransmitter associated with reward and pleasure, is also implicated in negative reinforcement. Drugs that modulate dopaminergic activity may provide emotional relief by altering the perception of aversive stimuli. The interplay between dopamine and stress pathways contributes to the reinforcing effects of substances during negative reinforcement (Koob & Volkow, 2010). Glutamate, the primary excitatory neurotransmitter in the brain, is involved in stress response modulation. Drugs that target glutamatergic receptors, such as N-methyl-D-aspartate (NMDA) receptor antagonists, may influence the perception of stress and emotional distress. This modulation contributes to the negative reinforcement aspect of substance use.

Corticotropin-releasing factor (CRF) is a neuropeptide involved in the stress response. Dysregulation of the CRF system is associated with heightened stress and anxiety. Drugs that modulate CRF receptors may influence the negative reinforcement loop by mitigating the impact of stressors on emotional well-being. Neurotransmitter modulation in negative reinforcement illustrates the complexity of the neural circuitry involved in seeking emotional relief through substance use. Understanding how different neurotransmitters contribute to stress modulation and mood regulation provides insights into the mechanisms that drive the reinforcing effects of substances in the context of negative reinforcement.

Conditioning and associative learning: Conditioning and associative learning are fundamental processes that shape human behavior. Exploring the principles of classical and operant conditioning, shedding light on how individuals form associations between stimuli and responses would make the picture clearer. Classical conditioning, famously demonstrated by Ivan Pavlov, involves the association between a neutral stimulus and an unconditioned stimulus to evoke a conditioned response. For example, Pavlov's dogs learned to associate the ringing of a bell (neutral stimulus) with the presentation of food (unconditioned stimulus), ultimately causing them to salivate at the sound of the bell alone. This process illustrates the power of pairing stimuli to produce learned responses (Pavlov, 2010). Operant conditioning, developed by B.F. Skinner, focuses on the relationship between behavior and its consequences. In this paradigm, behaviors are strengthened or weakened based on the positive or negative consequences that follow. For instance, a rat in a Skinner box learns to press a lever to receive a food pellet, illustrating how the consequence of receiving food reinforces the behavior of lever-pressing

Operant conditioning relies on reinforcement and punishment to modulate behavior. Positive reinforcement involves presenting a rewarding stimulus to strengthen a behavior, while negative reinforcement removes an aversive stimulus, also strengthening a behavior. Conversely, positive punishment presents an aversive stimulus, weakening a behavior, and negative punishment removes a rewarding stimulus, also weakening a behavior. Extinction occurs when a conditioned response weakens due to the absence of reinforcement. However, the phenomenon of spontaneous recovery suggests that, after a period of rest, the extinguished response may reappear in the presence of the conditioned stimulus. These dynamics highlight the complexities of learning and memory. Higher-order conditioning involves establishing new conditioned stimuli by pairing them with existing conditioned stimuli. This process allows for the formation of complex associations and the transfer of learned responses to novel stimuli. The principles of higher-order conditioning contribute to the richness and flexibility of learned behaviors (Kehoe & White, 2002).

The principles of conditioning and associative learning have wide-ranging applications in behavior modification. From therapeutic interventions to educational settings, understanding how stimuli and responses become associated enables the development of effective strategies for behavior change. Applied behavior analysis, rooted in operant conditioning principles, exemplifies the practical applications of these theories. Cognitive theories of conditioning, such as the Rescorla-Wagner model, integrate cognitive processes into the traditional behaviorist framework. These models emphasize the importance of cognitive factors in learning, challenging the behaviorist perspective that focuses solely on observable behaviors. Conditioning and associative learning form the bedrock of behavioral psychology, providing a comprehensive framework for understanding how individuals acquire new behaviors through the association of stimuli and responses. The exploration of classical and operant conditioning, alongside their applications and cognitive underpinnings, underscores the significance of these learning processes in shaping human behavior.

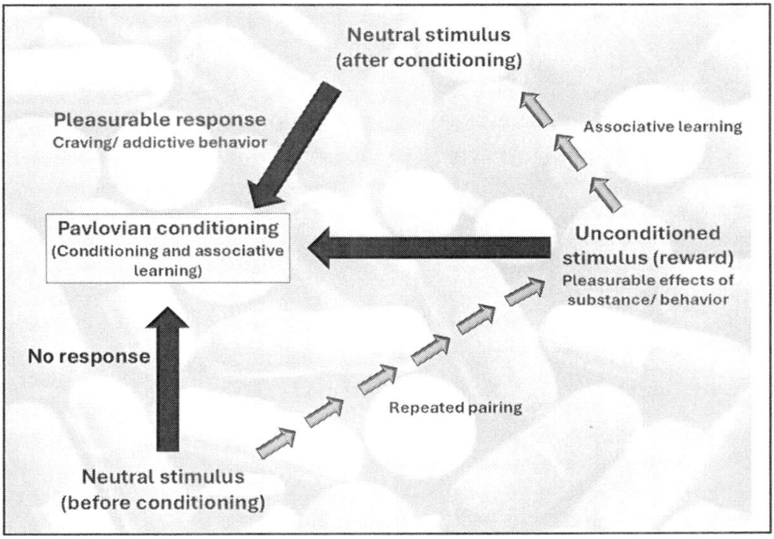

Conditioning and associative learning

Pavlovian and operant conditioning: Pavlovian and operant conditioning are two fundamental forms of learning that have shaped our understanding of behavior. There arises a need to explore the work of Ivan Pavlov and B.F. Skinner, along with others that have contributed to the evolution of behavioral psychology. Classical or Pavlovian conditioning, pioneered by Ivan Pavlov, involves the association of a neutral stimulus with an unconditioned stimulus to evoke a conditioned response. The classic example is Pavlov's dogs associating the ringing of a bell (neutral stimulus) with food (unconditioned stimulus), leading to salivation (conditioned response). Pavlov's work laid the foundation for understanding how stimuli could elicit reflexive responses through learned associations (Pavlov, 2010). Operant conditioning, developed by B.F. Skinner, centers on the relationship between behavior and its consequences. Behaviors are strengthened or weakened based on positive or negative consequences. For instance, a rat pressing a lever to receive a food pellet demonstrates operant conditioning. Skinner's operant chamber (Skinner box) became an iconic tool for studying behavior in controlled environments (Skinner, 1938).

Operant conditioning relies on reinforcement and punishment to shape behavior. Positive reinforcement involves presenting a rewarding stimulus to strengthen a behavior, while negative reinforcement removes an aversive stimulus, also strengthening behavior. Positive punishment introduces an aversive stimulus to weaken behavior, and negative punishment removes a rewarding stimulus, weakening behavior. These dynamics are fundamental to behavior modification. Extinction occurs when a conditioned response weakens due to the absence of reinforcement. Spontaneous recovery, on the other hand, suggests that after a rest period, the extinguished response may reappear. These phenomena showcase the intricate dynamics of learning and memory. Higher-order conditioning involves creating new conditioned stimuli by pairing them with existing conditioned stimuli. This process allows for the formation of complex associations and the transfer of learned responses to novel stimuli. Higher-order conditioning contributes to the flexibility and richness of learned behaviors (Kehoe & White, 2002).

Pavlovian and operant conditioning principles find applications in behavior modification. From therapeutic interventions to educational settings, these principles inform strategies for shaping and changing behaviors. Applied behavior analysis, rooted in operant conditioning, exemplifies the practical applications of these theories. Cognitive theories, such as the Rescorla-Wagner model, integrate cognitive processes into the traditional behaviorist framework. These models emphasize the importance of cognitive factors in learning, challenging the behaviorist perspective that focuses solely on observable behaviors. Pavlovian and operant conditioning stand as cornerstones in the field of behavioral psychology, providing comprehensive frameworks for understanding how learned associations shape behavior. The exploration of these conditioning paradigms, their applications, and cognitive underpinnings underscores their enduring significance in unraveling the mysteries of human learning and behavior.

Environmental factors influencing reward sensitivity: Reward sensitivity, a crucial component of motivation and decision-making, is influenced by a myriad of environmental factors. Key environmental elements that modulate reward sensitivity, shedding light on the intricate interplay between external factors and the brain's reward system would be explored briefly. This would provide a foundation for understanding the dynamic relationship between the environment and reward processing. Socioeconomic status significantly influences reward sensitivity. Individuals from lower SES backgrounds may exhibit altered neural responses to rewards. Neuroimaging studies suggest that socioeconomic disparities can affect the functioning of brain regions involved in reward processing, such as the nucleus accumbens and prefrontal cortex (Gianaros et al., 2008).

Early life adversity, including childhood trauma or neglect, can have enduring effects on reward sensitivity. Adverse experiences during critical developmental periods may shape the neural circuits involved in reward processing, contributing to altered reward sensitivity later in life (Dannlowski et al., 2012). The social environment, particularly peer relationships, plays a pivotal role in shaping reward sensitivity during adolescence. Peer influence can impact reward-related decision-making processes, as evidenced by studies highlighting the neural mechanisms underlying susceptibility to peer pressure and reward anticipation in social contexts (Chein et al., 2011). Cultural factors contribute to variability in reward sensitivity. Cross-cultural studies reveal that cultural norms and values shape individuals' responses to rewards. The cultural context influences how rewards are perceived and valued, impacting the neural substrates involved in reward processing. Environmental enrichment, characterized by exposure to stimulating and complex environments, can enhance reward sensitivity. Studies in animal models suggest that enriched environments promote neuroplasticity and modulate reward-related neurotransmitter systems, potentially influencing reward processing in humans.

The urban environment may impact reward sensitivity through interactions with dopaminergic systems. Urban living has been associated with altered dopamine functioning, potentially influencing reward-related behaviors. Factors such as chronic stress in urban settings may contribute to changes in reward sensitivity (Lederbogen et al., 2011). Understanding the environmental factors influencing reward sensitivity provides valuable insights into the intricate interplay between external conditions and the brain's reward systems. From socioeconomic status to early life experiences, the social environment, cultural factors, and even the nature of one's surroundings, each element contributes to the modulation of reward sensitivity. These insights have implications for comprehending individual differences in decision-making, motivation, and susceptibility to reward-related disorders.

Socioeconomic influences on reinforcement: Socioeconomic status (SES) plays a pivotal role in shaping reinforcement processes, influencing how individuals respond to rewards and punishments. Intricate interplay between socioeconomic factors and reinforcement mechanisms explores the impact of social and economic conditions on decision-making and behavior. Neuroscientific research has revealed that SES is associated with differences in neural responses to reinforcement. Individuals from lower SES backgrounds may exhibit altered activation patterns in brain regions linked to reward processing, such as the ventral striatum and prefrontal cortex. These neural differences contribute to variations in reinforcement sensitivity across different socioeconomic groups (Gianaros et al., 2008). Economic deprivation, a hallmark of lower SES, can influence reinforcement learning processes. Individuals facing economic challenges may show heightened sensitivity to rewards as a coping mechanism. Conversely, the uncertainty associated with economic instability may contribute to altered reinforcement learning strategies, impacting decision-making in reward-based scenarios (Glimcher, 2011).

Behavioral economics provides insights into how SES influences reinforcement processes from a decision-making perspective. Economic disparities can shape risk preferences, time discounting, and sensitivity to gains and losses. These behavioral economic factors contribute to variations in reinforcement-related choices among individuals with different SES backgrounds. Social reinforcement, rooted in social learning theory, is deeply influenced by SES. Social contexts within lower SES environments may expose individuals to different reinforcement contingencies, affecting the acquisition of behaviors through observational learning. The social environment can shape the reinforcement values attributed to specific actions, influencing subsequent behavior. Socioeconomic disparities are often associated with increased stress levels. Chronic stress, prevalent in lower SES populations, can impact reinforcement sensitivity. Stress-induced alterations in neurobiology and cognition may influence how individuals perceive and respond to rewards and punishments, contributing to variations in reinforcement processes (Evans & Schamberg, 2009).

Educational attainment, closely linked to SES, also plays a role in shaping reinforcement processes. Higher levels of education are associated with cognitive flexibility, which can influence how individuals adapt their behavior based on reinforcement feedback. Educational experiences contribute to variations in reinforcement learning strategies (Baker et al., 2016). Socioeconomic influences on reinforcement underscore the pervasive impact of social and economic conditions on how individuals perceive, seek, and respond to rewards and punishments. From neural correlates to behavioral economic perspectives and the role of education, understanding the intricate relationship between SES and reinforcement provides a nuanced perspective on decision-making processes within diverse socioeconomic contexts.

Challenges in breaking the reinforcement cycle: Breaking the reinforcement cycle, particularly in the context of maladaptive behaviors, presents a multifaceted challenge. Neurobiological factors contribute to the resilience of reinforcement cycles. The brain's reward system, involving structures like the nucleus accumbens and prefrontal cortex, can exhibit persistent changes in response to repeated reinforcement. Neuroplasticity and the establishment of strong synaptic connections pose challenges in rewiring these entrenched pathways. The process of conditioning and habit formation contributes to the durability of reinforcement cycles. Habits, once established, become automatic responses to specific cues. Disrupting these ingrained habits requires concerted effort, as behaviors become deeply embedded in daily routines. This poses a challenge for individuals attempting to break free from maladaptive reinforcement patterns (Wood & Rünger, 2016). Psychological resistance to change is a significant hurdle in breaking reinforcement cycles. Individuals may experience cognitive dissonance when attempting to adopt new behaviors that conflict with established patterns. Fear of the unknown, anxiety, and a preference for familiarity contribute to the challenge of overcoming psychological barriers to behavior change. Environmental triggers and contextual cues play a pivotal role in sustaining reinforcement cycles. The association between specific environments and reinforcing stimuli can be deeply ingrained. Breaking the reinforcement cycle requires identifying and modifying these environmental triggers, which can be challenging due to their ubiquity and the automatic nature of the associations (Neal et al., 2011).

Social and peer influences contribute to the perpetuation of reinforcement cycles. Social networks can either reinforce or undermine efforts to change behavior. Peer pressure, social norms, and the desire for social acceptance can create powerful reinforcing dynamics that challenge individuals attempting to break free from maladaptive cycles (Cialdini & Goldstein, 2004). The absence of external support systems poses a significant challenge in breaking reinforcement cycles. Support from family, friends, or professional networks is crucial for individuals seeking behavior change. Without a robust support system, individuals may struggle to maintain motivation and overcome obstacles in the process of breaking entrenched reinforcement patterns. Relapse and recidivism underscore the persistent challenge in breaking reinforcement cycles. Even after initial success in behavior change, individuals may revert to previous patterns due to various factors, including stress, triggers, or a lack of coping mechanisms. Ongoing efforts and continuous support are essential to address the risk of relapse (Marlatt & Donovan, 2005). The challenges in breaking reinforcement cycles are multifaceted, encompassing neurobiological, psychological, social, and environmental factors. Acknowledging these complexities is essential for designing effective interventions and support systems that address the diverse obstacles individuals face in their journey toward behavior change.

Treatment Approaches Targeting Reinforcement: Addressing maladaptive reinforcement patterns is a critical aspect of effective treatment for various behavioral and mental health issues. Diverse treatment approaches that specifically target reinforcement processes emphasize evidence-based strategies and interventions. Cognitive-Behavioral Therapy (CBT) is a widely used approach that targets reinforcement processes by addressing maladaptive thoughts and behaviors. CBT aims to restructure cognitive patterns that contribute to dysfunctional reinforcement cycles. Behavioral interventions within CBT help individuals identify, challenge, and modify their reinforcement associations, promoting healthier responses to stimuli. Contingency Management (CM) is an evidence-based intervention that utilizes positive reinforcement to encourage desired behaviors. This approach involves systematically reinforcing target behaviors with rewards, such as vouchers or privileges. By creating a reinforcement system aligned with treatment goals, CM has proven effective in various settings, including substance use disorders (Prendergast et al., 2006).

Dialectical Behavior Therapy (DBT) integrates acceptance and change strategies to address reinforcement dynamics, particularly in individuals with emotion dysregulation. DBT emphasizes skill-building in emotional regulation, distress tolerance, and interpersonal effectiveness. By fostering adaptive coping mechanisms, DBT helps individuals navigate challenging situations without relying on maladaptive reinforcement patterns. Aversion therapy aims to break maladaptive reinforcement cycles by pairing undesirable behaviors with aversive stimuli. This classical conditioning approach creates negative associations with behaviors that were previously reinforced. Aversion therapy has been utilized in the treatment of various conditions, including substance use disorders and certain behavioral addictions. Motivational Interviewing (MI) focuses on enhancing intrinsic motivation for behavior change. By exploring and resolving ambivalence, MI helps individuals identify their own reasons for change. MI recognizes the importance of reinforcement processes in decision-making and empowers individuals to align their goals with their values, fostering lasting behavioral change.

Exposure Therapy targets reinforcement processes associated with avoidance behaviors. Commonly used in anxiety and trauma-related disorders, exposure therapy involves systematically confronting feared stimuli. By breaking the reinforcement of avoidance, individuals learn to tolerate distress and reshape maladaptive reinforcement patterns. Mindfulness-Based Interventions (MBIs), such as Mindfulness-Based Stress Reduction (MBSR) and Mindfulness-Based Cognitive Therapy (MBCT), target automatic and habitual reinforcement patterns. By cultivating present-moment awareness, individuals learn to observe and respond to stimuli without automatic reactivity. MBIs have shown promise in reducing the impact of maladaptive reinforcement cycles. Treatment approaches targeting reinforcement processes are diverse, reflecting the complexity of behavior change. From cognitive restructuring to positive reinforcement strategies and exposure-based interventions, these approaches recognize the pivotal role of reinforcement in shaping behaviors. Integrating evidence-based treatments that specifically address maladaptive reinforcement cycles is essential for fostering lasting change in individuals across various clinical contexts.

CHAPTER 4

COMMON FEATURES OF DRUG ADDICTION

"All the suffering, stress and addiction comes from not realizing you already are what you are looking for."
~ Jon Kabat-Zinn

A reflection on the shared experiences of addiction, suggesting a path of self-discovery as a key to healing. Let's talk about why people feel lost and turn to addiction, and how knowing yourself can be the key to healing. Finding what we need inside us can help break free from addiction. This chapter examines the common features of drug addiction and provides a comprehensive lens through which we can understand the shared patterns, challenges, and underlying mechanisms that characterize the complex spectrum of substance use disorders. This exploration of the common features of drug addiction serves as a roadmap to identify the universal threads intertwining various substances' impact on individuals, revealing the overarching traits that transcend specific drugs in the realm of addictive behaviors.

Drug addiction, often referred to as substance use disorder in clinical contexts, is a chronic and relapsing condition characterized by compulsive drug seeking, continued use despite harmful consequences, and long-lasting changes in the brain's structure and function. Understanding the precise definition of drug addiction is crucial for effective prevention, intervention, and treatment strategies. Individuals with drug addiction exhibit an overwhelming urge to obtain and use substances, often to the detriment of their well-being and responsibilities. This compulsive behavior is a hallmark of addiction and reflects the powerful impact of drugs on the brain's reward system. Loss of Control: One defining feature of addiction is the inability to control drug use. Individuals may repeatedly attempt to quit or cut down but find themselves unable to resist the cravings and compulsions associated with drug-seeking behavior. This loss of control is indicative of neurobiological changes that undermine decision-making processes. Despite experiencing adverse consequences such as health problems, strained relationships, or legal issues, individuals grappling with addiction persist in their drug use. This persistence is fueled by changes in the brain's reward and stress systems, making it challenging to break the cycle of drug dependence. Addiction is associated with profound alterations in the brain's structure and function. These changes, including neuroplasticity, neurotransmitter imbalances (e.g., dopamine dysregulation), and disruptions in the reward circuitry, contribute to the persistence of addictive behaviors and the difficulty of achieving sustained recovery (Nestler, 2005).

The field of addiction medicine has evolved, and contemporary diagnostic manuals, such as the Diagnostic and Statistical Manual of Mental Disorders (DSM-5), use the term "substance use disorder" to encompass the spectrum of problematic substance use. The severity of the disorder is classified as mild, moderate, or severe based on the number of diagnostic criteria met. Drug addiction is a complex, multifaceted condition characterized by compulsive drug seeking, loss of control, continued use despite adverse consequences, and neurobiological changes in the brain. This definition acknowledges the chronic nature of addiction and emphasizes the need for comprehensive approaches that address both the behavioral and neurobiological aspects of the disorder. Understanding the nuanced definition of drug addiction is crucial for shaping effective public health policies, treatment strategies, and interventions aimed at mitigating the impact of substance use on individuals and society.

Understanding the common features of drug addiction holds immense significance in various domains, ranging from public health policies to the development of effective prevention and treatment strategies. This knowledge is crucial for addressing the complexities of addiction and mitigating its impact on individuals and society. A comprehensive understanding of the common features of drug addiction provides the foundation for the development of informed public health policies. By recognizing the shared characteristics across different substances and patterns of use, policymakers can design evidence-based interventions that address the root causes of addiction and allocate resources more effectively identifying the common features of drug addiction allows for the design and implementation of targeted prevention strategies. Prevention efforts can focus on addressing risk factors such as genetic predisposition, environmental influences, and specific behavioral patterns that contribute to the development of addiction. Tailored prevention programs can be more effective in reaching at-risk populations and reducing the incidence of substance use disorders.

A deeper understanding of the common features of drug addiction informs the development of more effective treatment approaches. Evidence-based therapies can be tailored to address the specific neurobiological, genetic, and environmental factors contributing to an individual's addiction. This personalized approach enhances the efficacy of treatment programs and improves long-term outcomes for individuals seeking recovery (Volkow et al., 2020). Education about the common features of drug addiction is instrumental in reducing stigma and discrimination associated with substance use disorders. When the public is informed about the neurobiological and genetic components of addiction, there is a greater likelihood of empathetic attitudes toward individuals struggling with substance abuse. This, in turn, facilitates access to treatment and support services without the fear of judgment or social isolation (Barry et al., 2014).

Understanding the common features of drug addiction promotes a holistic approach to addressing substance use disorders. Integrating knowledge from various disciplines, including neuroscience, genetics, psychology, and sociology, allows for a more comprehensive understanding of addiction. This interdisciplinary perspective is essential for developing holistic treatment models that consider the multifaceted nature of drug addiction. The significance of understanding the common features of drug addiction cannot be overstated. This knowledge is instrumental in shaping policies, prevention efforts, and treatment approaches that address the complex interplay of biological, psychological, and social factors contributing to substance use disorders. By embracing a comprehensive understanding of addiction, society can work towards creating a more compassionate and effective response to the challenges posed by drug addiction.

Drug addiction is a global public health concern that affects individuals from diverse backgrounds and communities. Understanding the prevalence of drug addiction is essential for shaping effective interventions, allocating resources, and developing targeted public health strategies to address this complex issue. Drug addiction transcends geographical boundaries, impacting populations worldwide. According to the World Drug Report 2021 by the United Nations Office on Drugs and Crime (UNODC), an estimated 275 million people aged 15-64 used drugs at least once in 2020. This report emphasizes the global nature of the drug abuse problem and highlights the need for coordinated international efforts to address its prevalence (United Nations Office on Drugs and Crime, 2021).

The prevalence of drug addiction varies based on the type of substance involved. Substance use disorders can involve legal or illegal drugs, prescription medications, and even legal substances like alcohol and nicotine. The Substance Abuse and Mental Health Services Administration (SAMHSA) in the United States reported that in 2020, approximately 21.3 million people aged 12 or older had a substance use disorder related to alcohol or illicit drugs, representing 7.8% of the population (Substance Abuse and Mental Health Services Administration, 2021).

Drug addiction often begins in adolescence, and early initiation increases the risk of long-term dependence. The Monitoring the Future Study, an ongoing survey of American youth behaviors, reported that in 2020, 7.7% of 12th graders in the United States had used illicit drugs other than marijuana in the past month. This highlights the importance of prevention efforts targeted at young populations to mitigate the prevalence of drug addiction (National Institute on Drug Abuse, 2021).

The opioid epidemic has contributed significantly to the prevalence of drug addiction, particularly in the United States. The National Institute on Drug Abuse (NIDA) reported that in 2019, an estimated 10.1 million people aged 12 or older misused opioids in the past year. This crisis has underscored the urgency of addressing both the illicit and prescription opioid use contributing to addiction rates (National Institute on Drug Abuse, 2020). The prevalence of drug addiction is a complex and multifaceted issue with global implications. Understanding the extent of drug addiction's reach is crucial for implementing targeted prevention, intervention, and treatment strategies. By staying informed about the prevalence of drug addiction, policymakers, healthcare professionals, and communities can work collaboratively to address the challenges posed by substance use disorders on a local, national, and global scale.

Development of compulsive drug-seeking behaviors: The development of compulsive drug-seeking behaviors is a hallmark of addiction, reflecting profound changes in the brain's reward and control systems. Understanding the neurobiological mechanisms involved is crucial for devising effective interventions to mitigate the impact of addiction. Compulsive drug-seeking behaviors are intricately linked to the brain's reward circuitry. The ventral tegmental area (VTA) and the nucleus accumbens (NAc) are key components of this circuit, where the neurotransmitter dopamine plays a central role. The initial rewarding effects of drugs are associated with elevated dopamine release in the NAc, creating a reinforcing loop that strengthens the association between drug use and pleasure. As drug use persists, the neurobiological landscape undergoes profound changes.

The prefrontal cortex, a region responsible for executive functions and impulse control, becomes compromised. This impairment contributes to a loss of control over drug use, as individuals struggle to inhibit the urge to seek drugs despite negative consequences. The insula, implicated in interoceptive awareness, also plays a role in the compulsivity associated with drug-seeking (Nock et al., 2017). The development of compulsive drug-seeking behaviors is influenced by the concept of incentive salience. Drugs acquire exaggerated motivational significance, driving individuals to seek them even in the absence of true reward. Pavlovian conditioning, where environmental cues become associated with drug use, further strengthens these compulsive tendencies. The sight of drug paraphernalia or specific settings can trigger intense cravings and automatic behavioral responses.

Neuroplasticity, the brain's ability to adapt and reorganize, plays a dual role in addiction. Initially, it contributes to the rewarding effects of drugs. However, with chronic drug use, neuroplastic changes become maladaptive, reinforcing compulsive drug-seeking behaviors. Synaptic plasticity in the mesolimbic dopamine system and alterations in glutamatergic transmission contribute to the persistence of addiction (Lüscher & Malenka, 2011). Stress is a potent modulator of compulsive drug-seeking behaviors. The hypothalamic-pituitary-adrenal (HPA) axis, activated in response to stress, interacts with the mesolimbic system, further reinforcing the compulsive cycle of drug seeking. Chronic exposure to stress can enhance vulnerability to addiction and contribute to relapse even after periods of abstinence. The development of compulsive drug-seeking behaviors is a complex interplay of neurobiological adaptations, reward circuitry dysregulation, and environmental influences. Recognizing these intricate processes provides a foundation for targeted interventions aimed at disrupting the compulsive cycle of addiction. By understanding the neural mechanisms underpinning compulsive drug seeking, researchers and clinicians can pave the way for more effective strategies to prevent and treat addiction.

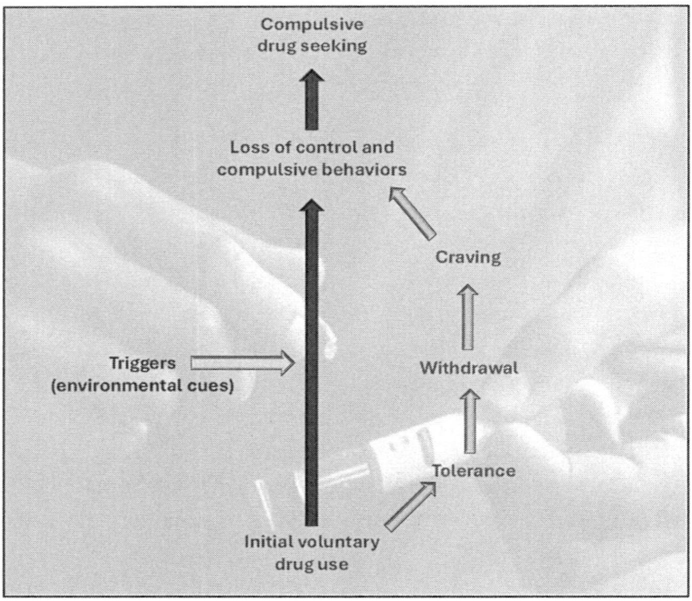

Compulsive drug-seeking behavior

Craving and withdrawal symptoms: Craving and withdrawal symptoms are pivotal components of the addiction cycle, reflecting the intricate interplay of neurobiological adaptations in response to repeated drug exposure. Craving in the context of drug addiction is characterized by an intense desire or urge to use a substance. It often manifests as a cognitive and emotional preoccupation with obtaining and using the drug, even in the absence of immediate availability. The neurobiology of craving involves the mesolimbic dopamine system, particularly the nucleus accumbens, where increased dopamine release reinforces the association between drug-related cues and pleasurable effects. Drug-associated cues, such as the sight of drug paraphernalia or specific environments linked to drug use, can trigger intense craving. This response is mediated by the mesocorticolimbic circuit, involving the prefrontal cortex, amygdala, and hippocampus.

Pavlovian conditioning, where these cues become strongly associated with drug use, plays a significant role in the development and persistence of craving. Withdrawal symptoms emerge when an individual dependent on a substance abruptly reduces or discontinues its use. These symptoms can be physiological, psychological, or both, reflecting the body's attempt to regain homeostasis in the absence of the drug (Koob, 2014). Neurotransmitter imbalances, especially in the gamma-aminobutyric acid (GABA) and glutamate systems, contribute to withdrawal symptoms, creating a powerful motivator for continued drug use to alleviate discomfort. The extended amygdala, including the bed nucleus of the stria terminalis (BNST) and central nucleus of the amygdala, plays a critical role in the expression of withdrawal symptoms. Activation of the extended amygdala is associated with negative affective states, anxiety, and dysregulation of stress responses, contributing to the motivation to relieve withdrawal through renewed drug use.

The concept of allostasis, the process by which the brain adapts to maintain stability in the face of chronic drug exposure, underlies the cycle of craving and withdrawal. The brain undergoes persistent changes to offset the effects of repeated drug use, contributing to the chronic relapsing nature of addiction. Allostatic changes in the reward circuitry, including the ventral striatum and prefrontal cortex, play a crucial role in the perpetuation of the addiction. Craving and withdrawal symptoms are integral components of the neurobiology of addiction. Understanding the neural mechanisms underlying these phenomena provides crucial insights for the development of targeted interventions aimed at breaking the cycle of compulsive drug use. By unraveling the intricate neurobiological processes involved in craving and withdrawal, researchers and clinicians can advance the development of more effective strategies for the prevention and treatment of drug addiction.

Escalation of drug use over time: The escalation of drug use over time is a characteristic pattern observed in individuals struggling with addiction. This phenomenon is deeply rooted in neurobiological adaptations that occur in response to chronic substance exposure. The journey of drug addiction often begins with initial exposure, where individuals experience the acute rewarding effects of the substance. Neuroadaptations, particularly in the mesolimbic dopamine system, occur as the brain attempts to maintain balance in the face of the foreign substance. This initial exposure sets the stage for the escalation of drug use, as the brain undergoes changes to accommodate the presence of the drug. Tolerance, a key factor in the escalation of drug use, develops as the body adapts to the presence of the drug, requiring higher doses to achieve the same effects. Neuroplasticity, the brain's ability to reorganize itself, plays a significant role in the development of tolerance. Changes in receptor sensitivity, neurotransmitter release, and neural circuitry contribute to the need for escalating drug doses to maintain the desired effects.

In addition to tolerance, sensitization is another neurobiological phenomenon observed in addiction. Sensitization involves an increased responsiveness to the drug over time, leading to heightened sensitivity to its effects. This dual process of tolerance and sensitization creates a cycle where individuals escalate their drug use to counteract diminishing effects while simultaneously experiencing an enhanced response to the drug, reinforcing the pattern of escalation (Robinson & Berridge, 2008). As drug use escalates, craving intensifies, becoming a driving force behind compulsive drug-seeking behaviors. Neurobiologically, this involves changes in the brain's reward circuitry, particularly the nucleus accumbens, where heightened dopaminergic activity reinforces the association between drug-related cues and pleasurable effects. The transition from controlled drug use to compulsive seeking marks a critical point in the escalation of addiction. Chronic drug use is associated with impaired inhibitory control and escalating impulsivity, contributing to the inability to regulate drug intake. Neurobiological changes in the prefrontal cortex, a region crucial for executive functions, undermine the ability to make decisions that prioritize long-term well-being over immediate drug-seeking desires. This compromised self-control further fuels the escalation of drug use (Goldstein & Volkow, 2011). The escalation of drug use over time is deeply rooted in neurobiological adaptations that alter the brain's reward circuitry, sensitivity to the drug, and inhibitory control mechanisms. Understanding these processes sheds light on the progression of addiction and informs interventions aimed at disrupting the cycle of escalating drug use. By addressing the neurobiological underpinnings of escalation, researchers and clinicians can develop targeted strategies to prevent and treat addiction effectively.

Loss of control over drug consumption: The phenomenon of losing control over drug consumption is a defining feature of addiction, reflecting profound neurobiological changes that compromise an individual's ability to regulate drug intake. The prefrontal cortex, a brain region crucial for executive functions and decision-making, plays a central role in regulating drug consumption. Chronic drug use is associated with impaired prefrontal cortex functionality, specifically in areas responsible for inhibitory control. This compromise in executive functions contributes to the diminished ability to regulate drug intake and is a key factor in the loss of control observed in addiction (Goldstein & Volkow, 2011). The mesolimbic dopamine system, a critical component of the brain's reward circuitry, undergoes significant alterations in addiction. Prolonged drug exposure leads to dysregulation of dopaminergic signaling, resulting in blunted responsiveness to natural rewards. This desensitization to non-drug rewards and exaggerated responses to drug-related cues contribute to a heightened motivation for drug consumption, overriding normal regulatory mechanisms.

Loss of control over drug consumption is closely linked to the transition from voluntary drug use to compulsive drug-seeking behaviors. Neurobiologically, this involves changes in the mesolimbic dopamine system, particularly in the nucleus accumbens. The persistent stimulation of this reward pathway by drugs of abuse creates a powerful motivational force that overrides the individual's capacity to control and limit drug intake. The concept of allostasis, the process by which the brain adapts to chronic drug exposure, sheds light on the loss of control in addiction. Initially, the brain undergoes adaptations to maintain balance in the presence of drugs. However, these adaptations become maladaptive over time, leading to a state of allostasis where the brain's new set point prioritizes drug-seeking and consumption at the expense of other behaviors.

The extended amygdala, including the bed nucleus of the stria terminalis (BNST) and central nucleus of the amygdala, is implicated in the loss of control over drug consumption. Activation of the extended amygdala is associated with negative affective states, stress, and heightened motivational responses to drug-related cues. Dysregulation of this region further contributes to the compulsive nature of drug-seeking behaviors (Heilig et al., 2016). The loss of control over drug consumption in addiction is intricately tied to neurobiological adaptations in key brain regions involved in reward processing, decision-making, and stress response. Understanding these neurobiological underpinnings is crucial for developing targeted interventions that can restore regulatory mechanisms and mitigate the compulsive cycle of drug-seeking behaviors. By unraveling the complexities of the loss of control, researchers and clinicians can pave the way for more effective strategies in the prevention and treatment of addiction.

Behavioral sensitization to abused drugs: Behavioral sensitization, a phenomenon characterized by an augmented response to a drug with repeated exposure, is a critical aspect of drug addiction. The mesolimbic dopamine system, particularly the nucleus accumbens, plays a central role in the development of behavioral sensitization. With repeated exposure to drugs of abuse, there is an increase in dopamine release in the nucleus accumbens. This heightened dopaminergic activity is associated with the reinforcing effects of drugs and contributes to the sensitized behavioral responses observed over time. Behavioral sensitization is intricately linked to neuroplasticity, the brain's ability to undergo structural and functional changes in response to repeated stimuli. Long-term potentiation (LTP) and long-term depression (LTD) in the synapses of the mesolimbic dopamine system contribute to the enduring changes associated with behavioral sensitization. These neuroplastic changes are thought to underlie the persistent nature of sensitized behaviors.

The incentive-sensitization theory proposes that repeated exposure to drugs leads to a hypersensitivity to drug-related cues, resulting in an enhanced incentive to seek and consume the drug. This theory posits that while the liking of the drug may remain stable or decrease, the incentive or craving for the drug increases with each exposure, contributing to the development of behavioral sensitization (Robinson & Berridge, 2008). Glutamatergic transmission, particularly involving the excitatory neurotransmitter glutamate, is implicated in the development of behavioral sensitization. Alterations in glutamate release and receptor activity in the nucleus accumbens and other reward-related brain regions contribute to the long-lasting changes in synaptic strength associated with sensitization. Glutamate's role in synaptic plasticity is a key factor in the enduring behavioral adaptations observed in addiction.

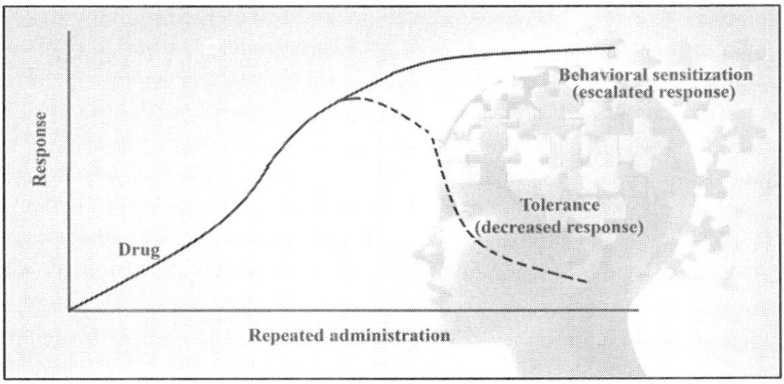

Behavioral sensitization to abused drugs

The prefrontal cortex, a region critical for executive functions and decision-making, is involved in the modulation of behavioral sensitization. Dysregulation of prefrontal cortical activity is observed in addiction, contributing to the impaired inhibitory control and heightened responsivity to drug-related cues associated with sensitization. The interplay between the prefrontal cortex and mesolimbic dopamine system is integral to the development and expression of sensitized behaviors (Kalivas et al., 2005). Behavioral sensitization to abused drugs involves intricate neurobiological processes centered around the mesolimbic dopamine system, synaptic plasticity, and glutamatergic modulation. Understanding these mechanisms provides valuable insights into the persistent nature of sensitized behaviors in addiction. By unraveling the complexities of behavioral sensitization, researchers aim to develop targeted interventions that can disrupt the neurobiological adaptations driving the escalation of drug-induced behaviors.

Features of commonly abused substances: The landscape of substance abuse is diverse, with various substances exerting unique effects on the human body and mind. Alcohol abuse is a pervasive issue with profound implications for public health. Alcohol, primarily ethanol, is a central nervous system depressant. It exerts its effects by enhancing the inhibitory neurotransmitter gamma-aminobutyric acid (GABA) and dampening the excitatory neurotransmitter glutamate, leading to relaxation, sedation, and impaired cognitive and motor functions. Alcohol consumption influences the brain's reward pathway, particularly the release of dopamine. This activation contributes to the reinforcing effects of alcohol, creating a pleasurable experience and motivating continued consumption. With chronic alcohol use, individuals often develop tolerance, requiring increased amounts of alcohol to achieve the desired effects. This escalation of consumption is a hallmark feature, leading to heightened health risks and the potential for alcohol use disorder (AUD). Alcohol abuse is associated with impaired decision-making and cognitive functions, particularly affecting the prefrontal cortex. This can result in risky behaviors, impaired judgment, and difficulties in controlling alcohol intake (Oscar-Berman & Marinković, 2007).

Alcohol abuse contributes to a myriad of physical and mental health consequences, including liver cirrhosis, cardiovascular issues, increased risk of accidents, and mental health disorders such as depression and anxiety (Rehm et al., 2009). Alcohol abuse extends beyond individual health, impacting social and interpersonal relationships. It can lead to strained family dynamics, impaired work performance, and increased societal burdens. Alcohol abuse is a multifaceted issue with far-reaching consequences. Understanding its features, encompassing neurobiological, psychological, and social dimensions, is essential for developing targeted interventions and public health strategies aimed at mitigating the impact of alcohol abuse on individuals and society.

Nicotine, the primary psychoactive component of tobacco, exerts a profound influence on the central nervous system, contributing to its addictive nature. Nicotine is a potent stimulant that belongs to the class of alkaloids. It exerts its effects by binding to nicotinic acetylcholine receptors (nAChRs) in the brain, leading to the release of neurotransmitters such as dopamine, norepinephrine, and serotonin. It is efficiently absorbed through the lungs when tobacco is smoked, rapidly reaching the brain within seconds. This quick delivery contributes to the reinforcing effects of nicotine, enhancing its addictive potential. Nicotine is highly addictive, and its repeated use leads to the development of dependence. The reinforcing properties of nicotine, coupled with its ability to enhance mood and concentration, contribute to the compulsive nature of tobacco use.

Nicotine withdrawal syndrome involves symptoms such as irritability, anxiety, and cravings which are a significant challenge for individuals attempting to quit smoking. Understanding the withdrawal syndrome is crucial for designing effective smoking cessation interventions (Picciott & Kenny, 2013). While nicotine itself is not responsible for the majority of health risks associated with tobacco use, the delivery method (smoking) exposes individuals to harmful chemicals and carcinogens. These risks include respiratory diseases, cardiovascular disorders, and an increased risk of various cancers. Nicotine influences multiple neurotransmitter systems, with a primary focus on acetylcholine, dopamine, and glutamate. These interactions contribute to the rewarding effects of nicotine and the neuroadaptive changes associated with chronic use. Nicotine, with its stimulant properties and addictive nature, plays a central role in tobacco dependence. Understanding the features of nicotine is crucial for developing effective smoking cessation strategies and addressing the broader public health implications associated with tobacco use.

Cannabis, derived from the Cannabis sativa plant, is one of the most widely used psychoactive substances globally. Cannabis contains over 100 cannabinoids, with delta-9-tetrahydrocannabinol (THC) being the primary psychoactive compound. THC interacts with cannabinoid receptors in the brain, primarily CB1 receptors, leading to the characteristic psychotropic effects associated with cannabis use (Di Marzo et al., 2015). The effects of cannabis use are diverse and can include relaxation, euphoria, altered perception of time and space, increased appetite, and intensified sensory experiences. However, individual responses can vary based on factors such as dosage, frequency of use, and an individual's susceptibility. Regular cannabis use can lead to the development of tolerance, requiring higher doses to achieve the same effects. Additionally, some individuals may experience dependence, characterized by cravings and a perceived need to continue cannabis use to avoid withdrawal symptoms.

Cannabis abuse is associated with cognitive impairment, particularly in areas such as attention, memory, and learning. Long-term and heavy use, especially during adolescence, may have lasting effects on cognitive function (Meier et al., 2012). Cannabis abuse has been linked to mental health issues, including anxiety, depression, and an increased risk of psychotic disorders, especially in vulnerable individuals. The relationship between cannabis use and mental health is complex and influenced by various factors. Smoking cannabis, a common method of consumption, poses respiratory health risks similar to tobacco smoking. Chronic cannabis smoking is associated with respiratory symptoms and an increased risk of bronchitis and other respiratory conditions (Tetrault et al., 2007). Cannabis abuse presents a multifaceted picture, with a range of pharmacological, psychological, and health-related features. Understanding these features is crucial for developing effective prevention and intervention strategies to address the complexities of cannabis use and its potential impact on individual well-being.

Cocaine, a powerful stimulant derived from coca leaves, has a profound impact on the central nervous system, contributing to its addictive potential. Cocaine is a potent stimulant that blocks the reuptake of neurotransmitters, particularly dopamine, norepinephrine, and serotonin, in the brain. This leads to an accumulation of these neurotransmitters in the synaptic cleft, intensifying signaling and resulting in the characteristic stimulant effects of cocaine. Cocaine use induces a rapid onset of intense euphoria, increased energy, and heightened alertness. Cocaine's effects are short-lived compared to some other substances of abuse. This short duration contributes to a pattern of repeated use, known as "binge" use, where individuals may consume multiple doses in a short period to maintain the desired effects.

Cocaine use poses a significant risk of dependence and addiction. The rapid and intense rewarding effects of cocaine can lead to compulsive drug-seeking behaviors, loss of control over use, and continued use despite negative consequences. Feature: Cocaine abuse is associated with cardiovascular risks, including increased heart rate, elevated blood pressure, and an increased risk of heart attacks and strokes. Additionally, the vasoconstrictive effects of cocaine can have detrimental effects on various organ systems. Chronic cocaine use is linked to psychiatric and behavioral consequences, including anxiety, paranoia, irritability, and aggression. Cocaine abuse can exacerbate pre-existing mental health conditions and contribute to the development of new psychiatric symptoms (Kosten & George, 2002). Cocaine abuse is characterized by its potent stimulant effects, short duration of action, and significant risks of dependence and health complications. Understanding these features is crucial for developing effective prevention, intervention, and treatment strategies to address the complex nature of cocaine abuse and its impact on individuals and public health.

Opioids, a class of potent analgesic drugs, have both therapeutic benefits for pain management and a high potential for abuse. Opioids are known for their powerful analgesic (pain-relieving) properties. They act by binding to specific receptors in the brain and spinal cord, modulating pain perception and producing a sense of relief (Ballantyne & Shin, 2008). Opioid use is associated with a sense of euphoria, relaxation, and sedation. These psychoactive effects contribute to the reinforcing properties of opioids and their potential for misuse. Prolonged use of opioids often leads to the development of tolerance, requiring individuals to increase the dosage to achieve the same level of pain relief or euphoria. Tolerance contributes to the risk of escalating opioid use. Opioid use can lead to both physical and psychological dependence. Physical dependence is characterized by the development of withdrawal symptoms when opioid use is reduced or stopped. Psychological dependence involves a perceived need for opioids to cope with emotions or stress. Opioids carry a substantial risk of addiction. The euphoric effects and the development of tolerance contribute to the compulsive drug-seeking behaviors and loss of control over use that are characteristic of opioid addiction (Rudd et al., 2016; Minozzi et al., 2011). Opioid use can lead to respiratory depression, a slowing or stopping of breathing, which is a primary cause of opioid overdose deaths. Overdose risk is heightened when opioids are used in excessive amounts or in combination with other substances. Opioid abuse is characterized by potent analgesic effects, the risk of tolerance and dependence, and a high potential for addiction and overdose. Understanding these features is essential for developing comprehensive strategies to address opioid abuse, improve pain management, and mitigate the public health impact of opioid-related issues.

Methamphetamine, a powerful central nervous system stimulant, has gained notoriety for its high potential for abuse and severe health consequences. Methamphetamine is a potent stimulant that increases the release of neurotransmitters such as dopamine and norepinephrine in the brain. This leads to intense feelings of euphoria, increased energy, and heightened alertness (Sulzer et al., 2005). Methamphetamine use is associated with intense euphoria and heightened focus. Users may experience a temporary improvement in mood, concentration, and a sense of increased productivity. Individuals who abuse methamphetamine often develop tolerance quickly, necessitating higher doses to achieve the desired effects. This pattern increases the risk of escalating use and the potential for adverse health outcomes.

Methamphetamine has a high potential for dependence and addiction. The reinforcing effects of the drug, coupled with the rapid development of tolerance, contribute to the compulsive drug-seeking behaviors characteristic of addiction. Chronic methamphetamine abuse is associated with a range of adverse psychological effects, including anxiety, paranoia, hallucinations, and violent behavior. Prolonged use may lead to long-lasting psychiatric issues (Salo & Nordahl, 2015). Methamphetamine abuse poses significant cardiovascular and physical health risks. Users may experience elevated heart rate, increased blood pressure, hyperthermia, and, in severe cases, cardiovascular collapse (Kevil et al., 2011). Methamphetamine abuse is characterized by its potent stimulant effects, rapid development of tolerance, high risk of dependence, and a range of adverse psychological and physical health consequences. Understanding these features is crucial for developing targeted prevention and intervention strategies to address the complexities of methamphetamine abuse and its impact on individuals and public health. Commonly abused substances exhibit diverse features, affecting various neurotransmitter systems and contributing to distinct patterns of use and addiction. Understanding the pharmacological and neurobiological characteristics of these substances is crucial for developing effective prevention and treatment strategies in the complex landscape of substance abuse.

Common neurochemical pathways shared by drugs of abuse: Various drugs of abuse, despite their diverse pharmacological profiles, often converge on common neurochemical pathways in the brain. Many drugs of abuse, including cocaine, amphetamines, opioids, and alcohol, exert their effects by influencing the mesolimbic dopamine system. This system, originating in the ventral tegmental area (VTA) and projecting to the nucleus accumbens, is central to reward processing and reinforcement. The mesolimbic dopamine system, a neural circuit central to reward and reinforcement, serves as a common pathway through which various drugs of abuse exert their effects. The mesolimbic dopamine system is comprised of a cluster of neurons in the midbrain, and projects to the nucleus accumbens (NAc) in the forebrain. This pathway is a critical component of the brain's reward system, playing a pivotal role in motivation, reinforcement, and the experience of pleasure. Upon exposure to rewarding stimuli, including drugs of abuse, the VTA neurons release dopamine into the NAc. This dopamine release is associated with the perception of reward and reinforces behaviors that lead to the stimuli, creating a powerful motivational force (Schultz, 2016; Wise, 2004). Various drugs, such as cocaine, amphetamines, opioids, and alcohol, act on the mesolimbic dopamine system, leading to an increase in dopamine release. This shared mechanism contributes to the reinforcing properties of these substances and their potential for misuse. Chronic exposure to drugs of abuse induces neuroplastic changes in the mesolimbic system, leading to adaptations that contribute to the development of addiction. These adaptations may include alterations in receptor sensitivity, synaptic strength, and connectivity within the circuit. Environmental cues associated with drug use can trigger dopamine release in the mesolimbic system, creating conditioned responses and contributing to the persistence of addictive behaviors. This process is crucial in understanding relapse mechanisms. The mesolimbic dopamine system stands as a central and shared pathway in the neurobiology of drug abuse. Understanding the intricate workings of this system provides valuable insights into the mechanisms underlying addiction, paving the way for targeted interventions and treatment strategies.

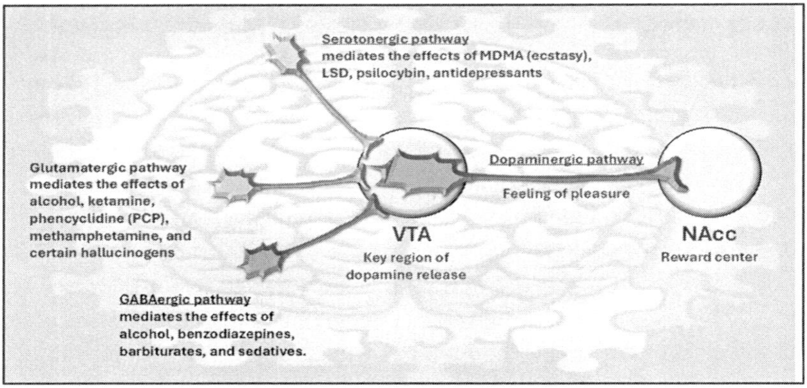

Common neurochemical pathways shared by drugs of abuse

Glutamate, the primary excitatory neurotransmitter in the brain, plays a crucial role in the neurobiology of drug abuse. The glutamatergic system is fundamental to synaptic communication and excitatory signaling in the central nervous system. It regulates various physiological processes, including learning, memory, and reward. Several drugs of abuse impact the glutamatergic system, influencing glutamate release, receptor activation, and downstream signaling. This modulation contributes to the reinforcing properties and behavioral effects associated with drug use (Gipson & Kalivas, 2014). The nucleus accumbens (NAc), a key component of the brain's reward system, receives glutamatergic input. Drugs of abuse, including cocaine and amphetamines, enhance glutamatergic transmission in the NAc, contributing to the rewarding effects of these substances. Long-term potentiation, a form of synaptic plasticity associated with learning and memory, is modulated by glutamatergic transmission. Drugs of abuse, such as opioids, can induce synaptic adaptations through alterations in glutamatergic signaling. Abrupt cessation of drug use can lead to a hyperglutamatergic state during withdrawal. This heightened glutamatergic activity is implicated in the negative emotional states and craving associated with withdrawal, contributing to the risk of relapse (Reissner & Kalivas, 2010). The glutamatergic system stands as a common and critical pathway in the neurobiology of drug abuse. Understanding the intricate role of glutamate in drug-induced synaptic adaptations provides valuable insights for the development of targeted interventions and therapeutic strategies to address substance use disorders.

The endogenous opioid system, comprising endorphins and their receptors, plays a pivotal role in the neurobiology of drug abuse. The endogenous opioid system consists of endorphins, enkephalins, and dynorphins, which are endogenous ligands for opioid receptors, including mu-opioid receptors (MOR), delta-opioid receptors (DOR), and kappa-opioid receptors (KOR). This system is widely distributed in the central nervous system and is involved in pain modulation, reward processing, and mood regulation. Exogenous opioids, such as heroin and prescription opioids, activate the same opioid receptors as endogenous opioids. These drugs mimic the actions of endorphins, producing analgesia, euphoria, and a sense of reward, contributing to their addictive potential (Williams et al., 2013). Activation of the MOR in the mesolimbic dopamine system, particularly in the nucleus accumbens, contributes to the rewarding effects of opioids. This interaction between the endogenous opioid and dopaminergic systems is a common feature in the reinforcing properties of drugs of abuse (Koob & Le Moal, 2005). Repeated activation of the endogenous opioid system by exogenous opioids leads to the development of tolerance, requiring higher doses for the same effects, and physical dependence. These neuroadaptations contribute to the cycle of drug abuse and dependence. The endogenous opioid system is implicated in withdrawal symptoms and drug craving during abstinence. Dysregulation of this system contributes to the negative emotional states and persistent desire for the drug (Bodnar, 2018). Understanding the endogenous opioid system's role in drug abuse has therapeutic implications. Opioid replacement therapies, such as methadone and buprenorphine, target this system to mitigate withdrawal symptoms and cravings. The endogenous opioid system emerges as a central and shared pathway in the neurobiology of drug abuse. Understanding its intricate involvement in reward, reinforcement, and adaptation provides valuable insights for developing targeted interventions and treatment strategies for substance use disorders.

Gamma-aminobutyric acid (GABA) is the primary inhibitory neurotransmitter in the brain. Drugs like alcohol and benzodiazepines enhance GABAergic transmission, leading to sedative and anxiolytic effects. GABA inhibitory neurotransmitter system is integral to the neurobiology of drug abuse. GABA is the primary inhibitory neurotransmitter in the central nervous system, playing a crucial role in regulating neural excitability. GABAergic transmission is fundamental to maintaining the balance between excitation and inhibition in the brain. Various drugs of abuse, including alcohol, benzodiazepines, and barbiturates, modulate the GABAergic system. These substances enhance GABAergic transmission, leading to increased inhibitory effects, sedation, and anxiolysis (Olsen & Liang, 2017). The GABAergic system interacts with brain reward pathways, including the mesolimbic dopamine system. Drugs that enhance GABAergic transmission may indirectly influence the reward circuitry, contributing to the reinforcing properties of substances. GABAergic interneurons regulate the activity of dopaminergic neurons, particularly in the ventral tegmental area (VTA). Drugs of abuse, such as cocaine and opioids, may influence the GABAergic control of dopamine release, contributing to their addictive potential.

Chronic drug use can lead to adaptations in the GABAergic system, and abrupt cessation results in withdrawal. GABAergic dysregulation during withdrawal is associated with symptoms such as anxiety, seizures, and increased susceptibility to relapse (Kauer & Malenka, 2007). Medications that modulate GABAergic transmission, such as benzodiazepines and certain anticonvulsants, are used in the treatment of alcohol and sedative-hypnotic withdrawal. These medications help manage withdrawal symptoms and reduce the risk of complications. GABAergic inhibition emerges as a common and critical pathway in the neurobiology of drug abuse.

Understanding the complex interactions within the GABAergic system provides insights for developing targeted interventions and treatment strategies for substance use disorders. Serotonin (5-HT) plays a role in the regulation of mood and impulsivity. Drugs like MDMA (ecstasy) and hallucinogens impact the serotonergic system, contributing to their psychoactive effects. The serotonergic system, centered around the neurotransmitter serotonin (5-HT), plays a crucial role in the neurobiology of drug abuse. The serotonergic system originates in the raphe nuclei of the brainstem, releasing serotonin throughout the central nervous system. Serotonin acts as a neurotransmitter and neuromodulator, influencing mood, appetite, and various physiological functions. Several drugs of abuse, including MDMA (ecstasy), LSD, and hallucinogenic mushrooms, directly impact the serotonergic system. These substances often bind to serotonin receptors, leading to altered mood, perception, and cognition (Vollenweider & Kometer, 2010). The serotonergic system interacts with brain reward pathways, including the mesolimbic dopamine system. Drugs of abuse, such as cocaine and amphetamines, can influence serotonin levels, indirectly impacting the reward circuitry and contributing to the reinforcing properties of substances.

Serotonin is implicated in emotional regulation and mood stabilization. Dysregulation of the serotonergic system is associated with mood disorders, and individuals may turn to substance use as a means of self-medication (Ossipov et al., 2014). Chronic drug use can lead to adaptations in the serotonergic system, and withdrawal from certain substances may result in dysregulation of serotonin levels. This dysregulation contributes to negative emotional states during withdrawal. Understanding the role of serotonin in drug abuse has therapeutic implications. Medications that target the serotonergic system, such as selective serotonin reuptake inhibitors (SSRIs), are used in the treatment of mood disorders and certain substance use disorders. Serotonergic modulation emerges as a common and critical pathway in the neurobiology of drug abuse. Understanding the intricate interactions within the serotonergic system provides valuable insights for developing targeted interventions and treatment strategies for substance use disorders. Despite the diversity in their mechanisms of action, drugs of abuse often intersect at key neurochemical pathways, particularly those involved in reward, reinforcement, and synaptic transmission. Understanding these commonalities provides insights into the shared neurobiology of addiction and aids in the development of targeted interventions for substance use disorders.

The role of polydrug use in addiction: Polydrug use, the concurrent use of multiple substances, represents a pervasive and complex aspect of addiction. Polydrug use involves the simultaneous consumption of different substances, such as alcohol, cannabis, opioids, and stimulants. Users often engage in polydrug use to enhance or counteract the effects of one substance with another, leading to a variety of consumption patterns (Martinotti et al., 2015). Polydrug use is associated with a higher risk of addiction compared to single-substance use. The interaction between different substances can lead to synergistic effects, intensifying the rewarding properties and reinforcing the habit of simultaneous consumption. The combined use of different substances can lead to complex pharmacological interactions. For example, the simultaneous use of opioids and benzodiazepines may result in respiratory depression, highlighting the importance of understanding these interactions in the context of addiction. Polydrug use can complicate addiction treatment. The need to address multiple substances simultaneously, each with its withdrawal symptoms and treatment protocols, poses challenges for healthcare professionals. Integrated treatment approaches are often required for effective outcomes.

Polydrug use is often associated with increased mental health issues. The combined effects of different substances can exacerbate psychiatric symptoms, leading to conditions such as anxiety, depression, or psychosis (Fairbairn et al., 2017). Polydrug use significantly contributes to the complexity of addiction. Recognizing its role in increased addiction risk, treatment complications, pharmacological interactions, and impact on mental health is crucial for developing comprehensive interventions and improving outcomes for individuals struggling with substance use disorders.

Psychological factors in co-occurring mental health disorders: Co-occurring mental health disorders, often referred to as comorbidity or dual diagnosis, involve the simultaneous presence of two or more mental health conditions. Co-occurring mental health disorders often share common risk factors. Genetic predisposition, early life stressors, trauma, and environmental influences contribute to vulnerabilities that may manifest in multiple psychological conditions simultaneously (Kessler et al., 2011). The relationship between mental health disorders is often bidirectional. The presence of one disorder can influence the onset, course, or severity of another. For example, substance use disorders may exacerbate symptoms of mood or anxiety disorders, and vice versa. Individuals with co-occurring disorders may use substances or engage in certain behaviors as coping mechanisms or forms of self-medication. Substance use may temporarily alleviate symptoms of anxiety, depression, or trauma, creating a cycle of dependence.

The presence of co-occurring disorders can complicate treatment engagement and adherence. Psychological factors, such as stigma, shame, or feelings of hopelessness, may influence an individual's willingness to seek and participate in mental health and substance use treatment (Drake et al., 2008). Effective treatment for co-occurring disorders often involves integrated approaches that address both mental health and substance use issues simultaneously. Psychosocial interventions, medication management, and support systems are crucial components of integrated treatment. Understanding the psychological factors contributing to co-occurring mental health disorders is essential for designing effective prevention and intervention strategies. The complex interplay of shared risk factors, bidirectional influences, coping mechanisms, and treatment engagement underscores the need for holistic and integrated approaches to address the unique challenges of individuals with dual diagnoses.

Common social and environmental triggers for drug abuse: Drug abuse is often influenced by a myriad of social and environmental factors that shape an individual's vulnerability to substance use. Peer pressure is a significant social trigger for drug abuse, especially among adolescents and young adults. Social dynamics and the desire for acceptance may lead individuals to experiment with substances to fit in or be perceived as part of a particular social group (Simons-Morton & Farhat, 2010). The family environment, including family history of substance abuse, dysfunctional family dynamics, and lack of parental support, can contribute to drug abuse. A supportive family structure and open communication can act as protective factors (Brook et al., 2011). Socioeconomic factors, including poverty and lack of access to education and employment opportunities, contribute to drug abuse. Economic hardship and limited resources may drive individuals toward substance use as a coping mechanism. Media portrayal of substance use can influence attitudes and behaviors. Glamorizing or normalizing drug use in movies, music, and advertising may contribute to the perception that substance abuse is socially acceptable. The availability and accessibility of drugs within the community can significantly impact substance abuse rates. Easy access to illicit substances may increase the likelihood of experimentation and regular use (Ponicki et al., 2013). Understanding the social and environmental triggers for drug abuse is crucial for developing targeted prevention and intervention strategies. By addressing these factors comprehensively, communities can work towards creating environments that discourage substance abuse and promote healthier lifestyles.

Addressing drug abuse involves targeting various aspects of the addiction cycle, encompassing physical, psychological, and social dimensions. Alterations in neurotransmitter systems, including dopamine, serotonin, and glutamate, are central to drug abuse. Medications that modulate these neurotransmitters can help manage cravings, withdrawal symptoms, and the reinforcing effects of drugs. Utilization of agonists, antagonists, and partial agonists for treating opioid abuse is in practice and it often involves targeting the mu-opioid receptors. Medications such as methadone (agonist), naltrexone (antagonist), and buprenorphine (partial agonist) interact with these receptors to manage opioid dependence. Interventions that target neural circuitry associated with reward pathways and decision-making aim to disrupt the reinforcing effects of drugs. Cognitive-behavioral therapies and medications may impact these neural circuits. Chronic drug abuse can dysregulate stress response systems. Interventions targeting the HPA axis aim to restore balance, reducing stress-related cravings and withdrawal symptoms.

Cognitive-behavioral therapy targets maladaptive thought patterns and behaviors associated with drug abuse. Contingency management reinforces positive behaviors, encouraging abstinence. Social support is crucial for recovery. Involving family and peer interventions provides a network of support, improving treatment outcomes and reducing relapse risk. Effective treatment for drug abuse involves a holistic approach, addressing neurobiological, psychological, and social dimensions. Integrating diverse interventions targeting these common pathways provides a comprehensive strategy for managing and overcoming drug abuse. Personalized treatment plans that consider individual differences and needs are essential for optimal outcomes in the complex landscape of drug addiction.

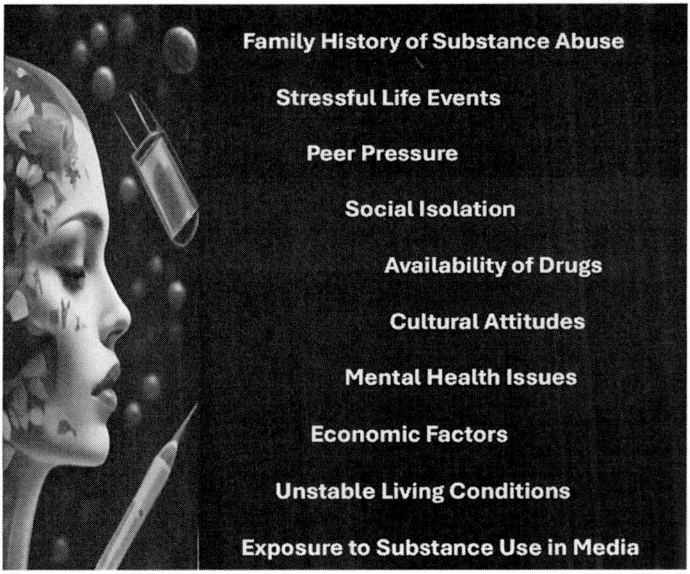
Family History of Substance Abuse
Stressful Life Events
Peer Pressure
Social Isolation
Availability of Drugs
Cultural Attitudes
Mental Health Issues
Economic Factors
Unstable Living Conditions
Exposure to Substance Use in Media

Common social and environmental triggers for drug abuse

Common features of relapse and recovery in drug abuse: Relapse and recovery are integral components of the complex journey individuals face during and after drug abuse treatment. This text delves into common features observed in relapse and recovery, shedding light on the challenges and strategies associated with these processes. Relapse often stems from a combination of internal and external factors. High-risk situations, exposure to drug-related cues, stress, and underlying mental health issues can trigger a return to substance use. Cognitive-behavioral strategies play a pivotal role in both relapse and recovery. Individuals learn to recognize negative thought patterns, develop coping skills, and implement relapse prevention techniques (Donovan, 2013). The presence or absence of a strong social support system significantly impacts the likelihood of relapse. Family support, peer connections, and involvement in recovery communities play vital roles.

Neurobiological changes contribute to both relapse vulnerability and recovery success. Persistent cravings and altered reward circuitry may increase susceptibility to relapse, while ongoing recovery efforts can gradually normalize brain function. The process of recovery is often characterized by stages of change. Individuals move from pre-contemplation to maintenance, with relapse sometimes occurring as part of the learning and growth process. Sustained recovery often involves ongoing care and relapse prevention efforts. Continued engagement in aftercare programs, counseling, and support groups contribute to maintaining recovery. Understanding the common features of relapse and recovery is essential for developing comprehensive and effective treatment approaches. Recognizing the dynamic nature of the recovery journey, addressing triggers, enhancing coping skills, and fostering resilience contribute to improved outcomes and the establishment of a sustainable recovery path. Integrated interventions that consider the multifaceted nature of addiction empower individuals to navigate challenges and achieve lasting recovery.

Common prevention strategies for drug abuse: Preventing drug abuse among adolescents is a critical public health goal, and school-based prevention programs play a pivotal role in achieving this objective. School-based prevention programs often incorporate evidence-based educational curricula designed to increase students' knowledge about the risks associated with drug abuse. These curricula typically cover topics such as the effects of drugs on the body, the risks of addiction, and effective refusal skills (Botvin et al., 2001). Life skills training programs aim to enhance students' personal and social skills, empowering them to resist peer pressure and make healthy decisions. These programs often focus on communication skills, problem-solving, decision-making, and stress management. Utilizing peer leaders or mentors is a common strategy in school-based prevention programs. Peers can effectively communicate prevention messages, share personal experiences, and serve as positive role models, influencing their classmates to make healthy choices.

Collaboration with community organizations and resources is a vital aspect of school-based prevention programs. Engaging parents, local agencies, and community leaders strengthens the impact of prevention efforts, creating a supportive environment for students. Interactive approaches, such as role-playing, group discussions, and interactive exercises, are commonly integrated into prevention programs. These methods actively engage students, facilitating a deeper understanding of the consequences of drug abuse and enhancing critical thinking skills (Ringwalt et al., 2003). School-based prevention programs are crucial in addressing the complex issue of drug abuse among adolescents. By incorporating evidence-based strategies, collaborating with communities, and fostering a positive and supportive school environment, these programs contribute significantly to reducing the risk of drug abuse and promoting the overall well-being of students. Ongoing evaluation and adaptation based on the latest research are essential for the continued effectiveness of school-based prevention initiatives. Public health initiatives play a pivotal role in preventing and addressing drug abuse at a population level. Public health initiatives often prioritize education and awareness campaigns to inform the public about the risks associated with drug abuse. These campaigns utilize various mediums, including social media, community events, and educational materials, to disseminate information and promote prevention (National Institute on Drug Abuse, 2018). Ensuring access to treatment and rehabilitation services is a fundamental aspect of public health initiatives. These services aim to support individuals struggling with drug abuse, providing a pathway to recovery and preventing further harm to both the individuals and the community. Public health initiatives often incorporate harm reduction strategies to minimize the negative consequences of drug abuse. This may include the distribution of clean needles, supervised injection sites, and education on safer drug use practices. Advocacy for evidence-based policies and legislation is a crucial component of public health initiatives. These efforts aim to create an environment that supports prevention, treatment, and harm reduction measures, contributing to the overall reduction of drug abuse.

Engaging communities in the prevention of drug abuse is essential. Community-based programs foster collaboration, address local needs, and empower community members to take an active role in prevention efforts (Hawkins et al., 2008). Public health initiatives for preventing drug abuse involve a multi-faceted approach that encompasses education, treatment, harm reduction, policy advocacy, and community engagement. By addressing the complex interplay of individual, social, and environmental factors, these initiatives contribute to creating healthier and safer communities. Ongoing research and evaluation are essential to refine strategies, adapt to emerging challenges, and enhance the overall effectiveness of public health efforts in preventing drug abuse.

Harm reduction is a public health approach that prioritizes minimizing the negative consequences associated with drug use without necessarily requiring abstinence. This text explores key harm reduction strategies and interventions, emphasizing their effectiveness in promoting health, safety, and overall well-being among individuals struggling with drug abuse. Needle exchange programs provide sterile needles and syringes to individuals who use drugs, reducing the risk of bloodborne infections such as HIV and hepatitis. These programs also serve as points of contact for education, counseling, and referrals to other health services. Supervised consumption facilities, or supervised injection sites, offer a safe and hygienic environment for individuals to use drugs under the supervision of trained staff. These facilities not only prevent overdose deaths but also provide opportunities for education, counseling, and access to healthcare services. Naloxone is an opioid antagonist that can reverse opioid overdoses. Harm reduction initiatives involve the widespread distribution of naloxone kits to individuals at risk of overdose, as well as training community members, including friends and family, on how to administer naloxone.

Harm reduction encourages safer substance use practices to minimize health risks. This includes educating individuals on proper injection techniques, safer smoking methods, and the potential dangers associated with different drugs. Providing education and counseling services is integral to harm reduction. These services aim to empower individuals with information about the risks and consequences of drug use while offering non-judgmental support and guidance. Harm reduction initiatives often link individuals to comprehensive healthcare services, including testing for infectious diseases, mental health support, and access to addiction treatment when individuals are ready to seek help (Larney et al., 2017). Harm reduction approaches for drug abusers prioritize compassion, health, and safety. By addressing the immediate risks associated with drug use, these strategies create pathways for individuals to engage with healthcare services, explore treatment options, and, ultimately, make choices that improve their well-being. Ongoing research, community engagement, and policy advocacy are essential to furthering the effectiveness and acceptance of harm reduction initiatives on a global scale (Feinberg et al., 2008). Community involvement is a cornerstone in the prevention of drug abuse, fostering a collective responsibility to create supportive environments and implement targeted interventions. Community coalitions bring together diverse stakeholders, including residents, schools, law enforcement, healthcare providers, and local organizations, to collaboratively address drug abuse. These coalitions play a vital role in developing and implementing comprehensive prevention strategies tailored to the specific needs of the community.

Community involvement often extends to schools, where parents, teachers, and local organizations collaborate to implement evidence-based prevention programs. These programs provide students with the knowledge, skills, and support systems necessary to resist drug use (Spoth & Greenberg, 2011). Community education campaigns raise awareness about the risks of drug abuse, reduce stigma, and provide information on available resources. These campaigns can use various mediums, including workshops, social media, and community events, to disseminate information effectively. Communities can initiate programs to promote the safe disposal of unused or expired medications, preventing their misuse. Drug take-back events and accessible disposal locations contribute to reducing the availability of prescription drugs for potential abuse. Neighborhood watch programs and safety initiatives create secure environments that deter drug-related activities. These efforts encourage community members to work together, fostering a sense of belonging and shared responsibility for the well-being of the neighborhood.

Building strong support systems within the community, such as mentorship programs, recovery support groups, and mental health services, enhances individuals' resilience and reduces the risk of drug abuse (Litt et al., 2009).

Community involvement is a powerful force in preventing drug abuse, creating a foundation for resilient neighborhoods. By fostering collaboration, implementing evidence-based programs, and promoting a supportive environment, communities can effectively address the complex factors contributing to drug abuse and work towards creating healthier and safer spaces for all residents. Ongoing community engagement and adaptive strategies are essential for sustained success in preventing drug abuse.

CHAPTER 5

COMMONLY ABUSED DRUGS

"The priority of any addict is to anaesthetize the pain of living to ease the passage of day with some purchased relief." – Russell Brand

A look at the diverse substances often misused, tied together by a common goal: to escape the daily struggles of life. Understanding why people use them to escape hard days and painful feelings. This chapter explains how the landscape of substance misuse unfolds as we explore commonly abused drugs, each with its unique effects and risks, contributing to the intricate tapestry of addiction and public health challenges. This examination of commonly abused drugs takes us through a spectrum of substances, shedding light on the diverse pharmacological and psychological factors that underpin their misuse, as we navigate the complex dynamics of substance-related disorders.

Drug abuse is a multifaceted phenomenon influenced by various factors, including cultural norms, peer dynamics, socioeconomic conditions, and media representation. Cultural attitudes play a pivotal role in shaping the social landscape of drug use. Ritualistic and traditional uses of certain substances, along with broader cultural values, contribute to the perception and acceptance of drug use within specific communities. The influence of peers and social networks is a powerful determinant of drug use behavior. Peer pressure, social acceptance, and the role of social networks in facilitating or discouraging drug use contribute significantly to the social aspects of substance abuse. Socioeconomic status is intricately linked to drug use patterns. Economic disparities can influence access to treatment, recovery resources, and the prevalence of substance abuse within different socioeconomic strata.

Media portrayal significantly shapes public perception of drug use. Anti-drug campaigns, media messaging, and cultural representations influence societal attitudes, contributing to the complex interplay between media and drug use (McGinty et al., 2018). Community-based interventions and support systems are pivotal in addressing the social aspects of drug abuse. These efforts aim to mitigate the impact of substance abuse, reduce stigma, and improve societal responses. In short, the social use of abused drugs is a dynamic and multifaceted phenomenon deeply intertwined with cultural, peer, socioeconomic, and media influences. Understanding these dynamics is crucial for developing effective prevention, intervention, and support strategies.

Alcohol: Alcohol abuse is a widespread and complex public health issue with significant social, economic, and health consequences. Alcohol abuse is characterized by the harmful or hazardous use of alcohol leading to significant impairment or distress. This includes patterns of drinking that result in negative consequences, such as health problems, social issues, or impaired daily functioning. Alcohol abuse is a global concern, with varying prevalence rates across regions. Understanding the scope of the issue is essential for developing targeted interventions. Global surveys, such as the World Health Organization's Global Status Report on Alcohol and Health, provide comprehensive data on alcohol consumption and related disorders.

Alcohol abuse varies significantly by region, influenced by cultural norms, policies, and socioeconomic factors. Some regions experience higher rates of alcohol-related harm, including Europe, Eastern Europe, and certain parts of Asia. Several factors contribute to the prevalence of alcohol abuse, including social, cultural, economic, and individual factors. Understanding these contributors is crucial for designing effective prevention and intervention strategies. Alcohol abuse is a multifaceted issue with significant global impact. Recognizing the prevalence and understanding the contributing factors are crucial steps toward developing effective policies and interventions to address this public health concern. Alcohol abuse has far-reaching health consequences, affecting various organs and systems in the body. One of the most well-known consequences of chronic alcohol abuse is liver damage, leading to conditions such as fatty liver, alcoholic hepatitis, and cirrhosis. Prolonged alcohol exposure can overwhelm the liver's ability to metabolize alcohol, resulting in inflammation, scarring, and impaired liver function (Gao & Bataller, 2011). While moderate alcohol consumption may have cardiovascular benefits, excessive and long-term use can lead to hypertension, cardiomyopathy, and an increased risk of heart failure. Balancing potential benefits with risks is crucial in understanding the complex relationship between alcohol and heart health (O'Keefe et al., 2018).

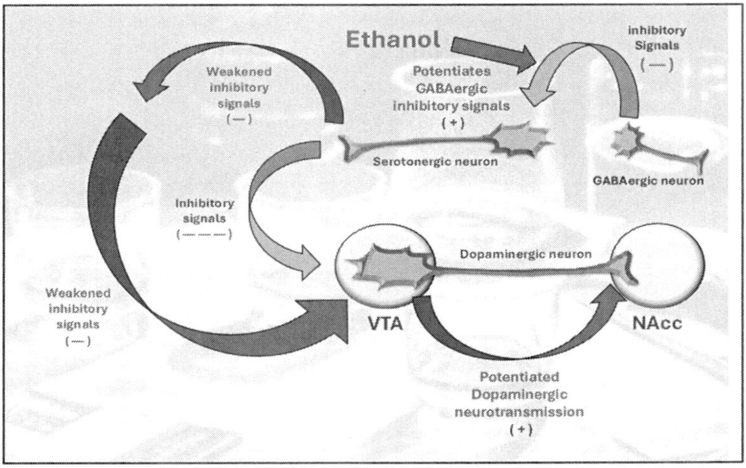

Alcohol acts via dysregulation of a GABAergic system

The central nervous system is particularly vulnerable to the effects of alcohol. Long-term alcohol abuse can result in neurological disorders such as Wernicke-Korsakoff syndrome, peripheral neuropathy, and cognitive impairments. These conditions often manifest due to nutritional deficiencies associated with heavy drinking. Alcohol abuse can lead to gastrointestinal issues, including gastritis, pancreatitis, and an increased risk of gastrointestinal cancers. Chronic irritation of the digestive tract by alcohol contributes to inflammation and damage to these vital organs. Alcohol abuse is closely linked to mental health disorders, including depression, anxiety, and an increased risk of suicide. Substance use disorders often co-occur with mental health conditions, forming a complex relationship that requires integrated treatment approaches (Boden et al., 2014). The health consequences and long-term effects of alcohol abuse are extensive and multifaceted. Recognizing these impacts is vital for public health efforts, prevention strategies, and the development of comprehensive treatment approaches.

Multifaceted social and economic impact of alcohol abuse has far-reaching consequences, affecting both individuals and society as a whole. Alcohol abuse often disrupts family dynamics, leading to strained relationships, domestic violence, and increased stress within households. Children of individuals with alcohol use disorders may experience adverse effects on their well-being and development. Alcohol abuse can significantly impact workplace productivity through absenteeism, presenteeism, and workplace accidents (Bennett & Lehman, 2001). Employees with alcohol use disorders may struggle with maintaining consistent job performance, affecting both individual careers and organizational outcomes. Alcohol misuse contributes to public safety concerns, including impaired driving incidents and an increased risk of accidents and injuries. The legal consequences of alcohol-related offenses, such as DUI (Driving Under the Influence), further strain legal systems and law enforcement resources.

Alcohol-related healthcare costs, including treatment for medical conditions arising from alcohol abuse, impose a substantial economic burden. This includes expenses related to emergency room visits, hospitalizations, and long-term medical care for individuals with alcohol use disorders. Children growing up in households affected by alcohol abuse may face long-term consequences, impacting their mental health, educational outcomes, and overall well-being. The intergenerational transmission of alcohol-related issues contributes to a cycle of social challenges. The social and economic impact of alcohol abuse is extensive, affecting individuals, families, workplaces, and society at large. Recognizing these consequences is essential for developing targeted interventions, policy initiatives, and support systems to mitigate the wide-ranging effects. Alcohol abuse is a complex and pervasive issue that requires a multifaceted approach to treatment. Various interventions and treatment options have been developed to address the diverse needs of individuals struggling with alcohol misuse. For individuals with severe alcohol dependence, the first step often involves medically supervised detoxification. This process helps manage withdrawal symptoms and ensures a safe transition to sobriety. Medications, such as benzodiazepines, may be prescribed under medical supervision. Inpatient rehabilitation programs provide a structured environment for individuals to focus on recovery. These programs typically offer a combination of counselling, group therapy, and medical supervision. The immersive nature of inpatient programs can be beneficial for those requiring intensive support. Outpatient counseling is a common and effective treatment option. Individuals attend therapy sessions while maintaining their daily routines. Cognitive-behavioral therapy (CBT), motivational enhancement therapy (MET), and contingency management are evidence-based approaches often used in outpatient settings.

Treatment of alcohol abuse involves the use of FDA-approved medications, such as disulfiram, naltrexone, and acamprosate, to complement behavioral therapy. These medications can help reduce cravings, prevent relapse, and support individuals in maintaining sobriety. Participation in mutual support groups, such as Alcoholics Anonymous (AA) or SMART Recovery, can provide individuals with a supportive community of peers. These groups offer a platform for sharing experiences, coping strategies, and fostering a sense of accountability. Relapse prevention strategies are crucial for maintaining long-term recovery. After completing initial treatment, individuals often engage in aftercare programs, which may include ongoing counseling, support groups, and periodic check-ins to address challenges and prevent relapse. The effectiveness of treatment options varies among individuals, and a personalized approach is often the most successful. Integrating a combination of these interventions, tailored to the individual's needs, can enhance the chances of sustained recovery.

Nicotine: Tobacco/nicotine abuse remains a global public health challenge with significant implications for individuals and societies. The prevalence of tobacco/nicotine use varies across regions, and understanding these patterns is crucial for developing effective interventions. Tobacco/nicotine use is a major contributor to the global burden of disease. According to the World Health Organization (WHO), tobacco use is responsible for more than 8 million deaths annually, with over 7 million of these deaths attributed to direct tobacco use, and around 1.2 million to non-smokers exposed to secondhand smoke (World Health Organization, 2021). Smoking prevalence varies across continents. According to the Global Burden of Disease Study, countries in Asia and Eastern Europe tend to have higher smoking prevalence rates, while some regions in Africa have lower rates. These disparities highlight the need for region-specific tobacco control measures.

In addition to smoking, the use of smokeless tobacco and other nicotine products contributes to the overall prevalence of nicotine abuse. Smokeless tobacco is particularly prevalent in some regions, including parts of Southeast Asia. The use of emerging nicotine products, such as e-cigarettes, has also increased globally, especially among youth. Tobacco/nicotine use often begins during adolescence. Global Youth Tobacco Surveys (GYTS) indicate that despite progress in some areas, many young people still initiate tobacco use at an early age. Targeted prevention efforts are essential to address this concerning trend. The implementation of comprehensive tobacco control policies has shown promising results in reducing tobacco use.

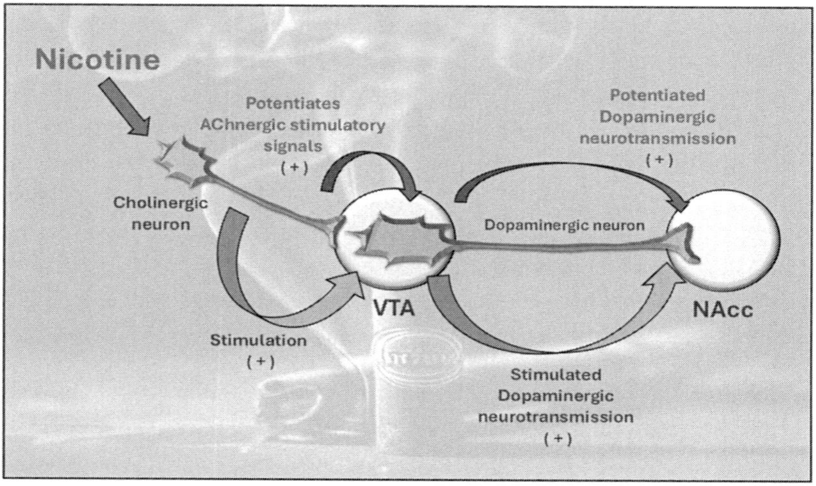

Nicotine acts via cholinergic system

Tobacco use, whether in the form of smoking or smokeless tobacco, poses significant health risks, contributing to a range of debilitating and often fatal conditions. Understanding these risks is crucial for public health initiatives and individual decision-making. Smoking is a leading cause of respiratory diseases, including chronic obstructive pulmonary disease (COPD) and lung cancer. It damages lung tissue, reduces lung function, and increases the risk of respiratory infections. Smoking significantly elevates the risk of cardiovascular diseases, including heart attacks and strokes. It contributes to the development of atherosclerosis and increases blood pressure. Cigarette smoking is a major cause of various cancers, including lung, throat, esophagus, and bladder cancers. It also increases the risk of pancreatic, liver, and colorectal cancers. Smokeless tobacco use is associated with severe oral health problems, including gum disease, tooth loss, and precancerous lesions in the mouth (leukoplakia).

Smokeless tobacco use increases the risk of cancers in the oral cavity, esophagus, and pancreas. It also contributes to an elevated risk of developing precancerous conditions. Both smoking and smokeless tobacco expose individuals to nicotine, leading to addiction and dependence. Nicotine is a highly addictive substance that contributes to continued tobacco use. Tobacco use during pregnancy, whether through smoking or smokeless tobacco, poses risks to fetal development, increasing the likelihood of preterm birth, low birth weight, and developmental issues. The health risks associated with smoking and smokeless tobacco are substantial and diverse, affecting multiple organ systems. Efforts to reduce tobacco-related harm require comprehensive strategies, including prevention, cessation support, and public health initiatives.

Nicotine withdrawal is a complex set of symptoms that individuals experience when attempting to quit smoking. The addictive nature of nicotine makes the withdrawal process challenging, both physically and psychologically. Physical symptoms include cravings such as intense desire for nicotine, often triggered by environmental cues or stress, headaches which are commonly reported during the initial withdrawal phase, fatigue and some may experience weight gain due to heightened appetite (Hughes, 2007). Psychological symptoms of nicotine withdrawal include irritability, mood swings and heightened irritability, feelings of restlessness and anxiety, some individuals may experience symptoms of depression and impaired focus and concentration (Piper et al., 2011). Nicotine withdrawal symptoms typically peak within the first few days after quitting and gradually subside over a few weeks. However, some psychological symptoms, such as cravings, can persist for more extended periods. Factors influencing the severity of nicotine withdrawal, include nicotine dependence. Individuals with higher levels of dependence may experience more intense withdrawal. Psychiatric comorbidities such as co-occurring mental health conditions can exacerbate withdrawal symptoms. The cessation method used to quit, such as cold turkey or gradual reduction, can impact withdrawal severity.

Nicotine Replacement Therapy (NRT) involves products like patches, gum, or lozenges can alleviate withdrawal symptoms by providing controlled doses of nicotine. Medications like varenicline and bupropion can help reduce cravings and withdrawal symptoms. Counseling and behavioral interventions can further enhance the effectiveness of pharmacological treatments (Stead et al., 2008). Nicotine withdrawal is a significant challenge faced by individuals attempting to quit smoking. Understanding the symptoms, duration, and available management strategies is crucial for both individuals and healthcare professionals involved in smoking cessation efforts.

Smoking cessation is a challenging but vital journey toward improved health. Various strategies and programs have been developed to assist individuals in quitting smoking, addressing both the physical and psychological aspects of nicotine addiction. One-on-one counseling sessions provide personalized support, helping individuals identify triggers, cope with cravings, and develop effective coping strategies. Group counseling sessions create a supportive environment where individuals can share experiences, receive encouragement, and build a sense of community. Smartphone applications offer personalized support, tracking progress, providing motivational messages, and offering interactive features. Text-based interventions send supportive messages, tips, and reminders to encourage abstinence and provide assistance during challenging times (Whittaker et al., 2016). Telephone-based quit lines provide counseling and support, connecting individuals with trained professionals to guide them through the quitting process. Local health programs and initiatives create awareness, offer resources, and engage communities in the fight against smoking (Stead et al., 2013). Interventions that consider cultural contexts and tailor support to individual needs can enhance engagement and effectiveness. Recognizing gender differences in smoking behaviors, gender-specific programs can address unique challenges faced by men and women. Smoking cessation programs in the workplace provide support, resources, and incentives for employees to quit smoking. Smoking cessation is a multifaceted journey that benefits from a combination of strategies and support systems. Combining behavioral interventions, pharmacotherapy, digital solutions, community engagement, and culturally competent approaches enhances the likelihood of successful quitting.

Marijuana/Cannabis: Marijuana, also known as cannabis, is a psychoactive substance that is widely used for recreational and medicinal purposes. While its legalization for medical and recreational use has increased in various regions, marijuana abuse remains a concern due to its potential negative effects on physical and mental health. Marijuana contains over 100 cannabinoids, with delta-9-tetrahydrocannabinol (THC) being the primary psychoactive compound responsible for its intoxicating effects. Marijuana can be smoked, vaporized, or consumed in various forms, including edibles and tinctures. Short-term effects include altered perception, impaired memory, increased heart rate, and altered judgment. Chronic marijuana abuse is associated with respiratory issues, cognitive impairments, and an increased risk of mental health disorders.

Marijuana Use Disorder (MUD) is characterized by problematic marijuana use leading to impairment or distress, often involving dependence and withdrawal symptoms. The prevalence of marijuana use disorder has increased, particularly among frequent and heavy users. Legalization has been associated with increased marijuana use, especially among certain age groups. Public health concerns include impaired driving, accidental ingestion by children, and potential long-term health effects. Cognitive-behavioral therapy and motivational enhancement therapy have shown efficacy in treating marijuana use disorder (Volkow et al., 2014). No FDA-approved medications specifically target marijuana use disorder, but research is ongoing. Marijuana abuse, despite its changing legal landscape, poses significant health risks. Understanding its effects, prevalence of use disorder, and available treatment options is essential for public health initiatives and individual well-being. Marijuana use spans both medical and recreational contexts, with evolving attitudes and legal frameworks shaping its accessibility and acceptance. This overview explores the dual nature of marijuana, highlighting its medicinal applications and recreational use, supported by references to key studies. Marijuana has been explored for its analgesic properties, offering relief from chronic pain conditions, such as neuropathy and arthritis. Cannabinoids in marijuana, particularly THC, have demonstrated antiemetic effects, providing relief for patients undergoing chemotherapy (Volkow et al., 2014). Marijuana shows promise in managing symptoms of neurological disorders, including epilepsy and multiple sclerosis. Research suggests potential benefits for certain mental health conditions, including anxiety and insomnia (Hall & Degenhardt, 2009).

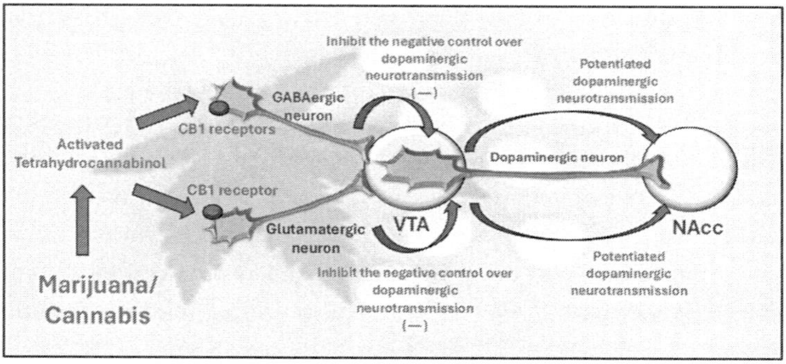

Marijuana potentiates dopaminergic neurotransmission via CB1 receptors

Tetrahydrocannabinol, the main psychoactive compound in marijuana, induces a range of effects, including euphoria, altered perception, and relaxation. Marijuana is often used recreationally in social settings for relaxation and enjoyment, with methods of consumption varying. Many regions have legalized medical marijuana, allowing patients to access cannabis for specific medical conditions under regulated frameworks (Pacula et al., 2015). Some jurisdictions have legalized recreational marijuana, allowing adults to use cannabis for non-medical purposes within specified limits. Concerns exist regarding the impact of marijuana legalization on youth consumption and potential adverse effects on brain. The association between marijuana use and impaired driving poses challenges for public safety and law enforcement (Budney & Borodovsky, 2017). The dual roles of marijuana, as a therapeutic agent and a recreational substance, continue to shape public discourse and policy. Balancing the potential benefits with associated risks is crucial for informed decision-making in both medical and recreational contexts.

Marijuana's legal status and public perception have undergone significant changes in recent years, reflecting evolving attitudes toward its medicinal and recreational use. Historically, marijuana faced strict legal restrictions, influenced by the prohibition era and moralistic attitudes. The Marijuana Tax Act of 1937 in the United States criminalized its use. The late 20th century witnessed a gradual shift in perspectives, with an increasing acknowledgment of marijuana's medicinal potential. Research highlighted its efficacy in managing pain, nausea, and other medical conditions. Changing societal attitudes toward marijuana became evident through public opinion polls, indicating a growing acceptance of its medical applications and a call for decriminalization (Dapari et al., 2022). States in the U.S. and various countries began passing laws allowing medical marijuana use, establishing regulated systems for patient access to cannabis-based medications.

In a groundbreaking shift, some jurisdictions, including certain U.S. states and entire countries, legalized recreational marijuana use, reflecting changing societal norms. Countries worldwide have reevaluated their marijuana policies, with some decriminalizing or legalizing it, signaling a departure from traditional punitive approaches. In regions where marijuana is legal at the state level, conflicts persist with federal laws that continue to classify it as a Schedule I controlled substance. Developing comprehensive regulatory frameworks remains a challenge, encompassing issues such as taxation, quality control, and age restrictions (Pacula et al., 2014). The legal status and public perception of marijuana continue to undergo transformative shifts, reflecting a nuanced understanding of its potential benefits and challenges. As the landscape evolves, ongoing research, comprehensive legislation, and public discourse will play pivotal roles in shaping the future of marijuana use.

Prescription Medications: Prescription drug abuse, the non-medical use of prescription medications, has emerged as a significant public health issue, leading to various physical, psychological, and societal consequences. Prescription medications, intended for therapeutic purposes, are sometimes misused for non-medical reasons, leading to various health risks. Opioid pain relievers, such as oxycodone and hydrocodone, are commonly abused for their pain-alleviating effects. Common medications include oxycodone (OxyContin), hydrocodone (Vicodin), and morphine. Opioids are frequently abused for their euphoric effects, contributing to the opioid epidemic. The risk of dependence and overdose is high. Benzodiazepines, like alprazolam and diazepam, central nervous system depressants prescribed for anxiety and sleep disorders but these are abused for their sedative and anxiolytic properties. Common medications include alprazolam (Xanax) and diazepam (Valium). Chronic use can lead to tolerance and dependence, necessitating careful prescribing.

Stimulants, like amphetamines and methylphenidate, are prescribed for attention deficit hyperactivity disorder (ADHD) and narcolepsy and abused for their cognitive-enhancing and euphoric effects. Common medications include Adderall and Ritalin. Stimulants are abused for their cognitive-enhancing and euphoric effects. Increased awareness of misuse in educational settings is crucial (McCabe et al., 2018). Prescription drug abuse has seen a rise globally, with opioids being a focal point of concern in many countries. Patterns of prescription drug abuse vary across demographics, with different age groups and genders showing distinct trends.

Overprescribing and easy access to prescription medications contribute to the greater risk of their abuse. Individuals with co-occurring mental health disorders are at an increased risk of prescription drug abuse. Long-term abuse of prescription drugs can lead to physical health issues, including respiratory depression and cardiovascular problems. Prescription drug abuse is associated with mental health challenges, including increased risk of depression and anxiety. Prescription monitoring programs help track and regulate the prescribing and dispensing of controlled substances. Public education and awareness campaigns are essential in preventing prescription drug abuse by promoting responsible use. Individuals may engage in polydrug abuse, combining opioids, benzodiazepines, and stimulants, amplifying the risks associated with each class. Prescription medications, when used appropriately, provide essential therapeutic benefits. However, the abuse of opioids, benzodiazepines, and stimulants poses significant public health challenges. Prescription drug abuse poses a multifaceted challenge with profound implications for public health. Comprehensive strategies, including effective regulation, targeted interventions, and increased awareness, are crucial in addressing this complex issue. Addressing the complex interplay of factors contributing to misuse is essential for effective prevention and intervention strategies. The misuse of prescription medications poses significant health risks, leading to various consequences that impact individuals physically, mentally, and socially. Opioid abuse can result in respiratory depression, constipation, and, in severe cases, overdose leading to respiratory failure. Consequences include opioid use disorder, increased risk of infectious diseases (e.g., HIV, hepatitis), and negative impacts on mental health (Volkow et al., 2019).

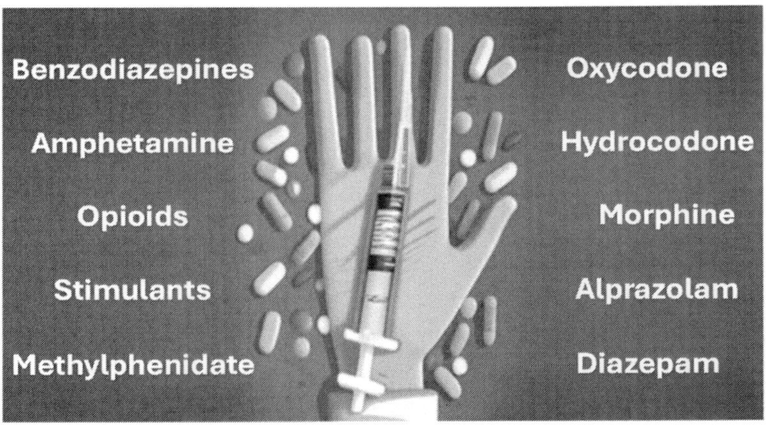

Commonly prescribed drugs with abuse potential

Benzodiazepine misuse can lead to sedation, drowsiness, and respiratory depression. Long-term use increases the risk of dependence (Lader, 2011) and may result in cognitive impairment, mental health issues, and an increased likelihood of accidents and injuries. Stimulant misuse can lead to cardiovascular issues, including elevated blood pressure, heart palpitations, and, in extreme cases, cardiac arrest (Volkow et al., 2007). Combining prescription medications, especially opioids, benzodiazepines, and stimulants, increases the risk of respiratory depression, overdose, and adverse drug interactions. Polydrug abuse exacerbates the health risks associated with individual classes of medications and poses challenges for effective treatment. Prescription drug abuse is linked to mental health issues such as depression, anxiety disorders, and an increased risk of suicidal ideation. Individuals abusing prescription medications may experience deteriorating mental health, further complicating the treatment process. The health risks and consequences of abusing prescription medications are far-reaching, impacting individuals physically, mentally, and socially. Recognizing these risks is crucial for developing effective prevention and intervention strategies.

Prescription drug abuse has become a critical public health issue, necessitating comprehensive efforts to curb its prevalence and mitigate associated risks. Abuse-deterrent formulations (ADFs) aim to make it more challenging to manipulate prescription drugs for non-medical use, deterring abuse. ADFs have demonstrated some effectiveness in reducing the abuse of certain prescription medications, although challenges persist. Educating healthcare providers on safe prescribing practices and implementing evidence-based guidelines can contribute to the responsible use of prescription medications. Studies show that provider education programs can lead to decreased opioid prescribing and improved adherence to guidelines. Legislation and regulations are implemented to control the availability and distribution of prescription medications, with a focus on minimizing opportunities for abuse. Regulatory measures, such as reclassifying certain medications, can contribute to a decline in their misuse. Public awareness initiatives aim to educate communities about the risks of prescription drug abuse, proper medication disposal, and available resources for those affected. Campaigns promoting awareness and prevention have shown positive outcomes in reducing prescription drug abuse among various age groups (Giga et al., 2021). Ensuring access to treatment and rehabilitation services is crucial for individuals struggling with prescription drug addiction. Expanding access to evidence-based treatment, including medication-assisted treatment, has proven effective in supporting recovery. Combating prescription drug abuse requires a multifaceted approach involving healthcare providers, policymakers, law enforcement, and the community. By combining strategies such as prescription monitoring, education, legislation, public awareness, and improved access to treatment, stakeholders can work collaboratively to address this complex public health challenge.

Opioids: The opioid epidemic is a complex public health crisis characterized by widespread misuse and addiction to opioid substances, leading to a surge in overdose deaths. The opioid epidemic gained prominence in the late 20th century and reached alarming proportions in the 21st century. Its roots can be traced back to the over-prescription of opioid painkillers, aggressive marketing by pharmaceutical companies, and a general lack of awareness about the potential risks associated with these medications. The widespread availability and prescription of opioid painkillers, such as oxycodone and hydrocodone, contributed significantly to the epidemic. Physicians often prescribed opioids for chronic pain conditions, leading to a surplus of pills in households and communities (Kolodny et al., 2015). Pharmaceutical companies played a role in fueling the epidemic through aggressive marketing of prescription opioids. Misleading claims about the safety and low risk of addiction associated with these medications contributed to their widespread use. As individuals became addicted to prescription opioids, some turned to heroin as a cheaper and more accessible alternative. The rise of synthetic opioids, particularly fentanyl, further exacerbated the crisis, leading to a spike in overdose deaths.

Limited access to effective addiction treatment and the stigma associated with substance use disorders hindered individuals from seeking help. This perpetuated the cycle of addiction and overdose (Saloner & Karthikeyan, 2015). Social and economic disparities, including poverty and lack of access to education and employment opportunities, contributed to the vulnerability of certain populations to opioid misuse and addiction. The opioid epidemic is a multifaceted crisis with origins deeply rooted in the healthcare system, pharmaceutical industry practices, and socioeconomic factors. Addressing this complex issue requires a comprehensive approach, involving policy changes, increased access to addiction treatment, and efforts to reduce the stigma associated with substance use disorders.

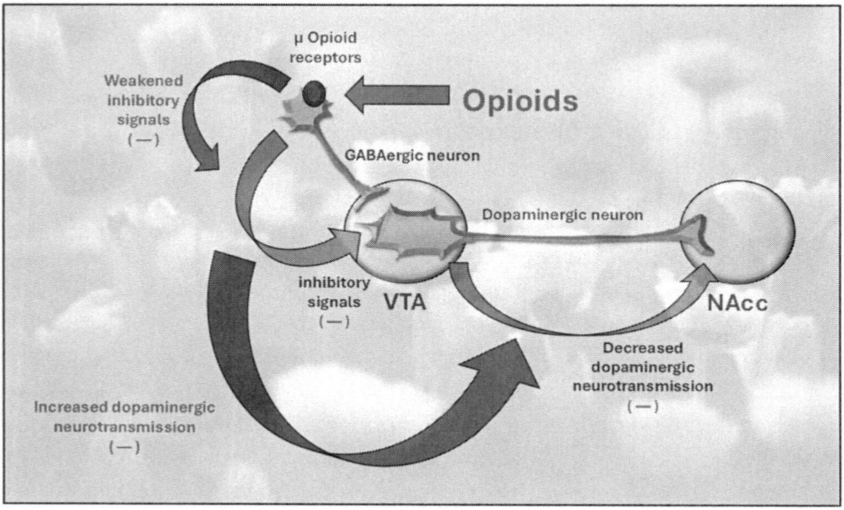

Opioids act via GABAergic interneurons

Opioids are a class of powerful pain-relieving drugs that can be classified into various categories, including prescription opioids, heroin, and synthetic opioids. Each type poses distinct risks and contributes to the overall opioid epidemic. *Prescription opioids* are medications typically prescribed by healthcare professionals to manage moderate to severe pain. They work by binding to opioid receptors in the brain and spinal cord, reducing the perception of pain. Common examples include hydrocodone (Vicodin, Norco), morphine, codeine, fentanyl patches (Duragesic) and tramadol. *Heroin* is an illicit opioid derived from morphine. It is usually sold as a white or brownish powder or as a black sticky substance known as "black tar heroin." Heroin is often injected, snorted, or smoked. Associated risks include increased risk of overdose, high addictive risk, transmission of infectious diseases through needle sharing. *Synthetic Opioids* are human-made substances designed to mimic the effects of natural opioids. They can be significantly more potent than prescription opioids and heroin. Common examples include fentanyl, carfentanil, U-47700 (Pink) and tramadol (in high doses). Increased risk of overdose due to high potency is observed and these are also involved in unintentional overdoses. Understanding the diverse landscape of opioids is crucial in addressing the complex challenges posed by the opioid epidemic. Prescription opioids, heroin, and synthetic opioids each contribute to the overall crisis, necessitating comprehensive strategies for prevention, treatment, and harm reduction.

Substance abuse, encompassing a range of substances including opioids, poses significant health risks, with overdose being a critical concern that can lead to fatalities. Understanding these risks is crucial for developing effective prevention, intervention, and harm reduction strategies. This overview explores the health risks, the dynamics of overdose, and the fatal consequences associated with substance abuse. Harm reduction strategies play a crucial role in minimizing the negative consequences associated with opioid use, while effective treatment options aim to address the root causes of addiction. Needle exchange programs provide sterile needles to individuals who use opioids, reducing the risk of infectious diseases like HIV and hepatitis. Naloxone, an opioid antagonist, is distributed widely to reverse opioid overdoses. Accessible naloxone kits empower individuals and communities to respond effectively in emergency situations. Supervised consumption sites offer a safe and monitored environment for individuals to use drugs. These sites reduce the risk of overdose and provide opportunities for healthcare professionals to engage with users (Strang et al., 2019).

Apart from medication-assisted treatment and cognitive-behavioral therapy (CBT), inpatient rehabilitation provides intensive, round-the-clock care, while outpatient programs offer flexibility and support for individuals to receive treatment while maintaining their daily routines. Peer support programs, including 12-step programs like narcotics anonymous, provide individuals with a supportive community of peers who understand the challenges of addiction. Combining harm reduction and treatment approaches creates a comprehensive strategy that addresses immediate risks while supporting individuals on their journey to recovery. Involving communities in the development and implementation of harm reduction and treatment programs fosters trust and encourages a collective effort in addressing opioid addiction. The integration of harm reduction strategies with evidence-based treatment approaches is vital in addressing the opioid epidemic. By acknowledging the immediate risks associated with opioid use and providing effective treatment options, communities can work towards reducing harm and supporting individuals on the path to recovery.

Benzodiazepines: Benzodiazepines (BZDs) are a class of psychoactive drugs commonly prescribed for their anxiolytic, sedative, and muscle relaxant properties. While effective when used as directed, the misuse and abuse of benzodiazepines have become a significant public health concern. Overprescription and prolonged use of benzodiazepines contribute to the potential for dependence and abuse. Individuals with mental health disorders may also misuse benzodiazepines as a form of self-medication. Benzodiazepines are often used in combination with other substances, amplifying their effects and increasing the risk of abuse.

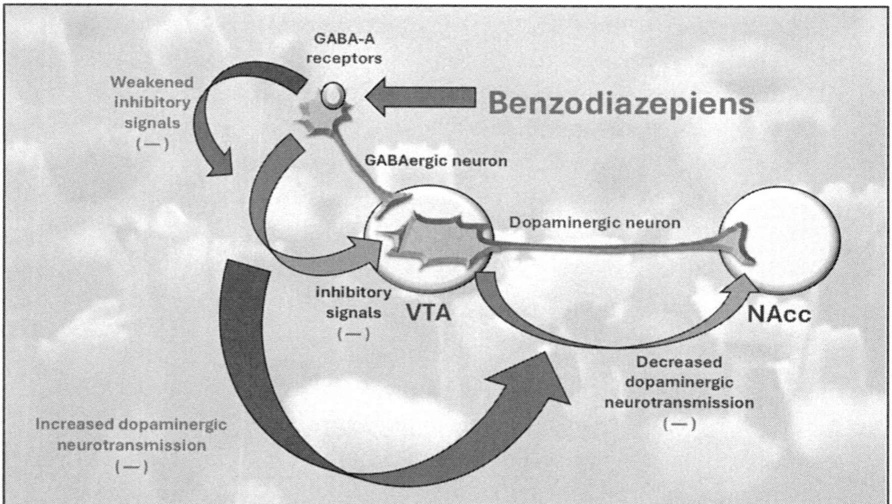

Benzodiazepine act via GABA-A receptors

Long-term benzodiazepine use is associated with cognitive impairment, respiratory issues, and increased risk of falls. Benzodiazepine abuse can lead to anxiety, depression, and worsening of pre-existing mental health conditions. The impact on relationships, employment, and overall quality of life can be profound. Medically supervised withdrawal is often necessary to manage benzodiazepine dependence. Cognitive-behavioral therapy (CBT) and motivational enhancement therapy are effective in addressing the psychological aspects of benzodiazepine abuse (Soyka, 2017). Gradual tapering of benzodiazepines and the use of alternative medications can support individuals in recovery. Benzodiazepine abuse poses serious health risks and societal challenges. Addressing the causes, understanding the consequences, and implementing effective interventions are crucial steps toward mitigating the impact of benzodiazepine abuse on individuals and communities.

Benzodiazepines, such as diazepam and lorazepam, are commonly prescribed to alleviate symptoms of anxiety disorders. They are also prescribed for sedative-hypnotic effects and certain benzodiazepines, like temazepam, are utilized for their sedative properties, aiding in the management of insomnia. Benzodiazepines such as diazepam and clonazepam are effective muscle relaxants, used in conditions like spasticity and muscle spasms (Bandelow et al., 2012). Ongoing research in benzodiazepines is focused on exploring novel compounds/ new benzodiazepine derivatives with potentially improved efficacy and reduced side effects. Immense focus is there on understanding the neurobiological pathways through which benzodiazepines exert their therapeutic effects. Current research also aims to enhance our understanding of benzodiazepine dependence, withdrawal mechanisms, and effective management strategies.

Special considerations and challenges target risk of dependence and ongoing research in this field explores strategies to minimize the risk of benzodiazepine dependence in long-term users. Benzodiazepines continue to play a significant role in the pharmacological management of various psychiatric and medical conditions. Ongoing research endeavors are essential to refine therapeutic approaches, address potential challenges, and contribute to the development of safer and more effective treatments. Prolonged use of benzodiazepines can lead to physical and psychological dependence, cognitive deficits, especially in older adults, affecting memory, attention, and psychomotor skills. When combined with other substances like alcohol or opioids, benzodiazepines increase the risk of respiratory depression and overdose. Providing comprehensive information about the risks and benefits of benzodiazepines helps empower patients to make informed decisions (Bandelow et al., 2012). Periodic assessments, including cognitive screenings, can aid in identifying early signs of dependence or cognitive impairment. Gradual tapering under medical supervision helps minimize withdrawal symptoms and reduce the risk of rebound effects. Prescribing benzodiazepines for short durations, when possible, helps reduce the likelihood of dependence and tolerance. Increasing awareness about the risks of benzodiazepine misuse within communities fosters a supportive environment. By implementing harm reduction strategies, fostering awareness, and promoting safer prescribing practices, the healthcare community can work towards minimizing the potential harm associated with benzodiazepine use.

Stimulants: Stimulants constitute a class of psychoactive substances that enhance alertness, attention, and energy while elevating mood. They are commonly used for medical purposes, such as treating attention deficit hyperactivity disorder (ADHD) and narcolepsy but are also subject to misuse due to their euphoric effects. Amphetamines, such as dextroamphetamine and methamphetamine, increase the release of neurotransmitters like dopamine and norepinephrine. Methylphenidate, commonly known as Ritalin, enhances dopamine and norepinephrine levels by blocking their reuptake. Cocaine inhibits the reuptake of dopamine, leading to its accumulation in the synaptic cleft.

Stimulants increase the release of neurotransmitters, particularly dopamine and norepinephrine, into the synaptic cleft. Some stimulants, like methylphenidate and cocaine, block the reuptake transporters, prolonging the presence of neurotransmitters in the synapse. Monoamine oxidase inhibitors, present in some stimulants, prevent the breakdown of neurotransmitters, further amplifying their effects. Stimulants enhance wakefulness and alertness by modulating the activity of neurotransmitters in the CNS. The release of dopamine contributes to the mood-elevating and euphoric effects associated with stimulant use. Stimulants can also enhance cognitive functions such as attention, concentration, and memory. Stimulants like methylphenidate and amphetamines are commonly prescribed for ADHD to improve focus and attention. Stimulants are used to manage symptoms of narcolepsy, promoting wakefulness. The euphoric effects of stimulants contribute to their misuse, leading to potential addiction and other health risks. Stimulants exert their effects on the CNS by modulating neurotransmitter systems, leading to enhanced alertness, mood elevation, and improved cognitive function. While invaluable for medical purposes, the potential for misuse underscores the importance of responsible prescribing and awareness.

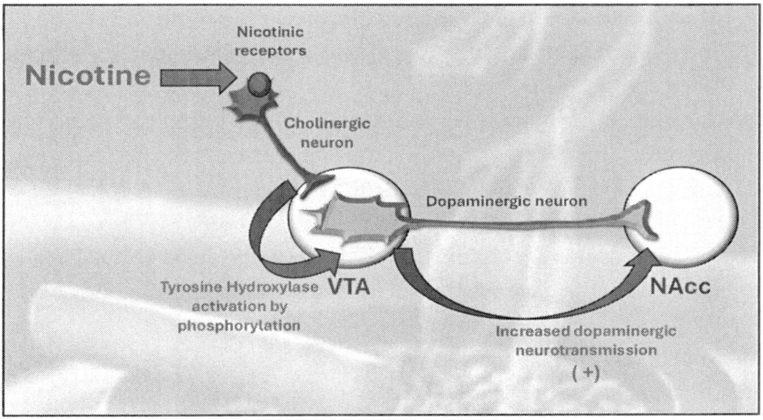

Nicotine acts via nicotinic receptors

Stimulants enhance alertness and energy levels by increasing the release of neurotransmitters such as dopamine and norepinephrine. Short-term use of stimulants is associated with enhanced cognitive functions, particularly improved focus and concentration. The release of dopamine contributes to feelings of euphoria and elevated mood in the short term. Stimulants can lead to a temporary increase in heart rate and blood pressure due to their stimulatory effects on the cardiovascular system. Short-term use may result in appetite suppression, contributing to weight loss (Berman et al., 2009). Prolonged stimulant use may lead to the development of tolerance, requiring higher doses to achieve the same effects, and dependence. Long-term stimulant use has been associated with cardiovascular complications, including hypertension and increased risk of heart disease. Chronic use may contribute to psychiatric consequences, including anxiety, paranoia, and increased risk of mood disorders (Frodl & Skokauskas, 2012). Prolonged stimulant use may lead to cognitive impairment, affecting memory, attention, and executive functions. Long-term use can result in neuroadaptations, altering the structure and function of the brain. Stimulants elicit a range of short-term and long-term effects, from increased alertness and euphoria to potential physiological and cognitive consequences. Balancing therapeutic benefits with potential risks is crucial for responsible use.

Stimulants, known for their cognitive-enhancing properties, find extensive therapeutic applications. Methylphenidate and amphetamines are widely used to manage ADHD symptoms, improving attention, focus, and impulse control. Stimulants help manage excessive daytime sleepiness in individuals with narcolepsy, promoting wakefulness. Ongoing research explores the use of stimulants as adjuncts in treating depression, especially in cases resistant to traditional antidepressants. Stimulants have been explored for their potential in enhancing cognitive functions in individuals without ADHD, but the ethical implications and risks warrant further investigation (Spencer et al., 2007). Research is ongoing to evaluate the use of stimulants in neurological disorders such as traumatic brain injury and cognitive impairment. Ongoing research explores the use of stimulants in managing ADHD with comorbid conditions, such as substance use disorders. Studies are underway to investigate the long-term effects of stimulant use, especially concerning cognitive function and psychiatric outcomes.

Research aims to delineate the balance between the potential cognitive benefits and risks associated with the use of stimulants. Stimulants play a vital role in therapeutics, addressing conditions like ADHD and narcolepsy (Lee et al., 2011). Ongoing research seeks to expand their applications, examining their potential in cognitive enhancement and neurological disorders, while ethical considerations guide the discourse around their broader use. Stimulant medications, commonly prescribed for conditions such as Attention-Deficit/Hyperactivity Disorder (ADHD), can be highly effective in managing symptoms and improving daily functioning. However, like any pharmacological intervention, the use of stimulants is not without potential risks. It is crucial to understand these risks and implement harm reduction strategies to ensure the safe and responsible use of these medications. Prolonged use of stimulants has been associated with potential cardiovascular risks. Elevated heart rate and increased blood pressure are common side effects that may pose risks, especially in individuals with pre-existing cardiovascular conditions. Stimulant use can exacerbate or trigger psychiatric conditions. Individuals may experience heightened anxiety, paranoia, or mood disorders, particularly at higher doses or in susceptible populations. While stimulants are prescribed to enhance focus and attention, there is a potential risk of developing substance use disorders, especially when used inappropriately or without proper medical supervision. Moderation in stimulant dosage is essential. Ensuring that individuals adhere to prescribed doses can minimize the risk of adverse effects while still providing therapeutic benefits (Greenhill et al., 2002). Periodic health check-ups, especially cardiovascular assessments, are vital for individuals using stimulants. Regular monitoring can help detect and address emerging issues early on. For individuals with a history of substance misuse or those at a higher risk of developing substance use disorders, supervised use of stimulants, especially in a healthcare setting, can enhance safety.

Individuals with co-occurring disorders, such as ADHD and substance use disorders, benefit from integrated treatment approaches. Combining medication with psychosocial interventions can address underlying issues more effectively (Wilens et al., 2006). Incorporating psychosocial interventions alongside stimulant treatment can provide additional support and address behavioral aspects, reducing the risk of misuse. Balancing the therapeutic benefits of stimulants with potential risks requires a comprehensive approach involving dose management, regular health monitoring, addressing co-occurring disorders, and community education.

Hallucinogens: Hallucinogenic drugs, including LSD (lysergic acid diethylamide), psilocybin (found in certain mushrooms), and PCP (phencyclidine), induce alterations in perception, mood, and cognitive processes. Understanding their mode of action provides insights into their effects on the brain and can inform discussions on their potential therapeutic applications. LSD primarily interacts with serotonin receptors, especially the 5-HT2A receptor subtype. Activation of these receptors is linked to the hallucinogenic effects of LSD. LSD's influence on serotonin receptors leads to altered sensory perception, including visual hallucinations and changes in the perception of time (Nichols, 2004). Psilocybin, like LSD, interacts with serotonin receptors, particularly the 5-HT2A subtype, contributing to its hallucinogenic effects. Psilocybin is known to modulate the DMN, a network associated with self-referential thoughts. This modulation may contribute to the drug's effects on introspection and ego dissolution (Carhart-Harris, et al., 2012).

PCP (Phencyclidine) acts as an antagonist at NMDA (N-methyl-D-aspartate) receptors, inhibiting the effects of glutamate, a major excitatory neurotransmitter. By blocking NMDA receptors, PCP disrupts normal glutamate signaling, leading to altered perception, dissociation, and cognitive impairment (Coelho et al., 2019). Hallucinogens, including LSD, psilocybin, and PCP, may induce neuroplastic changes and alter synaptic transmission, contributing to their long-lasting effects. Ongoing research is exploring the therapeutic potential of hallucinogens, particularly in the treatment of mental health. Hallucinogenic drugs, such as LSD, psilocybin, and PCP, induce profound alterations in perception and cognition. Understanding both short-term and long-term effects is crucial for assessing the risks and potential therapeutic applications of these substances.

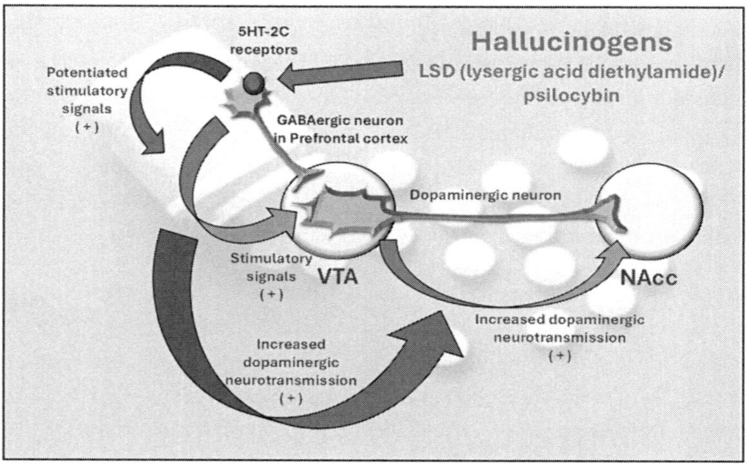

LSD and psilocybin act via 5HT-2C receptors

Short-term effects include intense hallucinations and LSD produces vivid visual, auditory, and sensory hallucinations, often referred to as a "trip."

Users may experience a distorted sense of time, with minutes feeling like hours. Physiological responses include increased heart rate and blood pressure. Intense emotions, both positive and negative, can be experienced, and users may undergo ego dissolution (Nichols, 2016). Psilocybin produces altered perceptions similar to LSD and induces visual and auditory hallucinations. Some users report heightened creativity and altered problem-solving abilities during the experience. Positive mood alterations and a sense of interconnectedness are common. Short-term side effects may include nausea and physical discomfort (Vollenweider & Kometer, 2010). PCP induces a state of dissociation from reality, leading to feelings of detachment from one's body and environment. PCP can cause analgesia, making users less sensitive to pain. Short-term effects may include restlessness, confusion, and aggressive behavior (Coelho et al., 2019).

Long-Term Effects produced by LSD include "flashbacks" or hallucinogen persisting perception disorder (HPPD) days, months, or even years after using LSD. Long-term psychological effects are less clear, with some studies suggesting positive outcomes, such as increased openness and decreased anxiety (Halpern et al., 2016). Psilocybin has long-term psychological benefits/ positive effects on mood, personality, and well-being. Psilocybin-assisted therapy is being explored as a potential treatment for depression, anxiety, and PTSD (Griffiths et al., 2016; Carhart-Harris et al., 2018). Long-term use of PCP (Phencyclidine) is associated with cognitive impairments, including memory and attention deficits. Chronic use may contribute to psychiatric symptoms such as depression, anxiety, and psychosis. While hallucinogenic drugs can induce intense short-term effects, ongoing research suggests that, under controlled conditions, they may have therapeutic potential, with possible long-term positive psychological outcomes. However, caution must be exercised due to the potential for adverse reactions and individual variability in response.

Once stigmatized as substances associated solely with recreational use, hallucinogens have gained renewed attention for their potential therapeutic benefits. Ongoing research is exploring their efficacy in treating various mental health conditions. Despite its classification as a Schedule I controlled substance, LSD has been studied for its therapeutic potential. Research has explored LSD-assisted psychotherapy for conditions such as anxiety, depression, and existential distress in patients facing life-threatening illnesses (Carhart-Harris et al., 2016; Gasser et al., 2014). Psilocybin, found in certain mushrooms, has shown promise in the treatment of depression, anxiety, and addiction. Clinical trials have explored psilocybin-assisted therapy for end-of-life distress, demonstrating significant reductions in anxiety and improvements in mood (Griffiths et al., 2016). MDMA, commonly known as ecstasy, has been investigated for its potential in treating post-traumatic stress disorder (PTSD). Clinical trials have reported significant reductions in PTSD symptoms following MDMA-assisted psychotherapy (V et al., 2018).

Hallucinogens are thought to modulate brain connectivity and induce neuroplastic changes, which may contribute to their therapeutic effects. Ongoing research aims to understand the neural mechanisms underlying these substances' impact on cognition and mood. Therapeutic benefits often stem from the integration of hallucinogenic experiences into an individual's life. Post-session integration sessions are crucial components of psychedelic-assisted therapy to maximize positive outcomes. Hallucinogens, when used in controlled settings, show promise in addressing mental health conditions. Ongoing research is shedding light on their therapeutic potential, with a focus on understanding the underlying mechanisms and optimizing treatment protocols. Ethical and rigorous exploration of these substances holds the key to unlocking their potential benefits.

While hallucinogenic substances like LSD, psilocybin, and MDMA have shown therapeutic potential, they also pose risks, especially when used without proper knowledge or in uncontrolled settings. Understanding these risks and implementing harm reduction strategies is crucial for promoting safer use. Risks associated with hallucinogenic substances include HPPD (Hallucinogen Persisting Perception Disorder. That means that some individuals may experience persistent visual disturbances or flashbacks after using hallucinogens (Halpern & Pope, 2003). Intense psychological experiences during a "bad trip" can lead to anxiety, panic, or even psychotic reactions. Hallucinogens can impair judgment, leading to accidental injuries or risky behaviors (Gouzoulis-Mayfrank & Daumann, 2006). Hallucinogens can interact negatively with certain medications, potentially leading to adverse effects. Harm reduction strategies therefore involve educating users and providing accurate information about the effects, risks, and potential consequences of hallucinogen use. A need also arises for encouraging the use of hallucinogens in controlled environments with experienced guides or therapists. Screening individuals for pre-existing mental health conditions is required to identify those at higher risk. Encouraging users to be aware of the dosage and purity of substances to avoid unintentional overdoses is pivotal for risk management. Integration sessions are needed to help individuals process and integrate their experiences. Risks associated with hallucinogens can be mitigated through informed use and harm reduction strategies. Continued research and responsible practices are essential to unlock the therapeutic potential of these substances while minimizing potential harms.

Designer Drugs: Designer drugs, also known as synthetic drugs or new psychoactive substances (NPS), refer to chemically engineered substances created to mimic the effects of controlled substances while evading legal restrictions. These drugs often emerge as analogs or derivatives of existing illicit substances. Designer drugs exhibit structural variations from existing controlled substances, allowing manufacturers to exploit legal loopholes. The rapid evolution of designer drugs involves constant modification of chemical structures to create novel compounds that are not yet regulated. Designer drugs are designed to mimic the effects of traditional illicit substances, providing users with a similar psychoactive experience. Manufacturers intentionally alter the chemical structure to avoid classification as controlled substances, allowing them to evade legal restrictions.

Designer drugs encompass a wide range of chemical classes, including synthetic cannabinoids, cathinones, phenethylamines, and tryptamines. Many designer drugs are readily available for purchase online, contributing to their accessibility and widespread use. Due to their novelty, designer drugs often lack adequate regulation, posing challenges for law enforcement and public health agencies. The rapid emergence and unpredictable nature of designer drugs can pose significant health risks, including unknown toxicity and potential for severe adverse effects. Designer drugs represent a dynamic and challenging category of substances due to their constantly evolving nature, legal complexities, and potential health risks. Continued research and vigilance are essential to address the impact of these substances on public health.

Designer drugs encompass a wide range of substances that are constantly evolving. Here are examples of notable designer drugs, highlighting their diversity and the challenges they pose:

- Synthetic Cannabinoids: Spice, K2, JWH-018, AMB-FUBINACA.
- Synthetic Cathinones (Bath Salts): Methylone, MDPV, Alpha-PVP
- Phenethylamines: 2C-B, N-BOMe compounds
- Piperazines: BZP (Benzylpiperazine), TFMPP (Trifluoromethylphenylpiperazine)
- Tryptamines: 5-MeO-DALT, AMT (Alpha-Methyltryptamine)
- Novel Opioids: U-47700, W-18
- Novel Benzodiazepines: Flubromazolam, Etizolam
- N-ethylamphetamine Derivatives: Ethylone, Butylone
- Novel Hallucinogens: 25I-NBOMe, 2C-EF
- Synthetic Stimulants: Naphyrone, MDPBP (3,4-methylenedioxy-α-pyrrolidinobutiophenone)

Designer drugs encompass a diverse array of substances, reflecting the constant innovation within the clandestine drug market. Monitoring and understanding these compounds are crucial for public health and regulatory efforts. Designer drugs pose significant health risks due to their unpredictable nature and constantly evolving formulations. Moreover, the legal implications surrounding these substances can vary widely. Designer drugs often have unpredictable compositions, making it challenging for users to gauge their potency and potential side effects. Limited research on many designer drugs means that their toxicity and long-term health effects remain largely unknown. Designer drugs can induce a range of adverse effects, including cardiovascular issues, seizures, hallucinations, and mental health disturbances (Corkery et al., 2017). Some designer drugs, particularly synthetic cannabinoids and cathinones, have shown potential for addiction, leading to compulsive use and dependence.

The rapidly changing formulations of designer drugs make it challenging for legal systems to keep up, leading to ambiguity in their classification.

Governments worldwide frequently update legislation to control and schedule specific designer drugs as they emerge. In some jurisdictions, the Analog Act allows authorities to prosecute substances that are structurally or pharmacologically similar to controlled substances, even if not explicitly listed. International collaboration is crucial to address the global nature of designer drug trafficking and to harmonize legal responses. Law enforcement faces challenges in identifying and prosecuting individuals involved in the production and distribution of designer drugs due to their constantly changing nature. Designer drugs present complex challenges at the intersection of public health and law enforcement. The ongoing collaboration between scientific communities, regulatory bodies, and legal systems is crucial to address the health risks and legal implications associated with these rapidly evolving substances.

The regulation and monitoring of designer drugs pose significant challenges due to their constantly evolving nature, diverse chemical structures, and global accessibility. Designers frequently modify the chemical structures of substances, creating new analogs that may not fall under existing regulatory frameworks. Legislative systems may struggle to keep pace with the emergence of new designer drugs, leading to gaps in legal frameworks. Designer drugs are often produced in one country and distributed globally, making it challenging for individual nations to regulate and monitor effectively. Analog laws, designed to regulate substances similar to controlled drugs, face challenges due to legal complexity and the need for continuous updates. Designer drugs are often accessible through online platforms and cryptomarkets, making it difficult for authorities to regulate and monitor transactions. The rapid emergence of new compounds may outpace the development of analytical methods, hindering timely identification and monitoring efforts. Inadequate research on the health effects of designer drugs complicates risk assessment and the development of targeted regulations. The lack of coordination among regulatory agencies at national and international levels hampers a unified approach to regulating and monitoring designer drugs. Limited public awareness about the risks associated with designer drugs can impede prevention efforts, requiring targeted educational initiatives. The dynamic and innovative nature of the designer drug market necessitates continuous adaptation of regulatory strategies. Effectively regulating and monitoring designer drugs demands a multi-faceted approach that addresses legal, technological, and international collaboration challenges. Ongoing efforts are essential to adapt regulatory frameworks to the evolving landscape of designer drug production and distribution.

Club Drugs: Club drugs are a category of psychoactive substances commonly associated with recreational settings like nightclubs, parties, and music festivals. They are known for their mood-altering and hallucinogenic effects. MDMA (3,4-Methylenedioxymethamphetamine), commonly known as "Ecstasy" or "Molly," is a synthetic drug that alters mood and perception. It is chemically similar to both stimulants and hallucinogens. It produces euphoria, heightened sensory perception, increased energy, sociability, distorted time perception and sensory distortions. Risk factors associated with chronic MDMA use include dehydration and overheating, hyponatremia (low sodium levels) due to excessive water consumption and serotonin syndrome at higher doses.

GHB (Gamma-Hydroxybutyrate), sometimes referred to as "Liquid Ecstasy" or "G," is a central nervous system depressant that can produce feelings of relaxation and euphoria. It exhibits euphoria, increased sociability, enhanced sensuality, reduced inhibitions, sedation and drowsiness in higher doses. Risk factors associated with chronic GHB use include respiratory depression, amnesia and loss of consciousness, dependence and withdrawal symptoms. Ketamine is a dissociative anesthetic that has hallucinogenic effects. It is often used in veterinary medicine but has gained popularity as a recreational drug. It produces these effects of dissociation from surroundings and altered perception of reality, euphoria, psychedelic experiences, analgesia and anesthesia at higher doses. Risk factors associated with ketamine abuse include hallucinations, vivid dreams, impaired motor function and coordination as well as potential for psychological dependence. Club drugs like MDMA, GHB, and ketamine carry both recreational and potential risks. Understanding their effects and risks is essential for harm reduction strategies and promoting informed decision-making among users. As far as mode of action is concerned, club drugs exert their effects on the central nervous system, leading to altered perception, mood, and cognition. MDMA (3,4-Methylenedioxymethamphetamine) primarily acts by increasing the release of neurotransmitters, particularly serotonin, dopamine, and norepinephrine, from presynaptic neurons. It inhibits the reuptake of these neurotransmitters, prolonging their presence in the synaptic cleft. The release of serotonin is especially significant and contributes to the characteristic empathogenic and entactogenic effects.

GHB (Gamma-Hydroxybutyrate) is a neurotransmitter and a precursor to GABA (gamma-aminobutyric acid), the primary inhibitory neurotransmitter in the central nervous system. It binds to GABA receptors, inducing inhibitory effects on neuronal activity. GHB also activates its own specific receptors, the GHB receptors, leading to additional central nervous system effects. Ketamine is an NMDA receptor antagonist, blocking the action of glutamate at the NMDA receptor. By inhibiting NMDA receptors, ketamine disrupts normal neurotransmission, leading to dissociative and anesthetic effects. It also interacts with other receptors, including opioid and monoaminergic receptors, contributing to its diverse effects. The mode of action of club drugs involves complex interactions with neurotransmitter systems, leading to a range of psychoactive effects. Understanding these mechanisms is crucial for both scientific research and harm reduction strategies associated with the use of these substances.

The prevalence of club drugs in party and nightlife scenes varies across regions and over time. MDMA (Ecstasy/Molly) is a popular club drug known for its euphoric and empathogenic effects. Its prevalence in party and nightlife scenes has been consistently documented, especially in electronic dance music (EDM) events and raves. GHB (Gamma-Hydroxybutyrate) has been associated with the party and club scenes, particularly due to its sedative and euphoric effects. However, its use is often less widespread compared to other substances like MDMA. Ketamine is commonly used in club and party settings, often for its dissociative and psychedelic effects. It has been documented at events where electronic and psychedelic music is prevalent. The prevalence of club drugs can be influenced by factors such as local drug cultures, law enforcement practices, and harm reduction efforts. Epidemiological studies often focus on specific regions or subpopulations within the party and nightlife scenes. Designer drugs, often synthetic analogs of controlled substances, pose significant health risks due to their unpredictable nature and potential for toxic effects.

Designer drugs frequently have variable and unpredictable compositions, making it challenging for users to know what substances they are consuming. This unpredictability increases the risk of adverse reactions and overdose. Designer drugs can have toxic effects on various organ systems, leading to acute and long-term health consequences. These effects may include cardiovascular issues, kidney and liver damage, and neurotoxicity (Prosser & Nelson, 2012). Designer drugs can induce severe psychiatric effects, including anxiety, paranoia, hallucinations, and mood disorders. Prolonged use may contribute to the development of mental health disorders. Due to their psychoactive nature, designer drugs can lead to the development of substance use disorders, with users experiencing cravings, tolerance, and withdrawal symptoms. The health risks associated with designer drugs are multifaceted and can range from acute toxic effects to long-term psychiatric consequences. Given the continuously evolving nature of these substances, understanding their potential risks is crucial for public health and harm reduction efforts.

Epidemiological Trends in Substance Abuse: The contemporary drug abuse landscape reveals alarming trends, with opioids, stimulants, and synthetic drugs dominating global substance misuse patterns. Prescription opioid misuse remains pervasive, particularly in North America, where fentanyl analogs now account for over 70% of overdose fatalities according to recent CDC reports. Methamphetamine use has surged across diverse demographics, with crystalline variants demonstrating unprecedented purity levels that amplify addiction potential and neurotoxicity. The synthetic cannabinoid market continues evolving rapidly, with new chemical formulations outpacing regulatory controls and presenting novel public health challenges. Cocaine consumption maintains steady prevalence worldwide, with European monitoring data showing increased availability of high-purity product alongside rising polydrug use combinations. Alcohol abuse persists as the most widespread substance disorder, contributing to 5% of global disease burden while often co-occurring with illicit drug use. Emerging concerns include the normalization of prescription stimulant misuse among young adults and the growing availability of novel psychoactive substances through cryptomarkets.

This complex scenario demands coordinated surveillance systems capable of tracking both established and emerging substance threats in real time. The psychosocial dimensions of contemporary drug abuse reveal troubling intersections with mental health crises and socioeconomic disparities. Cannabis legalization movements have paradoxically coincided with increased rates of cannabis use disorder, particularly among daily users of high-THC products. MDMA and psychedelic compounds are experiencing resurgence among millennials and Gen Z populations, often amid misguided perceptions of their safety profiles. Inhalant abuse persists as a hidden epidemic among marginalized youth populations, with neurological consequences remaining under-addressed in clinical settings. The COVID-19 pandemic exacerbated existing substance use trends, with WHO data indicating 25% increases in alcohol-related hospitalizations and relapses across multiple nations. Polysubstance use has become the norm rather than exception, creating complex clinical presentations that challenge traditional treatment paradigms. Dark web drug markets continue sophisticating their operations, utilizing encryption and cryptocurrency to circumvent law enforcement efforts. These developments underscore the urgent need for harm reduction strategies that address both the pharmacological realities of modern substances and their evolving cultural contexts.

CHAPTER 6

ROLE OF DOPAMINE IN DRUG ADDICTION

Abstinence is necessary to restore homeostasis, and with it, our ability to get pleasure from less potent rewards.
– Anna Lembke

Find out how a brain chemical called dopamine is involved in addiction. Stopping the use of drugs can help reset the brain's happiness levels. In this chapter the pivotal role of dopamine in drug addiction is illuminated as we unravel the neurochemical intricacies that drive reward-seeking behaviors and the formation of addictive patterns. Delving into the role of dopamine in drug addiction unravels a narrative of neurotransmitter influence, shedding light on how this key chemical messenger orchestrates the reinforcement mechanisms underlying the allure and persistence of substance use disorders.

Drug addiction is a complex phenomenon with a strong neurobiological basis. Dopamine plays a crucial role in the development and maintenance of addiction. Dopamine is a neurotransmitter associated with pleasure, reward, and reinforcement. In normal circumstances, it regulates motivation, mood, and the perception of pleasure. The mesolimbic and mesocortical pathways, particularly the projection from the ventral tegmental area (VTA) to the nucleus accumbens (NAc) and prefrontal cortex, are central to the rewarding effects of substances (Lewis et al., 2021). Addictive substances, including drugs of abuse, stimulate the release of dopamine in the mesolimbic pathway, creating a rewarding experience that reinforces drug-seeking behavior. Repeated drug use can lead to dysregulation of the dopamine system, altering its baseline function and contributing to the development of addiction.

The initial use of drugs often results in an acute increase in dopamine levels, contributing to the positive reinforcement associated with drug use. As addiction progresses, there is a shift from the acute effects of drugs to the development of tolerance and sensitization, both of which involve changes in dopamine transmission. Dopamine plays a crucial role in drug craving, and cues associated with drug use can trigger dopamine release, contributing to the high risk of relapse. Individual differences in dopamine receptor genes and the dopamine transporter gene contribute to variability in responses to drugs and susceptibility to addiction. Genetic factors influence the function of dopaminergic pathways, affecting an individual's vulnerability to addiction. Pharmacotherapies for addiction often target the dopamine system, aiming to normalize its function and reduce the reinforcing effects of drugs. Behavioral therapies also play a crucial role in addiction treatment by modulating dopamine release in response to non-drug rewards (Wise & Robble, 2020). Understanding the role of dopamine in addiction provides valuable insights into the neurobiology of substance abuse disorders. Targeting the dopamine system holds promise for developing effective treatments for addiction.

Dopamine release in response to natural rewards: Neuroimaging studies have been pivotal in elucidating the intricate relationship between dopamine release and natural rewards. Functional magnetic resonance imaging (fMRI) and positron emission tomography (PET) have allowed researchers to observe and quantify dopamine release in response to various natural rewards. Studies using fMRI have demonstrated a correlation between subjective feelings of pleasure and increased dopamine release. For instance, the consumption of palatable food or engagement in rewarding social interactions has been associated with heightened activity in dopamine-rich brain regions (Schultz, 2015). Animal studies, particularly using rodents, have provided valuable insights into the relationship between neural firing patterns, dopamine release, and behavioral responses to natural rewards. Microdialysis and electrophysiological recordings have enabled researchers to directly measure dopamine levels in response to specific rewarding stimuli (Salamone et al., 2009). Research in animals has demonstrated a direct link between dopamine release and behavioral responses to natural rewards. Dopaminergic neurons in the ventral tegmental area (VTA) and their projections to the nucleus accumbens play a crucial role in mediating these reward-related behaviors.

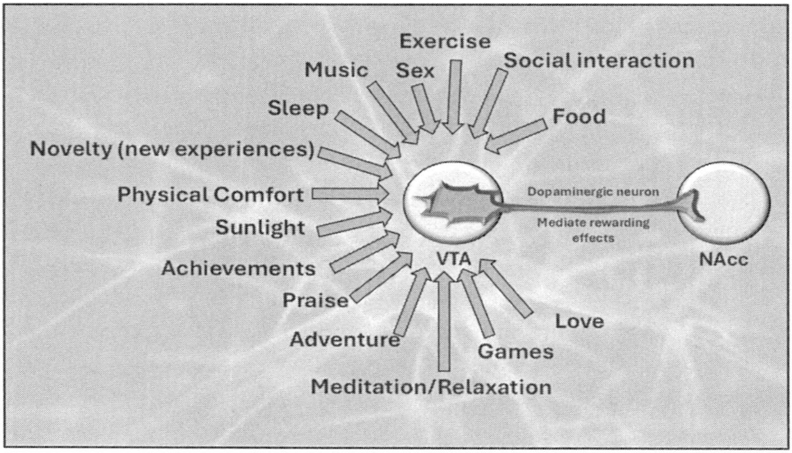

Natural reinforcers mediate the rewarding effects via dopaminergic pathway

Natural reinforcers refer to stimuli or experiences that are inherently rewarding to an organism, typically due to their association with survival, well-being, or pleasure. These reinforcers are not learned through conditioning; instead, they have intrinsic value that promotes the organism's survival and reproductive success. Natural reinforcers play a crucial role in shaping behavior and motivation. The consumption of food is a fundamental natural reinforcer. Nutrient-rich foods are essential for survival, and the pleasure associated with eating helps ensure that individuals maintain a healthy diet. Water is a primary natural reinforcer, crucial for maintaining hydration and sustaining life. The sensation of thirst motivates organisms to seek and consume water. Social interactions, including bonding, companionship, and positive social experiences, are powerful natural reinforcers. Human and many animal species exhibit a strong drive for social connection. Sexual activity is a natural reinforcer that is essential for the reproduction of many species.

Understanding the temporal dynamics of dopamine release is crucial. Studies employing fast-scan cyclic voltammetry have provided real-time insights into the dynamic changes in extracellular dopamine levels during the experience of natural rewards. This has shed light on the rapid and phasic nature of dopamine signaling (Howe & Dombeck, 2016). The temporal aspects of dopamine release have implications for reward prediction and reinforcement learning, contributing to our understanding of how the brain encodes the anticipation and receipt of natural rewards. Dopamine release in response to natural rewards is a multifaceted process, involving intricate neural mechanisms.

Neuroimaging studies and animal research collectively contribute to our understanding of how dopamine, as a neurotransmitter, participates in the complex orchestration of the brain's reward system in the face of natural rewards. The mesolimbic dopamine pathway, particularly the VTA-NAc axis, is a central player in reward processing in response to natural reinforcers. Dopamine, a neurotransmitter associated with pleasure and reinforcement, is released in the NAc in response to natural rewards, influencing motivation and learning (Schultz, 2015). The prefrontal cortex, especially the OFC and mPFC, is crucial for decision-making related to natural rewards. It integrates sensory information, emotional valence, and cognitive processes to guide adaptive behaviors (Wallis, 2007). The hippocampus is involved in encoding and retrieving contextual information associated with natural rewards (Shohamy & Adcock, 2010), contributing to memory formation and the contextual understanding of rewarding stimuli.

Dopamine-the neurotransmitter of reward: Dopamine, a monoamine neurotransmitter, has long been recognized as a central player in the brain's reward system. Its intricate role in mediating pleasure, motivation, and reinforcement makes it a cornerstone in understanding the neural basis of reward. It is primarily synthesized in the ventral tegmental area (VTA) and substantia nigra, and it exerts its effects through various pathways, notably the mesolimbic and mesocortical systems. Dopamine release is linked to reward prediction and reinforcement learning, forming the basis for associative learning and motivated behavior. The consumption of food, a fundamental natural reward, leads to dopamine release in brain regions such as the nucleus accumbens, reinforcing eating behavior. Positive social interactions, another natural reward, have been linked to dopamine release, emphasizing the role of this neurotransmitter in social motivation. Dysregulation of the dopaminergic system is implicated in addiction, where substances or behaviors lead to abnormal dopamine release, reinforcing addictive patterns (Lüscher& Malenka, 2011). Dopamine stands at the forefront of neurotransmitters governing reward processing. Its intricate involvement in natural rewards, social interactions, and the dysregulation seen in disorders underscores its central role in shaping behavior and motivation.

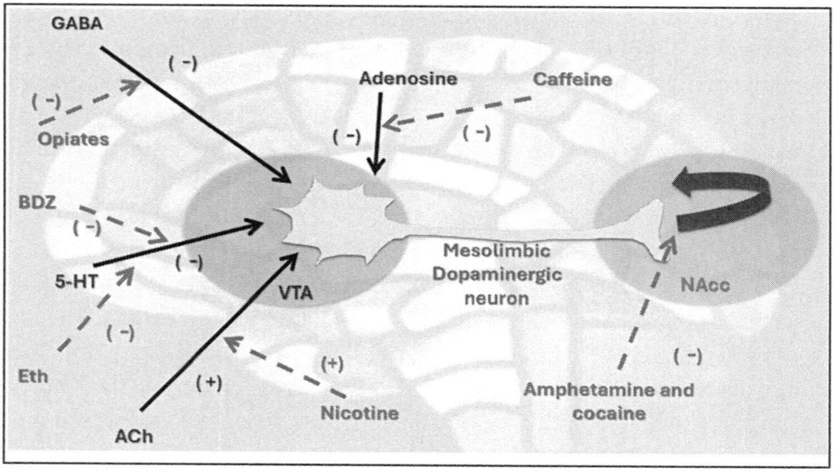

Dopamine-the neurotransmitter of reward

Psychostimulants such as amphetamine and methylphenidate, primarily target the central nervous system to enhance alertness, attention, and energy levels. One of the key mechanisms through which they achieve these effects is by increasing the levels of neurotransmitters, particularly dopamine, in the brain. Psychostimulants enhance the release of dopamine from presynaptic nerve terminals into the synaptic cleft. This increased availability of dopamine in the synapse leads to heightened stimulation of postsynaptic receptors, contributing to the drugs' stimulant effects (Sulzer, 2011). Additionally, some psychostimulants inhibit the reuptake of dopamine by presynaptic neurons. By blocking the reuptake transporters, these drugs prolong the presence of dopamine in the synapse, intensifying the signaling between neurons and enhancing dopaminergic activity. Amphetamines, for example, bind to the dopamine transporter, promoting the release of dopamine from synaptic vesicles. This process is mediated by the interaction of amphetamines with vesicular monoamine transporter 2 (VMAT2), leading to increased cytoplasmic dopamine levels (Volkow et al., 2007). Understanding the role of dopamine in the mechanism of psychostimulants has clinical implications, especially in the treatment of attention deficit hyperactivity disorder (ADHD) and narcolepsy, where drugs like methylphenidate and amphetamines are commonly used.

Benzodiazepines (BDZ) primarily interact with the GABA system, they do not directly modulate dopamine levels. It has been reported that benzodiazepines increase firing of dopamine neurons of the ventral tegmental area through the positive modulation of GABA(A) (gamma-aminobutyric acid type A) receptors in nearby interneurons (Tan et al., 2010). BDZ actions on the mesocorticolimbic dopamine system are similar to other drugs of abuse. Specifically, BDZs increase dopamine release from the ventral tegmental area onto target mesolimbic structures through a disinhibition mechanism, where BDZ binding to the GABA-A receptors expressed on the VTA GABAergic interneurons leads to inhibition of the interneurons and the subsequent increased activation of the dopaminergic projection neurons (Tan et al., 2011). Such a disinhibition-based mechanism is shared by some other drugs of abuse, such as opioids. In addition, like other drugs of abuse, a single injection of BDZs can cause VTA synaptic plasticity in the form of increased ratio of α-amino-3-hydroxy-5-methyl-4-isoxazolepropionic acid (AMPA) to N-methyl-D-aspartate (NMDA) receptor-mediated excitatory currents in the VTA for at least 3 days post-injection (Heikkinen et al., 2009).

These physiological data provide a mechanistic explanation for the above behavioral findings noting self-administration of α1-preferring compounds and reduced ability of α1-sparing compounds to sustain self-administration. Over the span of three decades, a substantial body of evidence has underscored the involvement of dopamine D3 receptors in opioid abuse disorders. Firstly, D3R is strategically distributed in key areas of the mesolimbic DA system, including the ventral striatum, midbrain, and ventral pallidum. These regions have been linked to behaviors governed by opioid-associated cues, implicating D3R in the neural circuitry underlying addiction. Secondly, the repeated exposure to opioids induces neuroadaptations in the D3R system, further emphasizing their role in the development and maintenance of addictive behaviors. Thirdly, the synthesis and characterization of highly potent and selective D3 receptor antagonists/partial agonists have reinforced the notion of D3 receptor as promising targets in the context of opioids abuse.

Building on extensive preclinical and preliminary clinical evidence, D3 receptor emerges as a promising target for the development of pharmacotherapies for opioid abuse. This potential is reflected in their ability to regulate the motivation to self-administer drugs and disrupt responsiveness to drug-associated stimuli, pivotal factors in the reinstatement of drug-seeking behavior triggered by re-exposure to the drug, drug-associated environmental cues, or stress. Notably, the discovery that highly selective D3 receptor antagonists, such as R-VK4-116 and R-VK4-40, do not adversely affect peripheral biometrics or cardiovascular effects, either alone or in the presence of substances like oxycodone or cocaine (Newman et al., 2023) suggests a promising safety profile for this class of drugs. This finding raises the prospect of using these compounds in the safe and effective treatment of opioid abuse disorders, providing a potential breakthrough in addiction medicine.

Dopaminergic Pathways involved in drug abuse: Understanding the neurobiological underpinnings of drug abuse is crucial for developing effective interventions. Neurochemical effects of abused drugs are mediated via mesolimbic and mesocortical pathways in the brain, involving intricate neural circuits that contribute to addictive behaviors. Mesolimbic pathway is a central component of the brain's reward system. Key structures involved include the ventral tegmental area and the nucleus accumbens (Wise, 2004). The mesolimbic pathway, a critical neural circuit in the brain, plays a pivotal role in mediating the experience of reward and reinforcement. Dopamine is the primary neurotransmitter involved in the mesolimbic pathway. It has a significant role in transmitting signals related to reward and reinforcement (Schultz, 2015). The ventral tegmental area (VTA) is a key region within the mesolimbic pathway. Dopaminergic neurons in the VTA project to various regions, including the nucleus accumbens (NAc), amygdala, and prefrontal cortex. Dopamine is implicated in motivation and the experience of pleasure associated with rewarding stimuli. Drugs of abuse, including cocaine, amphetamines, and opioids, exert their reinforcing effects by increasing dopamine levels in the mesolimbic system. This drug-induced dopamine release is a crucial factor in the development and maintenance of addictive behaviors. Dopamine in the mesolimbic pathway is involved in reinforcement learning, influencing behavior based on rewarding outcomes.

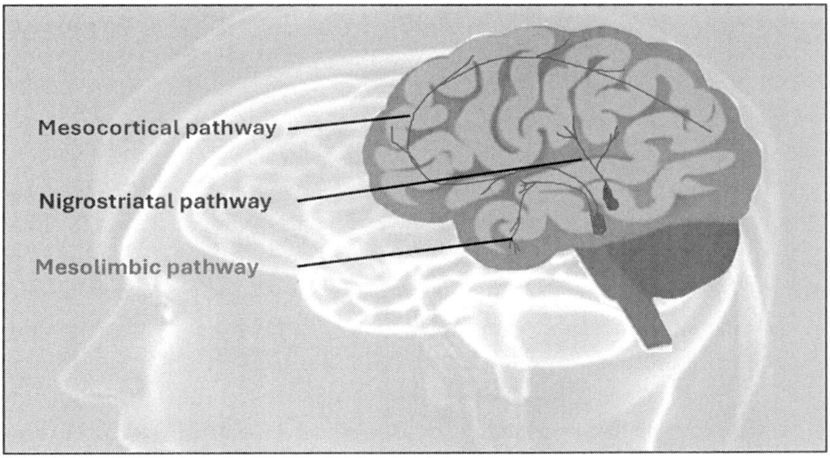

Dopaminergic pathways involved in addiction

Dopaminergic projections from the VTA to the NAc contribute to the encoding of reward prediction errors. In summary, dopamine is central to the function of the mesolimbic pathway, and its activity in this circuitry underlies the processing of reward, reinforcement, motivation, and the development of behaviors associated with addiction and pleasure. The nucleus accumbens is a key structure within the mesolimbic pathway, often referred to as its "pleasure center." The NAc is central to the processing of rewarding stimuli and the experience of pleasure. The NAc is implicated in motivation and the experience of pleasure associated with rewarding stimuli. The mesolimbic pathway stands as a crucial neural substrate in the intricate network of reward and reinforcement processing. Understanding its role in both natural and drug-induced rewards provides valuable insights into the fundamental mechanisms underlying behavior and holds potential for therapeutic interventions in disorders involving reward dysregulation. Mesocortical Pathway has an important role in executive functions, decision-making, and emotional regulation. Key structures include prefrontal cortex and the cingulate cortex. Modulation of dopamine in the mesocortical pathway has strong impact on cognitive processes and it is also involved in drug associated cognitive behavior (Grace, 2000).

Dysregulation in this pathway is implicated in cognitive deficits observed in drug addiction. Mesocortical pathway is involved in inhibitory control and decision-making, crucial factors in addiction. Discuss studies linking dysfunction in the mesocortical pathway to impulsive behaviors and poor decision-making observed in individuals with substance use disorders. Mesolimbic and mesocortical pathways communicate and integrate information demonstrating the reciprocal connectivity between the VTA, NAc, and PFC (Grace, 2016). Individual differences in the functioning of these pathways may contribute to addiction vulnerability. Studies investigating genetic and environmental factors influence the interplay between these pathways and their implications for susceptibility to drug abuse (Haile et al., 2007). The mesolimbic and mesocortical pathways play integral roles in the neurobiology of drug abuse, shaping reward processing, decision-making, and emotional regulation. A deeper understanding of these pathways provides a foundation for developing targeted interventions aimed at mitigating the impact of addictive substances on the brain.

The dopamine reward hypothesis: The dopamine reward hypothesis posits that the neurotransmitter dopamine plays a central role in the brain's reward system and is implicated in the experience of pleasure, reinforcement, and motivation. Dopamine is a key neurotransmitter involved in reward processing and reinforcement. It is associated with the hedonic aspects of reward, contributing to the subjective experience of pleasure. Dopamine is also implicated in reinforcement learning, influencing behavior based on rewarding outcomes. Dopamine is involved in the processing of natural rewards, such as food and social interactions. Drugs of abuse, such as cocaine and amphetamines, exert their reinforcing effects by increasing dopamine levels in the brain. Dysregulation of the dopamine system is implicated in addiction, with heightened dopamine release associated with drug-seeking behavior. Dopaminergic neurons are involved in signaling reward prediction errors, contributing to reinforcement learning. Dopamine is implicated in motivational processes, influencing goal-directed behavior.

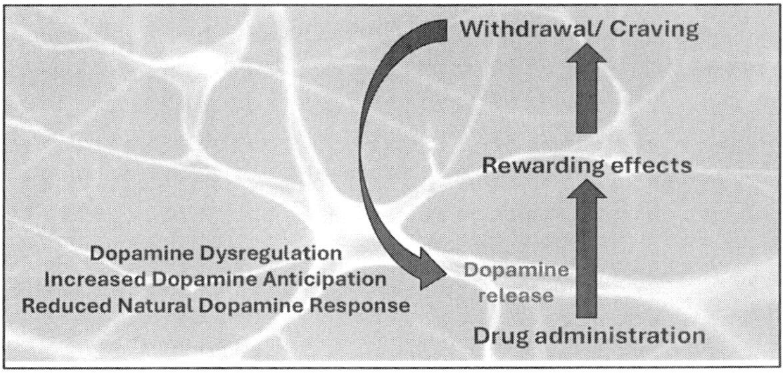

Dopamine hypothesis of addiction

Drug abuse significantly affects dopamine levels in the brain, and alterations in dopamine neurotransmission are often associated with the reinforcing effects of drugs. Cocaine is known to inhibit the reuptake of dopamine in the synapses, leading to increased dopamine levels in the brain. Amphetamines, such as methamphetamine, promote the release of dopamine and inhibit its reuptake, leading to elevated synaptic dopamine levels. Opioids can indirectly influence dopamine levels by modulating the activity of dopamine neurons in the mesolimbic pathway. Nicotine stimulates dopamine release, primarily in the mesolimbic pathway, contributing to the reinforcing effects of smoking. Alcohol can modulate dopamine release, although its effects are complex and can vary depending on the dose and brain region.

Various drugs influence dopamine release through different mechanisms, leading to alterations in the brain's reward system. Many drugs, such as cocaine, amphetamines (e.g., methamphetamine), and methylphenidate, block the reuptake of dopamine, leading to increased synaptic dopamine levels. Certain drugs, including direct dopamine agonists like apomorphine, stimulate dopamine receptors, mimicking the effects of dopamine. Drugs like amphetamines and MDMA (ecstasy) can increase the release of dopamine from presynaptic neurons, leading to elevated dopamine levels in the synaptic cleft (Rothman et al., 2001). Opioids, such as heroin and morphine, indirectly influence dopamine release by modulating the activity of dopamine neurons in the mesolimbic pathway. Nicotine, found in tobacco, stimulates dopamine release in the mesolimbic pathway, contributing to the rewarding effects of smoking. Alcohol can modulate dopamine release, although its effects are complex and can vary depending on the dose and brain region. These mechanisms demonstrate the diverse ways in which drugs can impact dopamine release, contributing to the reinforcing effects and addictive potential of these substances. Understanding these mechanisms is crucial for developing targeted interventions for substance use disorders.

Understanding the neurochemical changes resulting due to drug abuse can help explore the affecting neurotransmitter systems and neural circuits associated with reward, motivation, and control. It's important to note that the neurobiology of drug abuse is complex and involves interactions between multiple neurotransmitter systems and brain regions. Chronic drug abuse, especially of substances like cocaine and amphetamines, can lead to alterations in the dopamine system, including changes in dopamine release, receptor sensitivity, and reuptake. Drugs such as MDMA (ecstasy) and hallucinogens can impact the serotonin system, leading to changes in serotonin release and receptor function. Opioid drugs, including heroin and prescription opioids, can induce adaptations in the endogenous opioid system, affecting opioid receptor signaling. The glutamatergic system, particularly involving the neurotransmitter glutamate, undergoes adaptations during drug abuse, impacting synaptic plasticity and learning. Drugs like alcohol and benzodiazepines can affect the gamma-aminobutyric acid (GABA) system, leading to changes in inhibitory neurotransmission. Cannabis abuse can impact the endocannabinoid system, influencing endogenous cannabinoid receptor signaling. Chronic drug abuse can lead to dysregulation of stress-related systems, including changes in corticotropin-releasing factor (CRF) and the hypothalamic-pituitary-adrenal (HPA) axis.

Dopamine and Reinforcement: Dopamine release in the nucleus accumbens is associated with the rewarding aspects of drug use, contributing to the reinforcement of drug-seeking behavior. Dopamine plays a crucial role in associative learning, linking environmental cues with the rewarding effects of drugs and contributing to the development of drug-related behaviors. Dopamine is involved in the hedonic experience of pleasure, and drug-induced increases in dopamine levels contribute to the subjective rewarding effects of drugs (Berridge & Kringelbach, 2015). Understanding the intricate relationship between dopamine release and the reinforcing effects of drugs is crucial for comprehending the neurobiological basis of addiction. It involves complex interactions within the brain's reward circuitry and provides insights into potential targets for addiction treatment.

Dopamine mediating the abusive effects of different types of drugs: Dopamine plays a crucial role in mediating the abusive effects of stimulant drugs, contributing to their reinforcing properties and the development of addiction. Stimulant drugs, such as cocaine and amphetamines, increase extracellular dopamine levels in the brain, particularly in the mesolimbic pathway. Dopamine release in key reward-related areas, including the nucleus accumbens (NAc), is associated with the reinforcing effects of stimulant drugs. The mesolimbic dopamine pathway, originating in the ventral tegmental area (VTA) and projecting to the NAc, is critically involved in the rewarding effects of stimulants (Koob & Volkow, 2010). Dopamine release in response to stimulant use contributes to the associative learning between drug-related cues and the rewarding effects, promoting drug-seeking behavior. Chronic stimulant use induces neuroplastic changes in the dopamine system, including alterations in receptor sensitivity and signaling pathways. Dopamine mediates the hedonic experience of pleasure and euphoria associated with stimulant use, reinforcing the desire for repeated drug consumption.

Dopamine also plays a role in mediating the abusive effects of opioids, though the mechanism is distinct from stimulant drugs. Opioids primarily act on the endogenous opioid system, but their interaction with dopamine systems contributes to the reinforcing properties and addictive potential. Opioids, such as heroin and prescription opioids, can indirectly influence dopamine release in certain brain regions, including the nucleus accumbens, by modulating the activity of dopamine neurons. While opioids primarily act on the endogenous opioid system, their interaction with the mesolimbic dopamine pathway contributes to the rewarding effects and reinforcement of opioid use. Opioids, particularly during the initial use, can enhance dopamine release in the nucleus accumbens, a critical brain region involved in reward and reinforcement. Dopamine is implicated in reward-related learning processes, and the interaction between opioids and the dopamine system contributes to the formation of associations between drug-related cues and the pleasurable effects of opioids. Chronic opioid use can lead to dysregulation of the dopamine system, contributing to the development of addiction and drug-seeking behavior. Understanding the interplay between opioids and the dopamine system sheds light on the neurobiological mechanisms of opioid addiction. It also provides insights into potential targets for intervention and treatment strategies for opioid use disorders.

Benzodiazepines primarily act on the gamma-aminobutyric acid (GABA) system rather than directly interacting with the dopamine system. However, there are some indirect ways in which benzodiazepines may influence dopamine transmission, particularly in relation to the reward pathway. Benzodiazepines primarily enhance the inhibitory actions of GABA. This GABAergic modulation can indirectly affect the activity of dopamine neurons. The GABAergic system, under the influence of benzodiazepines, may indirectly influence the firing rates of dopamine neurons in certain brain regions where GABAergic and dopaminergic systems converge, such as the nucleus accumbens. Individuals using benzodiazepines may be at risk for co-abuse with substances that directly affect dopamine, such as alcohol or stimulants. It's important to note that while benzodiazepines themselves are not considered substances of abuse for their effects on the dopamine system, there is a risk of abuse and dependence due to their calming and anxiolytic effects. Moreover, co-abuse with substances that directly affect dopamine transmission may occur in some cases. The interaction between benzodiazepines and dopamine is a complex area that requires further research for a more comprehensive

While alcohol primarily interacts with the gamma-aminobutyric acid (GABA) system, it also influences the mesolimbic dopaminergic pathway, which plays a key role in reward and reinforcement. Acute alcohol exposure has been shown to increase dopamine release in the nucleus accumbens, contributing to the rewarding effects of alcohol consumption. Dopamine signaling in the mesolimbic system is involved in the motivational aspects of alcohol-seeking behavior, contributing to the development and persistence of alcohol use (Koob & Volkow, 2010). Dopamine release in response to alcohol consumption is associated with the positive reinforcement and pleasurable effects that contribute to the reinforcing properties of alcohol. Chronic alcohol use can lead to dysregulation of the dopamine system, contributing to the development of alcohol use disorder. Dopamine's role in reward processing is implicated in the positive reinforcement associated with alcohol consumption, contributing to the development of alcohol dependence. Understanding the involvement of dopamine in the abuse of alcohol provides insights into the neurobiological basis of alcohol use disorders and may inform strategies for treatment and intervention.

Hallucinogens, such as lysergic acid diethylamide (LSD), psilocybin (found in certain mushrooms), and dimethyltryptamine (DMT), have complex effects on neurotransmitter systems, including dopamine. While the precise mechanisms are not fully understood, dopamine modulation is thought to contribute to the subjective effects of hallucinogens. Hallucinogens, particularly those that interact with serotonin receptors (e.g., 5-HT2A), can indirectly influence dopamine release and transmission. Hallucinogens may activate the mesolimbic dopamine pathway, which is associated with reward and reinforcement (Gouzoulis-Mayfrank et al., 2002).

The primary action of hallucinogens is on serotonin receptors, but their influence on serotonin transmission can indirectly affect dopamine systems in interconnected brain regions (Halberstadt et al., 2010). The perceptual and cognitive effects induced by hallucinogens are believed to involve complex interactions between serotonin and dopamine systems. The alteration of perception and sensory experiences induced by hallucinogens may be related to changes in dopamine transmission in certain brain regions. It's important to note that while dopamine is involved, the primary action of hallucinogens is on serotonin receptors, and their effects are complex and multifaceted. The interplay between serotonin and dopamine systems contributes to the unique subjective experiences associated with hallucinogen use.

Dopamine and the development of tolerance: The role of dopamine in the development of tolerance to drugs of abuse is a complex and multifaceted process. Tolerance refers to a reduced response to a drug after repeated or prolonged exposure. Chronic exposure to drugs of abuse, such as stimulants or opioids, can lead to adaptations in the dopaminergic system. These adaptations may include synaptic plasticity involving changes in the strength and efficiency of synaptic connections between neurons. Long-term potentiation (LTP) and long-term depression (LTD) are forms of synaptic plasticity associated with learning and memory. Neurons can undergo structural changes, including alterations in dendritic branching, spine density, and axonal growth. These changes contribute to the remodeling of neural circuits. Changes in the expression of neurotransmitter receptors at synapses can occur in response to various stimuli. This includes upregulation or downregulation of receptors, affecting synaptic transmission (Nestler, 2001). Learning experiences induce adaptations in neuronal circuits, involving the strengthening or weakening of specific connections. This process is crucial for encoding and retrieving information. These adaptive changes contribute to the development and maintenance of addiction. Neuronal circuits can undergo homeostatic plasticity to maintain overall stability in activity levels. This may involve adjustments in synaptic strength to counterbalance prolonged changes in network activity. Understanding adaptations in neuronal circuits is fundamental to unraveling the mechanisms underlying learning, memory, and various neurological and psychiatric conditions, including addiction. Research in this area contributes to the development of therapeutic interventions aimed at modulating neural plasticity for beneficial outcomes.

Another mechanism involved in the development of tolerance is the downregulation of dopamine receptors. Prolonged exposure to drugs can result in a downregulation of dopamine receptors, reducing the expression of dopaminergic receptors. This could be mediated through decrease in the number of dopamine receptors in neuronal circuits. This phenomenon is observed in response to chronic exposure to certain substances, including drugs of abuse, and is a key aspect of neuroadaptations associated with addiction (Nestler, 2005). There are different types of dopamine receptors, including D1-like receptors (e.g., D1 and D5) and D2-like receptors (e.g.,

D2, D3, and D4) which could be downregulated. Downregulation can occur at various subtypes. Downregulation of dopamine autoreceptors leads to a decreased feedback inhibition of dopaminergic release resulting in an increased dopaminergic neurotransmission and potentiating addictive effects of drugs of abuse.

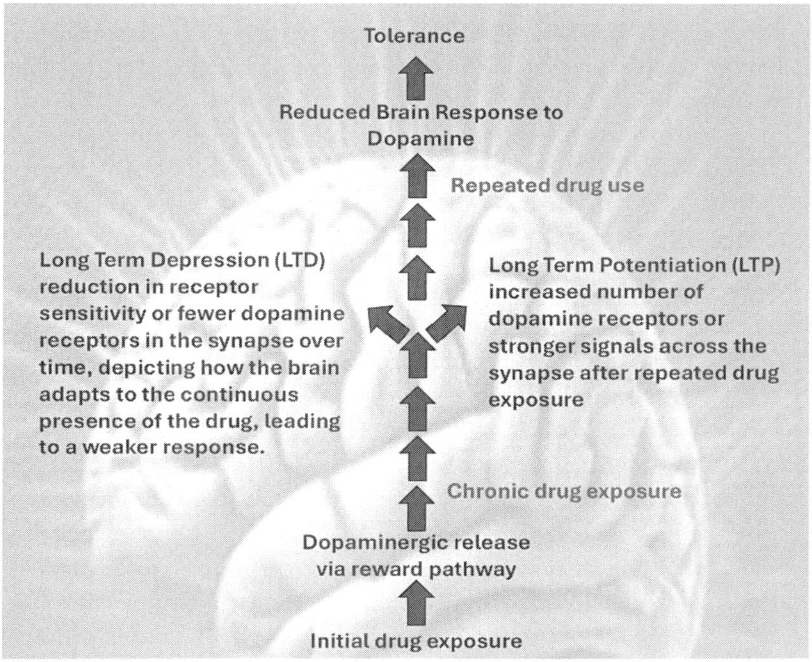

Dopamine in the development of tolerance

Downregulation is considered a compensatory mechanism in response to the increased levels of dopamine signaling induced by chronic drug use. It represents the brain's attempt to maintain homeostasis. This is implicated in the development of tolerance, a process where higher doses of a drug are required to achieve the same effect. Studying the downregulation of dopamine receptors provides insights into the neurobiological mechanisms of addiction and contributes to the development of therapeutic strategies aimed at restoring normal dopaminergic function in individuals affected by substance use disorders. Desensitization of dopamine receptors is another mechanism leading to the development of tolerance upon repeated administration of drugs of abuse. As a result of desensitization receptors become less responsive to the presence of dopamine. Desensitization of dopamine receptors refers to a process in which repeated or prolonged exposure to dopamine or dopamine-mimicking substances leads to a reduced responsiveness or sensitivity of the receptors. This phenomenon is a form of receptor adaptation and is observed in various contexts, including drug exposure and certain neurological and psychiatric conditions. Desensitization occurs when dopamine receptors are exposed to high levels of stimulation for an extended period. This can happen with chronic exposure to drugs of abuse or in response to persistent endogenous dopamine release (Gainetdinov et al., 2004).

Repeated stimulation of dopamine receptors triggers intracellular signaling pathways that lead to the phosphorylation of the receptors. This can result in the internalization of receptors, reducing their presence on the cell surface. Desensitization may involve the downregulation of dopamine receptors on the cell surface. Desensitization contributes to the development of tolerance, where an individual becomes less responsive to the effects of a drug over time. This is a common phenomenon observed in the context of substance use (Grace & Gomes, 2019). Understanding the mechanisms of dopamine receptor desensitization provides insights into potential therapeutic targets for conditions involving aberrant dopamine signaling. Desensitization of dopamine receptors is a complex process that can have significant implications for both normal brain function and the development of neuropsychiatric disorders.

Further research in this area is essential for developing targeted interventions for conditions associated with dysregulated dopamine receptor sensitivity. Repeated administration of abused drugs can alter the regulation of dopamine release, affecting the dynamics of neurotransmitter release and reuptake. Alterations in dopamine release refer to changes in the amount, pattern, or regulation of dopamine neurotransmitter release in the brain. These alterations can occur in response to various factors, including exposure to drugs, stress, or other environmental stimuli. Drug abuse can enhance dopamine release. Amphetamines, for example, increase the release of dopamine from presynaptic neurons into the synaptic cleft.

Chronic drug use or exposure to stressors can lead to impaired regulation of dopamine release. This can contribute to dysregulated reward processing and addiction. Dopamine release in reward pathways, such as the mesolimbic system, plays a crucial role in motivation and reinforcement. Alterations in this release can impact the experience of pleasure and reward. Neuroplastic changes could be induced upon repeated drug administration resulting in the regulation of dopamine release. These changes involve alterations in synaptic strength and connectivity (Kalivas & Volkow, 2005). Dopamine release is involved in reinforcement and conditioning processes, influencing learning and behavior. Alterations in dopamine release can impact these fundamental aspects of cognition. Understanding alterations in dopamine release is critical for unraveling the neurobiology of addiction, mental health disorders, and normal brain function. Research in this area informs the development of therapeutic strategies aimed at restoring balance in dopamine signaling for improved mental health outcomes. Chronic drug exposure can shift the threshold for experiencing reward, requiring higher doses of the drug to achieve the same level of pleasure or reinforcement. The development of tolerance involves a combination of molecular, cellular, and circuit-level adaptations, and dopamine plays a central role in these processes. These adaptations contribute to the progression of drug addiction and the challenges associated with treatment.

Dopamine and the development of behavioral sensitization: Sensitization, an increased response to a drug with repeated use, involves complex interactions within the dopaminergic system. Behavioral sensitization is a phenomenon where repeated exposure to a stimulus, such as a drug of abuse, leads to an amplified behavioral response over time. Dopamine plays a crucial role in the development of behavioral sensitization, particularly in the context of drug addiction. Dopaminergic neurotransmission via mesolimbic pathway, is central to the development of behavioral sensitization. It is implicated in the increased responsiveness to drugs of abuse and other stimuli with repeated exposure (Wang et al., 2023). Behavioral sensitization also induces changes in neural circuits involving dopamine, particularly within the mesolimbic and mesocortical pathways.

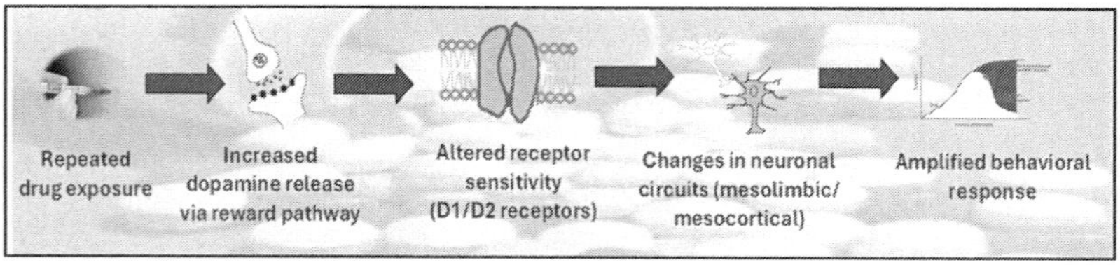

Dopamine and the development of behavioral sensitization

Chronic exposure to drugs induces changes in dopamine receptor sensitivity, contributing to the sensitized response. This involves alterations in D1-like and D2-like receptor signaling. Repeated exposure to drugs of abuse leads to sensitization of dopamine receptors. This involves an increased responsiveness to dopamine, often observed in both D1-like and D2-like receptor subtypes. Sensitization is associated with altered function of both D1 and D2 receptors. Changes in the balance between these receptor subtypes contribute to the sensitized behavioral response to stimuli. Behavioral sensitization is often accompanied by an increase in dopamine release in response to the drug or stimulus. This heightened release contributes to the sensitized behavioral response. Behavioral sensitization is associated with neuroplastic changes in dopaminergic circuits, including alterations in synaptic plasticity and neuronal activity. Behavioral sensitization is associated with neuroplastic changes in the brain, particularly within the mesolimbic dopamine system by forming new synaptic connections and modifying existing ones (Vanderschuren & Pierce, 2010). Chronic exposure to drugs of abuse can induce structural changes in neurons, including dendritic remodeling. This involves alterations in the branching and morphology of dendrites. Neuroplastic changes associated with sensitization include alterations in synaptic transmission, such as changes in the release of neurotransmitters like dopamine and glutamate. Long-term potentiation, a form of synaptic plasticity associated with learning and memory, may be involved in the neuroplastic changes underlying behavioral sensitization.

Behavioral sensitization is associated with changes in dopamine receptor sensitivity, including alterations in the expression and function of D1 and D2 receptor subtypes. Behavioral sensitization involves an increased response to a stimulus, often observed with repeated exposure to drugs of abuse. Dopamine receptor sensitivity plays a crucial role in this process, especially within the mesolimbic dopamine system. Behavioral sensitization is also associated with alterations in dopamine reuptake mechanisms. Increased dopamine release and impaired reuptake contribute to heightened receptor sensitivity. Both D1-like (e.g., D1) and D2-like (e.g., D2) receptor subtypes undergo sensitization. Changes in receptor sensitivity are observed in response to chronic exposure to drugs of abuse. Sensitization involves alterations in intracellular signaling pathways downstream of dopamine receptors. These changes contribute to long-lasting modifications in receptor sensitivity. D1 receptor signaling undergoes neuroadaptations, leading to enhanced sensitivity. This is particularly relevant to the development and expression of behavioral sensitization. D2 receptor sensitivity changes are also critical in the development of behavioral sensitization. Neuroadaptations in D2 receptor function contribute to the persistent effects of drug exposure. Dopamine receptor sensitivity changes occur at the circuit level, influencing the communication and integration of signals within the mesolimbic pathway (Lüscher & Malenka, 2011).

Sensitization involves circuit-level changes within the mesolimbic dopamine pathway, affecting the connectivity and communication between key brain regions. Behavioral sensitization, the heightened behavioral response to a stimulus with repeated exposure, is closely associated with circuit-level changes in the brain. These changes involve alterations in neural circuits, especially within the mesolimbic dopamine system. Behavioral sensitization causes adaptations and in the mesolimbic dopamine system, a key neural pathway involved in reward and reinforcement. The neural circuits within the mesolimbic pathway, undergo adaptations in response to repeated exposure to drugs of abuse, leading to long-lasting changes in behavior. Nucleus accumbens, the critical component of the mesolimbic system, is particularly implicated in circuit-level changes associated with behavioral sensitization. Repeated exposure to drugs of abuse leads to alterations in dopamine release and transmission, affecting the communication between neurons in the mesolimbic circuit. Circuit-level changes involve corticostriatal pathways, where communication between the prefrontal cortex and the striatum is modified during the development of behavioral sensitization. The amygdala and hippocampus, regions associated with emotional processing and memory, also play a role in circuit-level changes during behavioral sensitization (Ungless & Grace, 2012). These circuit-level changes associated with behavioral sensitization are crucial for comprehending the neurobiological mechanisms underlying addiction. These changes involve a complex interplay of neurotransmitter systems and contribute to the persistent behavioral alterations observed in individuals with a history of repeated drug exposure. Targeting these neuroplastic changes may offer potential therapeutic strategies for preventing or reversing the persistent behavioral responses associated with chronic drug exposure.

Dopamine also interacts with glutamate to play an integral role in the development of behavioral sensitization. Glutamate, the primary excitatory neurotransmitter in the brain, plays a crucial role in synaptic plasticity and learning. Glutamate transmission, particularly within the mesolimbic pathway, is involved in the neuroadaptive changes associated with behavioral sensitization. Changes in glutamate release and receptor function contribute to the long-lasting alterations in synaptic strength observed during sensitization (Wolf, 2016). The interaction between dopamine and glutamate systems is critical for the expression of behavioral sensitization. Dopamine and glutamate transmission in the NAc interact, and their combined effects contribute to the persistent changes in synaptic plasticity. N-methyl-D-aspartate (NMDA) receptors, a subtype of glutamate receptors, are also implicated in the development of behavioral sensitization. NMDA receptor activation is involved in the induction of synaptic plasticity and the modulation of dopamine release. Both dopamine and glutamate contribute to drug-induced plasticity in the NAc, leading to persistent changes in synaptic strength and behavior. This plasticity is considered a key mechanism underlying the expression of behavioral sensitization. This intricate interplay between dopamine and glutamate in the context of behavioral sensitization provides insights into the neurobiological mechanisms of addiction. Targeting these neurotransmitter systems may offer potential avenues for therapeutic interventions aimed at preventing or mitigating the persistent behavioral changes associated with repeated drug exposure. In short, behavioral sensitization is considered a form of neural plasticity that contributes to the progression of addiction, leading to increased drug-seeking and drug-taking behaviors. Understanding the role of dopamine in behavioral sensitization is essential for elucidating the neural mechanisms underlying addiction. It provides insights into potential targets for therapeutic interventions aimed at preventing or reducing the sensitized responses associated with chronic drug exposure.

Dopamine and the development of craving and relapse: Dopamine, craving, and relapse are interconnected elements in the context of addiction. Dopamine plays a central role in the development of craving—a strong desire or urge for the substance of abuse. Craving, in turn, is a significant predictor of relapse, marking the return to drug-seeking and drug-taking behaviors after a period of abstinence. Dopamine is a key neurotransmitter in the brain's reward system, particularly within the mesolimbic pathway. Craving and relapse to abused drugs might be mediated by a drop in dopamine release, creating compulsive desire of drug intake. Craving is associated with increased activity in brain regions involved in reward, such as the nucleus accumbens (NAc). Dopamine release in the NAc is heightened during craving, reinforcing the motivation to seek and consume drugs.

Drug cravings are mediated by neuroadaptations in the dopamine system, leading to persistent changes in receptor sensitivity and function. These neuroadaptations contribute to the enduring nature of craving, even during periods of abstinence. Neuroadaptations in the brain are fundamental processes that occur in response to repeated drug exposure and play a significant role in the development and persistence of drug cravings. These adaptations involve changes in the neural circuits, neurotransmitter systems, and molecular pathways, contributing to the enduring nature of cravings in individuals with substance use disorders. Chronic drug use leads to alterations in the dopamine system, including changes in dopamine release, receptor sensitivity, and signaling pathways. Enhanced dopamine release during drug use and withdrawal periods contributes to the reinforcement of drug-seeking behaviors and the development of cravings. The mesolimbic dopamine pathway, involving brain regions such as the nucleus accumbens, undergoes neuroplastic changes in response to drug exposure. Structural and functional adaptations within this pathway contribute to the persistence of drug cravings.

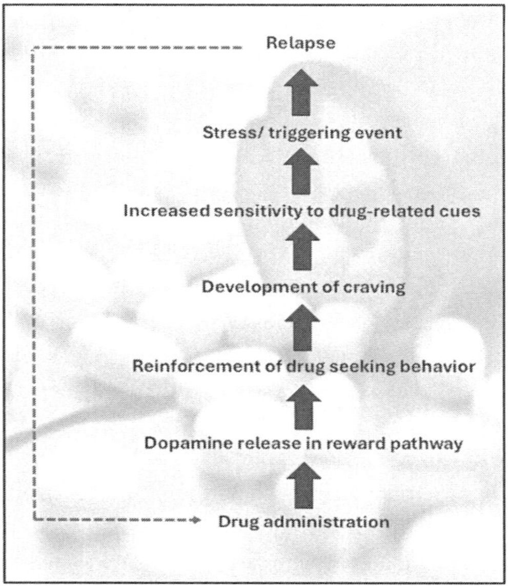

Dopamine and the development of craving and relapse

Long-lasting changes in synaptic plasticity occur in response to drug exposure, affecting the strength and efficacy of neuronal connections. Persistent synaptic alterations contribute to the encoding of drug-associated memories and the triggering of cravings in response to drug-related cues. Not only the drug but also the exposure to drug-related cues or contexts leads to cue-induced neuroadaptations, activating brain regions associated with cravings, such as the prefrontal cortex and amygdala. These neuroadaptations contribute to the heightened salience of drug cues and the persistence of cravings even in the absence of the drug. Apart from dopamine, dysregulation of various neurotransmitters, including dopamine, glutamate, gamma-aminobutyric acid (GABA), and serotonin, contributes to an imbalance that supports the maintenance of drug cravings. These neuroadaptations associated with drug cravings are crucial for developing effective strategies for addiction treatment and relapse prevention. Targeting these neurobiological changes may offer potential avenues for therapeutic interventions aimed at reducing the intensity and persistence of drug cravings in individuals recovering from substance use disorders. Craving is a significant predictor of relapse, and the intensity of craving often correlates with the likelihood of returning to drug use. Dopamine dysregulation, along with other neurobiological factors, contributes to the vulnerability to relapse. Understanding the relationship between craving and relapse is essential for developing effective strategies for addiction treatment and relapse prevention. Craving refers to an intense desire or urge to use a substance, often triggered by environmental cues, stress, or other factors associated with past drug use. Craving is a subjective experience that reflects the motivation to seek and consume the substance of abuse. Craving can persist long after the acute withdrawal phase, contributing to the chronic and relapsing nature of addiction. Persistent craving is a significant challenge for individuals in recovery, as it may continue even during periods of abstinence.

Environmental cues associated with drug use, such as places, people, or objects linked to past drug experiences, can trigger intense cravings. These cues can create a conditioned response, activating neural circuits associated with the anticipation of drug reward. Craving is closely linked to the dysregulation of dopamine, a neurotransmitter associated with reward and reinforcement. Environmental cues associated with drug use can lead to dopamine release in reward-related brain regions, contributing to the experience of craving (Volkow et al., 2008). Craving involves both psychological and physiological components. Psychologically, individuals may experience obsessive thoughts about using the substance. Physiologically, changes in heart rate, blood pressure, and stress hormones may accompany cravings.

The presence and intensity of craving are strong predictors of relapse. Higher levels of craving are associated with an increased likelihood of returning to drug use. Craving serves as a warning sign that an individual is at risk for relapse, highlighting the need for timely intervention. Recognizing and addressing craving is a key component of relapse prevention programs. Therapeutic interventions often focus on developing coping strategies to manage and reduce cravings. Cognitive-behavioral therapy and mindfulness-based approaches are commonly used to help individuals navigate and overcome cravings. Some medications target the neurobiological mechanisms underlying craving, aiming to reduce its intensity and frequency. Medications, such as those affecting dopamine, glutamate, or opioid receptors, may be used in conjunction with behavioral therapies. Recognizing the role of craving as a precursor to relapse underscores the importance of a comprehensive and individualized approach to addiction treatment. Strategies that address both the psychological and physiological aspects of craving, combined with ongoing support and relapse prevention efforts, are critical for improving long-term outcomes in individuals recovering from substance use disorders. Environmental cues associated with drug use can trigger conditioned responses that activate the dopamine system, leading to craving and an increased risk of relapse. Medications targeting the dopamine system, such as dopamine receptor agonists or antagonists, are explored as potential interventions for relapse prevention. Modulating dopamine function may help attenuate craving and reduce the likelihood of relapse. Coordination of dopamine, craving, and relapse provides insights into the neurobiology of addiction. Targeting dopamine-related mechanisms may offer potential therapeutic strategies for preventing and treating relapse in individuals with substance use disorders.

Dopamine system sensitivity following repeated drug abuse: Following repeated drug abuse, the sensitivity of the dopamine system undergoes significant changes, contributing to the development and persistence of addiction. These changes are part of the neuroadaptations that occur in response to chronic drug exposure. Chronic drug abuse leads to increased dopamine release in the brain's reward pathway, particularly in the nucleus accumbens. Over time, the brain adapts to the constant presence of the drug by altering dopamine release patterns. Prolonged exposure to drugs can lead to desensitization of dopamine receptors, specifically D2-like receptors (e.g., D2, D3, D4). Desensitization refers to a reduced responsiveness of receptors to dopamine signaling, requiring higher levels of dopamine to produce the same effect. Repeated drug exposure can lead to a downregulation of dopamine receptors, resulting in a decrease in the overall number of available receptors. Downregulation contributes to the development of tolerance, where higher doses of the drug are required to achieve the same effects. The downregulation of dopamine receptors is a complex process involving various molecular and cellular mechanisms.

Downregulation occurs as an adaptive response to prolonged exposure to elevated levels of dopamine, often resulting from chronic drug use.

Chronic exposure to high levels of dopamine leads to the internalization of dopamine receptors. Internalization involves the removal of receptors from the cell surface and their relocation to intracellular compartments. This process reduces the number of functional receptors available on the cell surface for dopamine binding. Prolonged activation of dopamine receptors by excessive dopamine levels results in receptor desensitization. Desensitization involves a reduction in the responsiveness of receptors to dopamine signaling, making the cells less sensitive to the neurotransmitter. Ubiquitination is a process by which small protein molecules called ubiquitins are attached to the dopamine receptors. Ubiquitinated receptors are then targeted for degradation by the proteasome, a cellular machinery responsible for breaking down and recycling proteins. This ubiquitin-proteasome system contributes to the removal of dopamine receptors from the cell membrane (Beaulieu et al., 2005). Dopamine receptors phosphorylation by protein kinases also causes their desensitization. Phosphorylated receptors can recruit arrestin proteins, which further contribute to receptor desensitization and internalization. These processes play a role in reducing the responsiveness of dopamine receptors to subsequent stimulation.

Persistent activation of dopamine receptors can trigger negative feedback mechanisms that downregulate dopamine receptor gene expression. Reduced synthesis of new receptors contributes to a decrease in the overall receptor population. Chronic exposure to drugs of abuse induces neuroadaptations in various intracellular signaling pathways associated with dopamine receptors. Altered signaling cascades contribute to changes in receptor sensitivity and expression levels. There are several molecular and cellular changes that occur in the brain following repeated drug abuse, contributing to the downregulation of dopamine receptors. These adaptations play a significant role in the development of tolerance, dependence, and addiction. The dopamine transporter, responsible for reuptake of dopamine from the synapse, may undergo changes following repeated drug use. Altered transporter activity can impact the duration and intensity of dopamine signaling in the synaptic cleft. Altered dopamine transporter (DAT) activity is a key aspect of the neuroadaptations that occur in response to chronic drug use. The dopamine transporter is responsible for reuptake of dopamine from the synapse, regulating the duration and intensity of dopamine signaling. Chronic exposure to drugs of abuse, such as psychostimulants (e.g., cocaine, amphetamines), can lead to a downregulation of dopamine transporter expression. Reduced dopamine transporter expression results in fewer transporters available to clear dopamine from the synaptic cleft, prolonging the presence of dopamine in the synapse (Mazei-Robison et al., 2008).

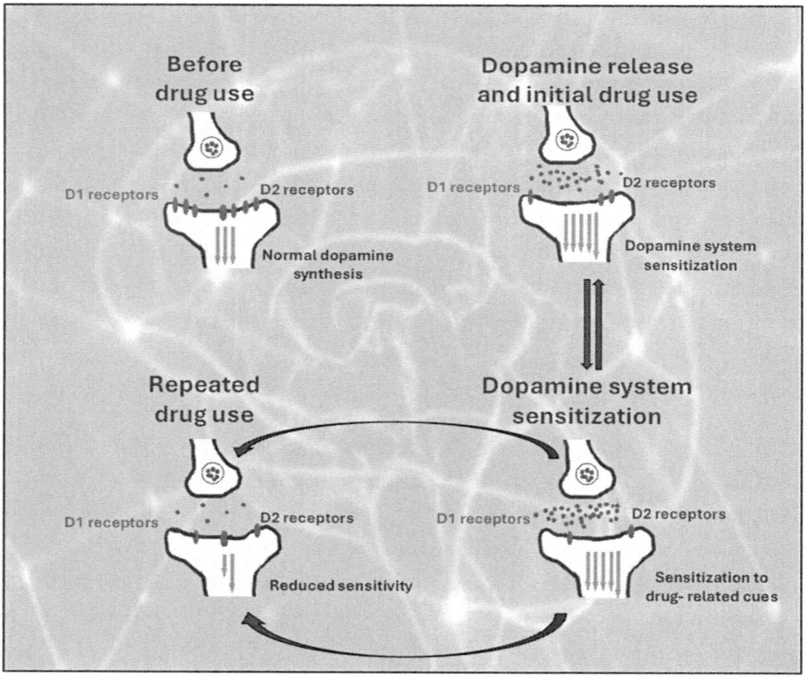

Dopamine system sensitivity following repeated drug abuse

Repeated exposure to drugs can also lead to the internalization and altered trafficking of the dopamine transporter (DAT). Internalization involves the removal of DAT from the cell surface, reducing its availability for dopamine reuptake. Altered trafficking may affect the subcellular distribution of DAT, impacting its function. Post-translational modifications, such as phosphorylation, ubiquitination, and palmitoylation, play a role in regulating DAT activity. Phosphorylation can influence DAT function, affecting its surface expression and reuptake capacity. Ubiquitination may target DAT for degradation, impacting its overall abundance. Palmitoylation can influence DAT membrane association and localization. Chronic drug exposure can lead to changes in the kinetic properties and affinity of the DAT for dopamine. Altered kinetics may affect the rate of dopamine reuptake, while changes in affinity may impact the transporter's sensitivity to dopamine concentrations. Chronic drug exposure can modulate the transcriptional and post-transcriptional regulation of the DAT gene. Changes in gene expression levels influence the overall abundance of DAT in the cell membrane. Interactions with intracellular proteins, including those involved in the regulation of vesicular trafficking and cytoskeletal dynamics, can influence DAT activity. Proteins such as syntaxin and α-synuclein have been implicated in modulating DAT function. This could explain how chronic drug exposure can lead to dysregulation of dopamine transporter activity, contributing to altered dopamine signaling and the neurobiology of addiction. Targeting these mechanisms may offer potential avenues for therapeutic interventions in substance use disorders. Chronic drug abuse induces persistent changes in synaptic plasticity within the reward pathway. These changes contribute to long-lasting alterations in the strength and efficacy of neuronal connections, maintaining the learned association between drug-related cues and the rewarding effects of the drug.

Neurotoxic effects on dopaminergic neurons are produced by the abused drugs, leading to structural damage and further impacting dopaminergic function. Neurotoxicity may contribute to persistent changes in the dopamine system even after cessation of drug use. Sensitivity changes in the dopamine system following repeated drug abuse provides insights into the neurobiology of addiction. Targeting these neuroadaptations may be crucial for developing effective interventions to prevent and treat substance use disorders. Several drugs of abuse, environmental toxins, and certain medications can induce neurotoxicity in the dopamine-rich regions of the brain. Neurotoxic substances can induce oxidative stress by generating reactive oxygen species (ROS) and free radicals. Increased oxidative stress can lead to damage to cellular components, including lipids, proteins, and DNA, within dopamine neurons. Reactive Oxygen Species (ROS) are chemically reactive molecules containing oxygen that are generated as natural byproducts of cellular metabolism. While they play essential roles in various cellular functions, an imbalance in ROS production and elimination can lead to oxidative stress, causing damage to cellular components. The majority of ROS in cells are produced in the mitochondria during oxidative phosphorylation. Electron leakage from the mitochondrial electron transport chain (ETC) complexes, particularly complexes I and III, can generate superoxide radicals (O2−). NADPH oxidases are a family of enzymes dedicated to ROS production and are present in various cell types, including immune cells. NADPH oxidase enzymes transfer electrons across biological membranes to molecular oxygen, producing superoxide (Bedard & Krause, 2007). These enzymes are involved in purine metabolism and can generate superoxide as byproducts.

Xanthine oxidase is converted from xanthine dehydrogenase under certain conditions, promoting ROS production. Certain members of the cytochrome P450 enzyme family, involved in drug metabolism and detoxification, can produce ROS. ROS generation occurs during the metabolism of specific substrates by these enzymes (Hlavica, 2010). Reactive oxygen species, especially hydroxyl radicals (•OH), can initiate lipid peroxidation in cell membranes. Lipid peroxidation produces lipid hydroperoxides and additional ROS, contributing to a chain reaction. Disruption of protein folding in the endoplasmic reticulum can lead to the accumulation of misfolded proteins and induce ROS production. Endoplasmic reticulum stress activates signaling pathways, including those involving ROS, to restore cellular homeostasis. Sources and regulation of ROS production are essential for maintaining cellular redox balance. Excessive ROS can lead to oxidative stress, contributing to various pathological conditions, including neurodegenerative diseases, cardiovascular disorders, and cancer. The body employs antioxidant defense systems to neutralize ROS and mitigate oxidative damage.

Mitochondrial dysfunction could be induced by neurotoxins or abused drugs, impairing energy production and increasing the production of ROS.

Dopamine neurons are particularly vulnerable to mitochondrial dysfunction, as dopamine metabolism itself generates oxidative stress. Mitochondrial dysfunction is a key mechanism involved in oxidative stress. Mitochondria, the energy-producing organelles within cells, are a major source and target of reactive oxygen species (ROS). The electron transport chain, located in the inner mitochondrial membrane, is responsible for generating ATP through oxidative phosphorylation. Dysfunction in the ETC can lead to electron leakage, resulting in the production of superoxide radicals (O2−). Complex I and complex III are common sites of electron leakage. Uncoupling proteins (UCPs) in the mitochondrial inner membrane can disrupt the coupling between electron transport and ATP synthesis. Uncoupling increases the production of superoxide radicals as electrons bypass ATP synthesis. Mitochondria have their own DNA (mtDNA), and it is particularly susceptible to oxidative damage due to its proximity to ROS production sites. Accumulation of mtDNA mutations and deletions can impair mitochondrial function and contribute to ROS generation (Ballinger & Bailey, 2019). Oxidative stress can induce the opening of the Mitochondrial Permeability Transition Pore (mPTP) in the inner mitochondrial membrane. mPTP opening disrupts the mitochondrial membrane potential, leading to ATP depletion and release of pro-apoptotic factors Imbalances in mitochondrial fusion and fission processes can contribute to dysfunction. Excessive fission can lead to the formation of fragmented and damaged mitochondria. Abnormal mitochondrial dynamics can impact energy production and ROS generation. Mitochondrial dysfunction-induced oxidative stress plays a significant role in various diseases, including neurodegenerative disorders, cardiovascular diseases, and metabolic disorders. Understanding these mechanisms provides insights into potential therapeutic targets for mitigating oxidative stress and preserving mitochondrial function.

Impaired mitochondrial biogenesis also contributes to oxidative stress can impair the process of mitochondrial biogenesis, which involves the synthesis and incorporation of new mitochondria. Reduced biogenesis leads to a decline in the number of functional mitochondria (Scarpulla, 2011). Mutations in nuclear or mitochondrial DNA can affect genes involved in mitochondrial biogenesis. For example, mutations in the peroxisome proliferator-activated receptor gamma coactivator 1-alpha (PGC-1α) gene, a master regulator of mitochondrial biogenesis, can lead to impaired mitochondrial function. Chronic inflammation can disrupt mitochondrial biogenesis. Inflammatory signals, such as cytokines, may interfere with the function of key regulators like PGC-1α, leading to reduced mitochondrial biogenesis. Insufficient cellular energy, such as during prolonged nutrient deprivation secondary to abused drug administration can reduce the cell's capacity to generate new mitochondria. Dysregulation of mitochondrial dynamics, specifically an imbalance in mitochondrial fission and fusion processes, can disrupt mitochondrial biogenesis. Optimal fission and fusion events are essential for maintaining a healthy mitochondrial network. Changes in the epigenetic regulation of mitochondrial biogenesis-related genes, such as DNA methylation and histone modifications, can ALSO influence the expression of key regulators. Impaired mitophagy, the selective removal of damaged mitochondria, can lead to the accumulation of dysfunctional mitochondria, negatively impacting mitochondrial biogenesis. Along with drug abuse, aging is associated with a decline in mitochondrial function and biogenesis. Age-related changes, including altered signaling pathways and increased oxidative stress, which further potentiates drug-induced impaired mitochondrial biogenesis.

Mitochondrial-ER crosstalk is crucial for cellular homeostasis. Disruption in this crosstalk can lead to increased oxidative stress and impaired cellular function causing drug craving and relapse. Mitochondrial dysfunction-induced oxidative stress plays a significant role in various diseases, including neurodegenerative disorders, cardiovascular diseases, and metabolic disorders. Understanding these mechanisms provides insights into potential therapeutic targets for mitigating oxidative stress and preserving mitochondrial function (Bravo-Sagua et al., 2017). Excitotoxicity occurs when excessive stimulation of glutamate receptors leads to an influx of calcium ions, causing neuronal damage. Overactivation of glutamate receptors, especially NMDA receptors, can result in excitotoxicity in dopamine-rich regions. Aggregation of alpha-synuclein, a protein abundant in dopaminergic neurons, is a hallmark of neurodegenerative disorders like Parkinson's disease. Neurotoxicants may contribute to the misfolding and aggregation of alpha-synuclein, leading to cellular dysfunction. Exposure to neurotoxic substances can trigger an inflammatory response in the brain, involving microglial activation. Chronic inflammation and activated microglia contribute to neuronal damage in dopaminergic regions. Dysregulation of protein degradation pathways, such as the ubiquitin-proteasome system and autophagy, can result in the accumulation of misfolded proteins in dopamine (McGeer & McGeer, 2008). Neurotoxicants may disrupt the homeostasis of dopamine by affecting synthesis, release, or reuptake. Imbalances in dopamine levels can contribute to cellular stress and vulnerability. These mechanisms are crucial for developing interventions that may mitigate the neurotoxic effects on dopamine neurons, potentially offering avenues for neuroprotective strategies in substance-abuse neurotoxicity.

Genetics and Individual Differences in dopamine-mediated effects of abused drugs: Individual differences in the dopamine-mediated effects of abused drugs are influenced by genetic factors. Genetic variations can affect the functioning of neurotransmitter systems, including the dopamine system, leading to variability in how individuals respond to drugs of abuse. Dopamine receptor polymorphisms can influence the density and sensitivity of dopamine receptors, affecting an individual's susceptibility to drug reward. Genetic variations in dopamine receptor genes, such as DRD2 and DRD4, have been associated with differences in drug response. The dopamine receptors D2 gene is one of the most widely studied in the context of drug abuse. Polymorphisms in the Taq1A and -141C Ins/Del regions of the dopamine receptors D2 gene have been associated with altered D2 receptor density and availability (Blum et al., 2023). Individuals carrying certain variants may exhibit reduced D2 receptor availability, which has been linked to increased vulnerability to drug addiction

Genetic variations in the dopamine receptors D3 gene have been implicated in susceptibility to drug abuse, particularly substances like cocaine and opioids. The Ser9Gly polymorphism in the D3 gene has been associated with altered receptor function and increased risk for addictive dopamine receptors behaviors (Xuan et al., 2008). The dopamine receptors D4 gene contains a variable number of tandem repeats (VNTR) polymorphism, with the 7-repeat allele being the most studied in relation to drug abuse. Carriers of the 7-repeat allele have been associated with novelty-seeking behaviors and increased vulnerability to substance abuse, including alcohol and illicit drugs (Skowronek et al., 2006).

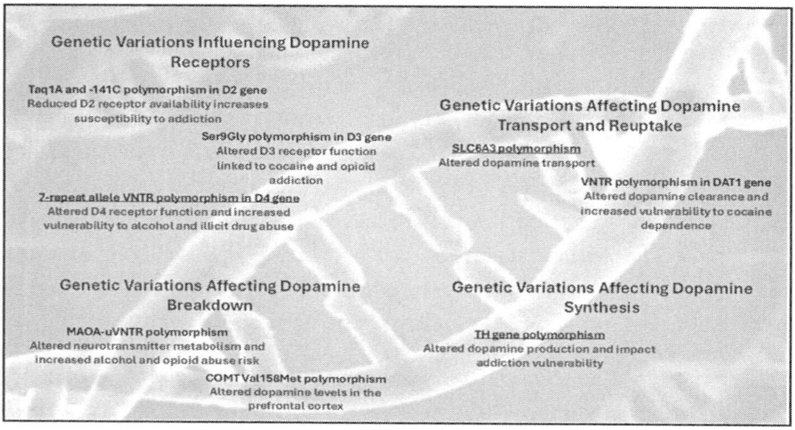

Genetic factors influencing dopaminergic system and reward sensitivity

Although less studied than other dopamine receptor subtypes, variations in the drug receptor D5 gene have been investigated in the context of drug abuse. Polymorphisms in this gene may influence individual responses to drugs affecting the dopamine system (Yang et al., 2008). These polymorphisms can influence several aspects of dopamine receptor function, including receptor density, affinity, and downstream signaling pathways. The variations in receptor function can, in turn, impact an individual's reward sensitivity, reinforcement learning, and susceptibility to addictive behaviors. Altered expression of dopamine transporter gene (SLC6A3) is responsible for reuptake of dopamine from the synapse. Polymorphisms in the SLC6A3 gene that codes for dopamine transporters have been linked to variations in dopamine clearance and response to stimulant drugs like cocaine and amphetamines. The dopamine transporter gene (SLC6A3) contains a variable number of tandem repeats (VNTR) polymorphism, known as the dopamine transporter1 polymorphism. This polymorphism has been associated with individual differences in dopamine transporter density and has been investigated in the context of drug abuse vulnerability (Fuke et al., 2001). Studies have explored the relationship between the DAT1 polymorphism and susceptibility to cocaine abuse. The 9-repeat allele, in particular, has been associated with altered dopamine transporter expression and an increased risk of cocaine dependence (Olasore et al., 2023). Investigations into the DAT1 polymorphism have extended to its role in various substance use disorders. The polymorphism's impact on dopamine transporter function and dopamine clearance may contribute to susceptibility to a range of addictive behaviors. There is a strong relationship between the dopamine transporter gene and its polymorphisms in the susceptibility to drug abuse. However, it's crucial to note that the relationship between genetics and drug abuse is complex, involving interactions with environmental factors and other genetic components.

COMT is an enzyme that degrades dopamine. Genetic variations in the COMT gene can influence dopamine levels in the prefrontal cortex, impacting individual responses to drugs affecting dopamine transmission. While the COMT gene is primarily known for its role in neurotransmitter metabolism and has been extensively studied in various psychiatric conditions, the direct link between COMT genetic variations and drug abuse is not as well-established as with other genes. However, some studies have explored associations between COMT polymorphisms and susceptibility to substance use disorders. Research has investigated the association between COMT polymorphisms, especially the Val158Met variant, and susceptibility to substance use disorders. Some studies suggest that variations in COMT may contribute to individual differences in vulnerability to addictive behaviors (Colzato et al., 2010). Studies have explored the influence of COMT genetic variations on cognitive effects induced by drugs of abuse, such as cannabis.

The Val158Met polymorphism has been implicated in the modulation of cognitive performance following drug exposure (Rabinak et al., 2014). Some investigations have explored the role of COMT in opioid addiction. Genetic variations in COMT may contribute to differences in the response to opioid medications and susceptibility to opioid use disorders (Baker et al., 2005). Genetic variations in COMT have been considered in the context of response to pharmacotherapy for substance use disorders. Individual differences in the efficacy of medications may be influenced by COMT polymorphisms (Yuferov et al., 2010). While these studies provide insights into potential associations between COMT genetic variations and aspects of drug abuse, it's essential to note that the field is dynamic, and more research is needed to establish clear and consistent links. Additionally, individual responses to drugs and susceptibility to substance use disorders are multifaceted, involving complex interactions between genetic, environmental, and neurobiological factors.

Tyrosine hydroxylase (TH) gene variations may affect the rate of dopamine production, influencing the responsiveness to drugs that act on dopamine pathways. Tyrosine Hydroxylase is an enzyme involved in dopamine synthesis. The Tyrosine Hydroxylase (TH) gene is involved in the synthesis of dopamine, norepinephrine, and epinephrine, making it a crucial component of the catecholamine biosynthetic pathway. While the direct association between TH genetic variations and drug abuse is not as extensively studied as some other genes, research has explored the role of TH in the context of addiction-related behaviors. Some studies have investigated the relationship between genetic variations in the TH gene and susceptibility to alcohol dependence. Variants in TH may influence dopamine levels in the brain, potentially impacting alcohol-related behaviors (Huang et al., 2007).

Research has explored the role of TH gene polymorphisms in nicotine dependence. Dopaminergic pathways, regulated in part by TH, are implicated in the reinforcing effects of nicotine (Guindalini et al., 2008). While not exclusively focused on TH, some studies examining the genetic basis of opioid dependence have investigated genes involved in dopamine synthesis, including TH. TH variations may contribute to individual differences in opioid-related behaviors (Gondré-Lewis et al., 2022). Dopaminergic systems, influenced by TH, are implicated in the reinforcing effects of psychostimulants like methamphetamine. Genetic variations in TH may contribute to individual differences in vulnerability to methamphetamine dependence (Richards et al., 2006). It is important to note that while these studies provide insights into the potential role of TH genetic variations in drug abuse, the field is dynamic, and more research is needed to establish clear and consistent links. The genetic basis of drug abuse involves complex interactions between various genes and environmental factors.

MAO enzymes are involved in the breakdown of dopamine. Variations in genes encoding MAO enzymes can influence the clearance of dopamine from synapses, affecting drug responses. Monoamine oxidase (MAO) genes, particularly MAOA and MAOB, are involved in the metabolism of monoamine neurotransmitters, including dopamine, norepinephrine, and serotonin. Variations in these genes have been studied in relation to various psychiatric and behavioral conditions, including drug abuse. The MAOA gene has been implicated in the susceptibility to substance use disorders.

Variations in MAOA may influence the metabolism of neurotransmitters involved in reward pathways, impacting an individual's vulnerability to drug abuse. The MAOA-uVNTR (variable number of tandem repeats) polymorphism has been studied in relation to alcoholism. The allelic variations in this region may influence the risk of developing alcohol dependence (Baker et al., 2005). Some investigations have explored the association between the MAOA gene and susceptibility to opioid dependence. Variations in MAOA may contribute to individual differences in opioid-related behaviors (Lötsch et al., 2014). The MAOB gene has been examined in the context of nicotine dependence. Genetic variations in MAOB may impact the metabolism of neurotransmitters involved in the reinforcing effects of nicotine (Ray et al., 2009). These studies provide insights into the potential role of MAO genes, particularly MAOA and MAOB, in the susceptibility to drug abuse. However, it's essential to acknowledge the complexity of genetic interactions and the multifactorial nature of substance use disorders. The field continues to evolve, and further research is necessary to establish more precise relationships between MAO gene variations and drug abuse.

Epigenetic factors, such as DNA methylation and histone modifications, can dynamically regulate gene expression in response to drug exposure. Epigenetic changes may contribute to long-term individual differences in drug effects. Understanding the interplay between genetics and the dopamine system is crucial for unraveling the basis of individual variations in drug response and susceptibility to addiction. It's important to note that genetic factors interact with environmental influences on shape drug-related behaviors, and research in this field is ongoing. DNA methylation involves the addition of methyl groups to cytosine residues, usually resulting in the suppression of gene expression. In drug abuse, alterations in DNA methylation patterns have been associated with changes in the expression of genes involved in addiction-related pathways, including those related to synaptic plasticity and reward (Poisel et al., 2023). Histone modifications, such as acetylation and methylation, play a crucial role in regulating chromatin structure and gene expression. In drug abuse, changes in histone modifications have been linked to alterations in the expression of genes related to addiction, affecting synaptic plasticity and reward pathways (Cheng et al., 2023). These references provide insights into the role of DNA methylation and histone modifications in the context of drug abuse. The studies mentioned highlight the dynamic nature of epigenetic processes and their impact on gene expression, ultimately influencing the development and persistence of addiction-related behaviors. For the most up-to-date information, it's recommended to refer to current literature in the field of epigenetics and drug abuse research.

Future Directions: Future research must investigate how dopamine interacts with other neuromodulators like orexin and endocannabinoids to create the precise neural signatures underlying different stages of addiction. Cutting-edge techniques such as single-cell RNA sequencing could reveal how chronic drug exposure alters dopamine receptor expression patterns in specific neuronal populations throughout the reward circuitry. Advanced computational models should be developed to predict how individual variations in dopamine system genetics interact with environmental stressors to determine addiction vulnerability. Researchers need to employ multi-electrode array technology to decode how dopamine-mediated synaptic plasticity differs between casual drug use and compulsive addiction states at the neural circuit level. The development of novel PET tracers capable of distinguishing between tonic and phasic dopamine release could transform our understanding of dopamine dynamics in human addiction. Longitudinal studies tracking dopamine system recovery during abstinence may identify critical windows for targeted neurorestorative interventions. Investigations into dopamine's role in drug-related memory reconsolidation could yield breakthrough therapies that weaken pathological reward memories without affecting normal learning. These approaches require integration across molecular, systems, and behavioral neuroscience to develop a unified theory of dopamine's multifaceted role in addiction.

Emerging technologies offer unprecedented opportunities to manipulate dopamine systems with precision for therapeutic benefit. Optogenetic and chemogenetic tools should be optimized to selectively target dopamine neuron subpopulations projecting to distinct brain regions, potentially allowing dissociation of their roles in craving versus consumption behaviors. Nanotechnology-based drug delivery systems could be engineered to release dopamine-modulating compounds in response to specific neural activity patterns associated with craving states. Research must explore how next-generation brain-computer interfaces could detect and disrupt pathological dopamine signals in real time while preserving normal reward processing. The development of dopamine-sensitive wearable devices may enable continuous monitoring of addiction-related neurochemical fluctuations in natural environments. Studies should investigate how novel psychedelic compounds with unique dopamine receptor binding profiles might reset maladaptive dopaminergic signaling patterns. Parallel research needs to examine how gut microbiome-derived metabolites influence dopamine neuron activity and susceptibility to addiction. These technological advances must be paired with rigorous ethical frameworks to ensure their responsible translation to clinical applications.

Future clinical research should focus on translating basic dopamine discoveries into personalized treatment strategies for addiction. Precision medicine approaches could utilize dopamine-related genetic biomarkers to predict individual responses to different pharmacological treatments and behavioral therapies. Trials should test whether combining dopamine-targeting medications with neuromodulation techniques like TMS or tDCS yields synergistic benefits for different addiction subtypes. Research must clarify how developmental changes in dopamine systems from adolescence through aging influence addiction vulnerability and treatment outcomes. Studies should explore whether dopamine system measurements could serve as objective biomarkers for diagnosing addiction severity and monitoring treatment progress. Investigations into nutritional interventions that support dopamine system homeostasis may reveal accessible adjuncts to conventional addiction treatments. The development of dopamine-aware digital therapeutics that adapt in real-time to users' neurochemical states could revolutionize relapse prevention. These clinical directions must be pursued with particular attention to reducing health disparities in addiction treatment access and outcomes. Ultimately, this research trajectory promises to move addiction medicine beyond symptom management toward genuine neural circuit repair.

CHAPTER 7

ROLE OF SEROTONIN IN DRUG ADDICTION

"Addiction begins with the hope that something 'out there' can instantly fill up the emptiness inside."
~ Jean Kilbourne

Learn how our feelings and brain chemicals are connected in addiction. Get to know more about another brain chemical, serotonin. Discover why we sometimes feel empty and try to fill that feeling with addictive things. This chapter covers the intricate role of serotonin in drug addiction comes into focus as we explore the profound impact of this neurotransmitter on mood regulation, impulse control, and the intricate web of addictive behaviors. Unveiling the significance of serotonin in drug addiction opens a window into the complex interplay between brain chemistry and addictive tendencies, highlighting the crucial role this neurotransmitter plays in modulating the emotional and behavioral aspects of substance use disorders.

The role of serotonin in drug addiction is a complex and multifaceted topic, involving the intricate interplay of neurotransmitters, neural circuits, and behavioral responses. This chapter explores the involvement of serotonin in various aspects of drug addiction, including reward pathways, behavioral manifestations, withdrawal symptoms, and comorbidities. By examining the serotonin system's contribution to addiction, we aim to deepen our understanding of the neurobiology underpinning substance use disorders and identify potential targets for therapeutic interventions. Drug addiction is a chronic, relapsing disorder characterized by compulsive drug-seeking, continued use despite adverse consequences, and long-lasting changes in the brain. Serotonin, a neurotransmitter known for its role in mood regulation and emotional processing, has emerged as a key player in the neurobiology of addiction (Belujon & Grace, 2017). The serotonin system, with its intricate network of pathways and receptors, plays a crucial role in modulating mood, emotion, and behavior. Serotonin is synthesized in the raphe nuclei and released into various brain regions, influencing a wide array of physiological processes (Haleem & Nawaz, 2013). The interaction between serotonin and other neurotransmitters in reward pathways is central to understanding addiction. Serotonin modulates the brain's response to rewarding stimuli and influences reinforcement mechanisms that are crucial in the development of addiction (Müller & Homberg, 2015).

Research has shown alterations in serotonin levels or receptor sensitivity contributing to various substance use disorders. Understanding the specific role of serotonin in each disorder provides insights into potential targeted treatments (Koob & Le Moal, 2001). The impact of serotonin on behavioral aspects such as impulsivity, craving, and relapse is crucial for understanding the dynamics of addiction. Studies in animal models provide valuable insights into serotonin's role in shaping addictive behaviors (Bari & Robbins, 2013). The involvement of serotonin in withdrawal symptoms associated with drug dependence is a critical aspect of addiction research. Serotonin's influence on the severity and duration of withdrawal contributes to the overall understanding of substance dependence (Koob & Volkow, 2016).

Serotonin, scientifically known as 5-hydroxytryptamine (5-HT), is a monoamine neurotransmitter that plays a crucial role in the central nervous system. First discovered in the gastrointestinal tract, serotonin is primarily synthesized in the raphe nuclei of the brainstem and is involved in various physiological processes (Haleem & Nawaz, 2013). Serotonin synthesis begins with the conversion of tryptophan to 5-hydroxytryptophan, a process catalyzed by the enzyme tryptophan hydroxylase. Subsequently, aromatic L-amino acid decarboxylase converts 5-hydroxytryptophan to serotonin. Once synthesized, serotonin is stored in vesicles and released into the synaptic cleft upon neuronal stimulation. Serotonin exerts its effects by binding to specific receptors, classified into seven main families (5-HT1 to 5-HT7). These receptors are widely distributed throughout the central and peripheral nervous systems, mediating diverse physiological and behavioral responses (Hoyer et al., 2002). Serotonin is often referred to as the "feel-good" neurotransmitter due to its role in regulating mood. Imbalances in serotonin levels have been linked to mood disorders such as depression and anxiety (Cowen & Browning, 2015). Serotonin is involved in the regulation of sleep-wake cycles. It promotes wakefulness and plays a role in the onset and maintenance of sleep. Serotonin is a key player in the regulation of appetite and digestion. It modulates the feeling of satiety and influences gastrointestinal motility (Mawe & Hoffman, 2013). Serotonin contributes to the regulation of cardiovascular function, including vasoconstriction and blood clotting. Dysregulation of serotonin neurotransmission is implicated in major depressive disorder. Selective serotonin reuptake inhibitors (SSRIs) are commonly prescribed to alleviate depressive symptoms (Stahl, 2013). Serotonin imbalance is associated with various anxiety disorders. Medications targeting serotonin receptors are frequently used in anxiety treatment. Disruptions in serotonin signaling are associated with gastrointestinal disorders such as irritable bowel syndrome and inflammatory bowel disease (Gershon et al., 2012). Serotonin, as a multifaceted neurotransmitter, plays a pivotal role in various physiological and behavioral processes. Its involvement in mood regulation, sleep-wake cycles, appetite, and cardiovascular function underscores its significance in maintaining overall well-being. Dysregulation of serotonin is associated with a range of disorders, highlighting the need for targeted therapeutic interventions.

The interplay between serotonin and various drugs of abuse has been a subject of extensive research, shedding light on the intricate mechanisms underlying addictive behaviors. Serotonin exerts a modulatory influence on dopaminergic reward pathways. This interaction is crucial in the context of addiction, where the dopaminergic system is a key player in reinforcing drug-seeking behaviors. Serotonin is implicated in regulating impulsive behaviors and decision-making processes. Dysregulation of serotonin levels may contribute to impaired impulse control seen in addiction (Bari et al., 2013). Serotonin's involvement in the neurobiological processes of drug withdrawal is critical for understanding the persistence of addictive behaviors (Kosten & George, 2002). Serotonin is implicated in the modulation of craving, a core component of addiction. Understanding how serotonin influences these cravings is essential for targeted treatment approaches (Dahchour & Ward, 2023). Genetic variations in the serotonin transporter gene have been linked to vulnerability to addiction and altered responses to drugs of abuse. Medications targeting the serotonergic system, such as selective serotonin reuptake inhibitors (SSRIs), have shown promise in the treatment of substance use disorders. Understanding the intricate interplay between serotonin and drug addiction is essential for developing effective therapeutic strategies. From modulating reward pathways to influencing withdrawal and craving, serotonin's role in addiction is multifaceted. Continued research into the serotonin system holds promise for advancing our understanding of addiction mechanisms and improving treatment outcomes.

Serotonergic agents abuse: Serotonergic agents, which directly influence the serotonin system, encompass a range of substances including hallucinogens, empathogens, and certain prescription medications. The abuse of these agents can lead to various psychological and physiological effects, and understanding their impact is crucial for addressing mental health and addiction concerns. Hallucinogens such as LSD and psilocybin exert their effects primarily through the serotonin receptor system, leading to altered perception and mood. While not typically associated with addiction, their misuse can have profound psychological consequences. MDMA, known as ecstasy, enhances the release of serotonin and other neurotransmitters, producing feelings of euphoria and increased sociability. However, chronic use can lead to neurotoxicity and mood disorders. While not typically abused for recreational purposes, SSRIs are commonly prescribed for various mental health conditions. However, misuse or abrupt discontinuation can lead to adverse effects (Sansone & Sansone, 2010). Certain opioids, through their interaction with serotonin receptors, may be associated with serotonin syndrome when used in combination with serotonergic agents. The abuse of serotonergic agents presents a complex scenario involving hallucinogens, empathogens, and prescription medications. Understanding the neurobiological mechanisms and potential consequences of misuse is crucial for both clinical treatment and public health initiatives.

Serotonin and reward pathway: Serotonin, a neurotransmitter primarily associated with mood regulation, also plays a crucial role in modulating the brain's reward pathway. The interaction between serotonin and the reward system is complex and involves various receptors, neural circuits, and feedback mechanisms. Serotonin can modulate dopamine release through 5HT-2 receptors, especially 55HT-2A and 5HT-2C. Activation of these receptors influences the activity of dopamine neurons in key areas of the brain involved in reward processing, such as the ventral tegmental area and nucleus accumbens. Serotonin helps maintain a balance in dopaminergic activity. Dysregulation of dopamine release is implicated in various psychiatric disorders, including addiction and mood disorders (Müller & Homberg, 2015). Activation of 5HT-1 receptors, particularly 5HT-1A, can influence reward-related behaviors. These receptors are distributed in brain regions associated with emotional processing and motivation, impacting the overall reward circuitry. Serotonin's role in mood regulation also contributes to its impact on reward-related behaviors. Mood disturbances can influence an individual's response to rewarding stimuli (Dayan & Huys, 2009). Serotonin, through 5HT-2C receptors, influences reward-related learning and decision-making processes. These receptors are densely expressed in areas involved in cognitive functions related to reward. Dysregulation of serotonin in these circuits may contribute to addictive behaviors by altering the processing of rewarding stimuli and influencing decision-making. Through 5HT-1B receptors, serotonin is involved in the regulation of impulsive behavior. Dysregulation of serotonin levels may contribute to impulsivity, a trait linked to various psychiatric disorders, including substance abuse (Dalley et al., 2011).

Serotonin, a neurotransmitter with diverse functions in the central nervous system, has long been implicated in the pathophysiology of mood disorders, such as depression, where alterations in reward processing contribute to symptoms (Cowen & Browning, 2015). Serotonin is a key neurotransmitter involved in mood regulation, emotional processing, and sleep-wake cycles. The monoamine hypothesis suggests that a deficiency in serotonin and other monoamines contributes to the development of depressive symptoms. Selective serotonin reuptake inhibitors (SSRIs) are widely used in treating depression by increasing serotonin levels in the synaptic cleft. Genetic variations in the serotonin transporter gene (SLC6A4) have been associated with vulnerability to depression (Trivedi et al., 2006).

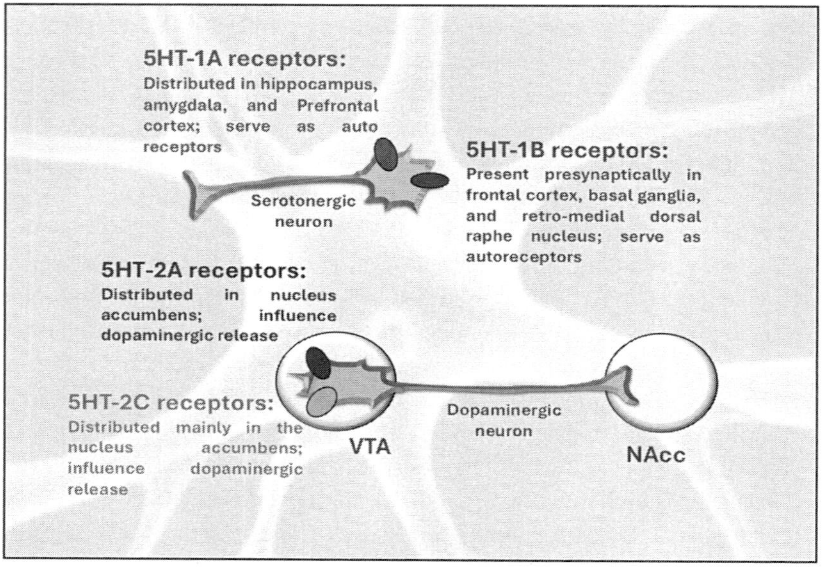

Serotonergic modulation of reward pathway

Impaired function of 5HT-1A receptors, which mediate serotonin's inhibitory effects, has been associated with depressive symptoms. Altered activity of 5HT-2 receptors, particularly 5HT-2A, has been implicated in mood disorders (López-Giménez & Vilaró, 2008). Serotonin is implicated in the regulation of neurotrophic factors, such as brain-derived neurotrophic factor (BDNF), which play a role in neuroplasticity and neuronal survival. Depression is associated with alterations in hippocampal structure and function, influenced by serotonin's impact on neurogenesis (Duman & Monteggia, 2006). Enteric Serotonin: The gut produces and releases serotonin, influencing the gut-brain axis. Dysregulation in this axis may contribute to mood disorders. Understanding serotonin's role in depression informs the development of novel antidepressant strategies targeting various aspects of serotonin regulation (Cipriani et al., 2018). Combined interventions targeting serotonin, such as medication and psychotherapy, are often employed for more comprehensive treatment. Serotonin dysregulation is a multifaceted contributor to the complex etiology of depression. As ongoing research delves deeper into the intricacies of serotonin's role in the brain and body, novel therapeutic approaches aiming to modulate serotonin function continue to emerge. Targeting serotonin receptors is explored as a potential avenue for developing treatments for addiction and other disorders involving reward dysregulation. Understanding how serotonin regulates the reward pathway is crucial for developing targeted interventions for conditions characterized by reward dysfunction. Further research is needed to uncover the precise mechanisms and potential therapeutic strategies.

Serotonin intricately modulates the reward system through various receptor subtypes, notably the 5HT-1A, 5HT-1B, and 5HT-2 receptors. 5HT-1A receptors are widely expressed in various brain regions, including the hippocampus, amygdala, and prefrontal cortex. Activation of 5HT-1A receptors, particularly in the mesolimbic pathway, can modulate dopamine release, influencing the hedonic aspects of reward (Müller & Homberg, 2015). 5HT-1B receptors, predominantly located on presynaptic terminals, inhibit the release of various neurotransmitters, including dopamine. Through modulation of dopamine release in the nucleus accumbens, 5HT-1B receptors influence reinforcement processes (Filip & Bubar, 2010). 5HT-2 receptors comprise subtypes such as 5HT-2A and 5HT-2C, distributed in brain regions associated with reward and motivation. 5HT-2 receptors play a crucial role in regulating dopamine release, impacting the salience and reinforcing aspects of rewards (Howell et al., 2015).

The combined activation of 5-HT1A, 5-HT1B, and 5-HT2 receptors creates a complex interplay that regulates the overall impact on reward processing (Cunningham et al., 2011). Chronic drug exposure can lead to adaptive changes in serotonin receptor expression, influencing the sensitivity of the reward system. Understanding the specific contributions of 5-HT1A, 5-HT1B, and 5-HT2 receptors opens avenues for developing targeted pharmacotherapies for addiction and mood disorders. Ongoing research is exploring the nuanced roles of serotonin receptors in reward processing, shedding light on novel therapeutic possibilities. The intricate orchestration of serotonin receptor subtypes, particularly 5-HT1A, 5-HT1B, and 5-HT2 receptors, plays a pivotal role in shaping the rewarding effects associated with various behaviors. A deeper understanding of their specific contributions holds promise for advancing our comprehension of reward processing and developing targeted therapeutic interventions.

Serotonin-Dopamine Interactions: Serotonin and dopamine, two prominent neurotransmitters, collaboratively regulate various physiological and behavioral functions, including the intricate aspects of the reward system. This exploration focuses on the dynamic interplay between serotonin and dopamine. Serotonergic projections from the raphe nuclei interact with dopaminergic neurons in the ventral tegmental area (VTA), a crucial component of the mesolimbic reward pathway. Serotonin also influences dopamine release in the prefrontal cortex, contributing to cognitive and executive functions (Puig & Gulledge, 2011).

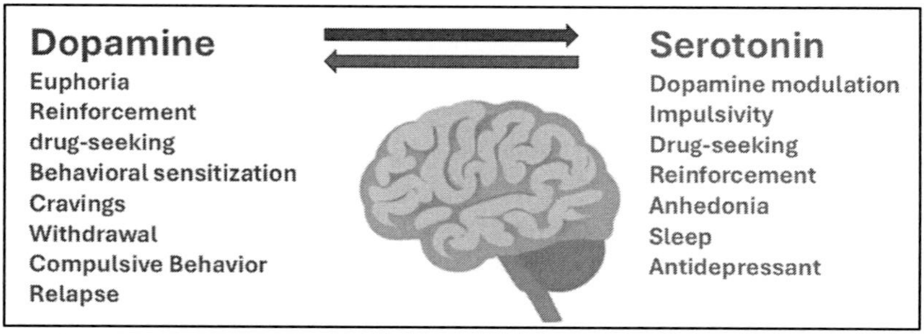

Serotonin-dopamine interactions in mediating addictive effects of drugs

The activation of presynaptic 5HT-1A receptors inhibits dopamine release, exerting a regulatory influence on the balance between serotonin and dopamine. 5HT-2C Receptors: These receptors, predominantly located in the mesolimbic pathway, modulate dopamine release and are implicated in reward-related behaviors. Serotonin neurons possess 5HT-1A autoreceptors that, when activated, inhibit serotonin release and indirectly influence dopamine transmission (Guiard et al., 2005). Serotonin neurons can directly or indirectly affect dopamine neurons through complex synaptic interactions in the VTA. Serotonin's impact on dopamine release contributes to the regulation of reward processing and reinforcement learning (Howell et al., 2015). Dysregulation of the serotonergic modulation of dopamine is implicated in addiction, where maladaptive reward-seeking behaviors emerge. Targeting serotonin receptors offers potential therapeutic avenues for disorders involving dysregulated dopamine transmission, including addiction and mood disorders (Baik, 2013). Understanding individual differences in serotonergic modulation of dopamine may pave the way for personalized treatment strategies. The interplay between serotonin and dopamine, with serotonin's modulation of dopamine release, intricately shapes the neural circuits governing reward and reinforcement. This dynamic interaction is a critical determinant of various behaviors, and unraveling its complexities holds promise for advancing our understanding of neuropsychiatric disorders and developing targeted therapeutic interventions.

Serotonin, a neurotransmitter classically associated with mood regulation, has garnered increasing attention for its intricate involvement in motivation. This exploration delves into the nuanced ways serotonin influences motivational processes, encompassing neural circuits, receptor subtypes, and behavioral outcomes. Serotonin neurons originating from the raphe nuclei intricately project to various brain regions implicated in motivation, including the prefrontal cortex, striatum, and hippocampus. Serotonin's interactions with the mesolimbic dopamine system play a pivotal role in reward processing and motivation (Salamone et al., 2009). Activation of presynaptic 5HT-1A receptors can influence motivation by modulating serotonin release, particularly in regions like the prefrontal cortex. 5HT-2C receptors are implicated in the modulation of motivation and reinforcement processes, and their activation can have divergent effects on behavior. Serotonin's role in mood regulation is intricately linked to motivation, with alterations in serotonin levels affecting approach behaviors (Daw et al., 2002).

Serotonin's influence on the BAS, a system associated with goal-directed behavior and positive affect, underscores its motivational significance. Serotonin's role in evaluating costs and benefits is crucial for effort-based decision-making, influencing whether an individual engages in a particular behavior. Alterations in serotonin levels can impact an individual's willingness to expend effort for rewards. Understanding serotonin's role in motivation provides insights into the motivational deficits seen in mood disorders. Developing interventions that selectively modulate serotonin for conditions characterized by motivational impairments. Serotonin's involvement in motivation is a multifaceted interplay encompassing neural circuits, receptor subtypes, and behavioral outcomes. As research continues to unveil the complexities of serotonin's role in motivation, the potential for novel therapeutic interventions targeting motivational disorders becomes increasingly promising. This intricate relationship between serotonin and motivation serves as a critical avenue for advancing our understanding of neuropsychiatric conditions and developing targeted treatment strategies. Apart from being associated with mood and emotional well-being, serotonin also has implications for reward processing. The role of serotonin in reward processing is complex and multifaceted, and research in this area is ongoing. It is known to modulate the activity of the brain's reward circuitry, which includes regions such as the nucleus accumbens, ventral tegmental area, and prefrontal cortex. A study by Cools et al. (2011) suggests that serotonin can influence reward processing by modulating the balance between inhibitory and excitatory inputs in the prefrontal cortex. Serotonin has been implicated in decision-making processes related to reward. Research by Seymour et al. (2012) suggests that serotonin may influence the processing of rewards and punishments, affecting the evaluation of different options during decision-making.

Social rewards are an important aspect of human behavior, and serotonin has been implicated in social decision-making. Research by Crockett et al. (2008) suggests that serotonin influences social behavior and cooperation by modulating responses to social rewards and punishments. Alterations in serotonin function have been linked to impulsivity and risk-taking behavior, which are integral components of reward processing. The work of Bevilacqua and Goldman (2013) discusses the role of serotonin in regulating impulsive behavior and its relevance to reward-related decision-making. It's important to note that the role of serotonin in reward processing is highly context-dependent, and its effects can vary based on factors such as the specific brain regions involved, the presence of other neurotransmitters, and individual differences.

Serotonin and Behavioral Rewards: Serotonin, a neurotransmitter primarily associated with mood regulation, also plays a role in the regulation of food intake and sexual behavior. The influence of serotonin on these behaviors is complex, involving various brain regions and interacting neural pathways. Serotonin has been implicated in the regulation of appetite and satiety. Increased serotonin levels are associated with a feeling of fullness, which can lead to a reduction in food intake. A pivotal role of serotonin in the control of appetite suggests potential use of serotonin agonists in the treatment of obesity. Serotonin is involved in the regulation of carbohydrate consumption, and alterations in serotonin levels may contribute to carbohydrate cravings. The link between serotonin and carbohydrate consumption suggests increased carbohydrate intake which may lead to increased serotonin synthesis.

Serotonin plays a crucial role in modulating various aspects of behavioral rewards, influencing motivation, reinforcement, and decision-making. There exists a strong relationship between serotonin and behavioral rewards. Serotonin is involved in regulating motivation and approach behavior towards rewards. Changes in serotonin levels can impact an individual's willingness to engage in goal-directed behavior (Boureau et al., 2015). Serotonin contributes to reinforcement learning processes, influencing how individuals learn from rewards and punishments in their environment. Serotonin is implicated in decision-making, particularly in the evaluation of rewards and risks. Altered serotonin levels can influence risk assessment during decision-making (Daw et al., 2002). Serotonin plays a role in modulating responses to social rewards and punishments, influencing social behavior and cooperation (Crockett et al., 2008). Serotonin is associated with mood regulation and can impact hedonic processing, affecting the experience of pleasure and reward. The interplay between serotonin and other neurotransmitter systems further adds complexity to the understanding of reward-related behaviors. Ongoing research continues to uncover the specific mechanisms and neural circuits through which serotonin modulates behavioral rewards.

Serotonin and substance abuse disorders: Serotonin, a neurotransmitter, plays a crucial role in the neurobiology of substance abuse disorders. The interaction between serotonin and various substances of abuse is complex, influencing aspects such as reward processing, mood regulation, and impulsivity. Serotonin is involved in modulating the mesolimbic dopamine system, which plays a key role in the rewarding effects of drugs of abuse. Dysregulation of serotonin function is associated with impulsivity, a trait linked to an increased risk of substance abuse. Alterations in serotonin neurotransmission have been implicated in alcohol abuse disorder and medications targeting serotonin receptors have been explored for alcohol abuse disorder treatment (Heinz & Beck, 2011).

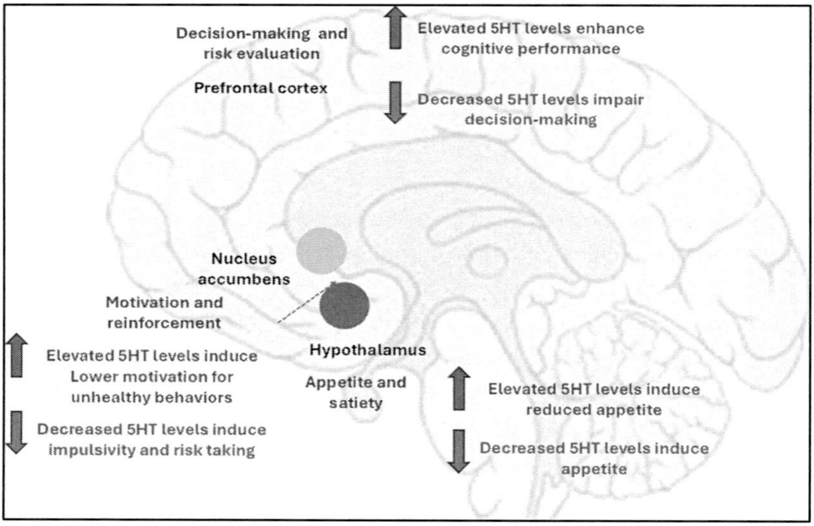

Serotonin and behavioral rewards

Cocaine use affects serotonin levels, and the interplay between serotonin and dopamine systems is relevant in cocaine addiction. Serotonin pathways are involved in the reinforcing effects of opioids, and medications targeting serotonin receptors have been studied for their potential in opioid use disorder treatment (He et al., 2011). Some serotonergic medications, such as selective serotonin reuptake inhibitors (SSRIs) and serotonin-norepinephrine reuptake inhibitors (SNRIs), have been explored for their potential in treating substance abuse disorder. It's important to note that while these references provide insights into the relationship between serotonin and substance abuse disorders, the field is dynamic, and ongoing research is essential to further understand the neurobiological mechanisms and develop effective treatments for substance use disorders.

The therapeutic targeting of serotonin in the context of drug abuse is a complex area of research, and various medications that influence serotonin pathways have been explored for their potential in treating substance use disorders. Serotonin is involved in the neurobiology of addiction, affecting reward, motivation, and impulsivity. Dysregulation of serotonin function is associated with various substance use disorders. Several medications that influence serotonin neurotransmission have been investigated for their potential in treating substance use disorders. These include selective serotonin reuptake inhibitors (SSRIs) and serotonin-norepinephrine reuptake inhibitors (SNRIs). Serotonergic medications, such as ondansetron (a 5-HT3 receptor antagonist), have been studied for their potential in the treatment of opioid use disorder, showing promise in reducing cravings and withdrawal symptoms (Kenna & Nielsen, 2018). The interplay between serotonin and dopamine systems is relevant in cocaine addiction. Medications targeting serotonin receptors have been explored for their potential in reducing cocaine-seeking behavior. Serotonergic medications, particularly ondansetron and selective serotonin reuptake inhibitors (SSRIs), have been investigated for their potential in reducing alcohol consumption (Johnson et al., 2003). It's important to note that while these studies suggest a potential role for serotonin modulation in the treatment of substance use disorders, the field is still evolving, and further research is needed to establish the effectiveness and safety of these approaches. Individual responses to medications can vary, and a comprehensive approach to addiction treatment may involve a combination of pharmacotherapy, behavioral interventions, and support services.

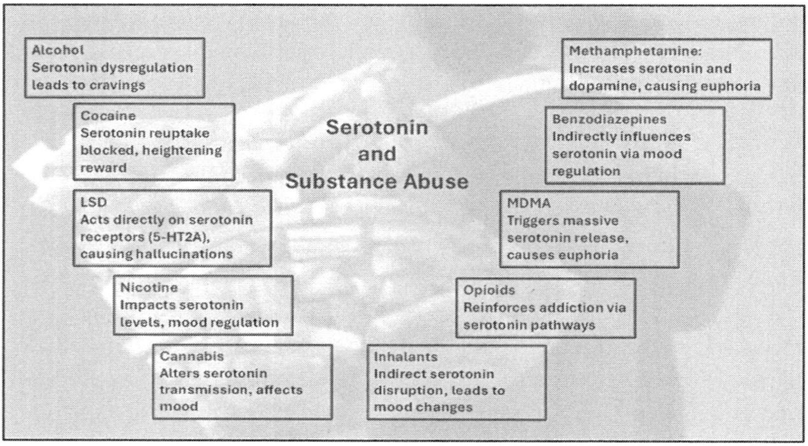

Serotonin and substance abuse

Serotonin and behavioral aspects of addiction: The involvement of serotonin in the behavioral aspects of addiction is complex and multifaceted. Serotonin influences various aspects of behavior, including reward processing, impulsivity, and mood regulation, all of which are relevant to addiction. Serotonin has been implicated in the regulation of impulsivity, a trait associated with an increased risk of addiction (Dalley & Roiser, 2012). Serotonin plays a role in mood regulation, and alterations in serotonin levels may contribute to cravings and negative affect during withdrawal, influencing relapse. Serotonin modulates reward processing and motivation, influencing an individual's responsiveness to drug-related cues and the reinforcing effects of substances. Serotonin has been implicated in the regulation of craving in cocaine addiction, influencing the subjective experience of drug-related cues (Kosten & George, 2002).

Serotonin pathways are involved in the modulation of opioid craving, and medications targeting serotonin receptors have been studied for their potential in opioid use disorder treatment. Some antidepressants that influence serotonin, such as selective serotonin reuptake inhibitors (SSRIs), have been explored for their potential in treating addiction by addressing mood-related symptoms. These references provide insights into the multifaceted role of serotonin in the behavioral aspects of addiction. The interplay between serotonin and other neurotransmitter systems contributes to the complexity of addiction-related behaviors. Ongoing research continues to deepen our understanding and inform the development of targeted interventions for addiction. Animal studies have shown a significant role of serotonin in animal models of addiction, contributing to various aspects of the addictive process, including reward processing, motivation, and impulse control. Animal models allow researchers to investigate the neurobiological mechanisms underlying addiction and test potential interventions. Animal models of addiction often involve assessing the rewarding effects of substances of abuse. Serotonin is implicated in modulating reward processing and reinforcement, influencing an animal's response to drugs (Rocha et al., 2010). Serotonin is associated with the regulation of impulsivity and risky decision-making, which are key behavioral aspects of addiction.

Animal models can be used to study how serotonin modulates these behaviors. Animal models allow researchers to study the role of serotonin in withdrawal and the negative affective states that contribute to drug-seeking behavior (You et al., 2016). Cocaine, a psychostimulant, affects serotonin levels. Animal models help elucidate how changes in serotonin function contribute to cocaine addiction and relapse. Animal models of opioid addiction provide insights into the role of serotonin in the reinforcing effects of opioids and the development of dependence. Animal models are used to test the efficacy of medications targeting serotonin receptors for the treatment of addiction. These studies highlight the importance of studying serotonin in animal models to understand the neurobiological mechanisms underlying addiction. Animal models provide a controlled environment for investigating specific aspects of addiction and evaluating potential therapeutic interventions.

Serotonin and drug withdrawal: Serotonin plays a significant role in drug withdrawal, influencing various aspects of the withdrawal syndrome such as mood, anxiety, and physiological symptoms. Serotonin is involved in the regulation of mood, and alterations in serotonin levels during drug withdrawal can contribute to negative affective states and increased anxiety (Staley & Krishnan-Sarin, 2015). Serotonin is implicated in the regulation of sleep, and changes in serotonin levels during drug withdrawal can contribute to sleep disturbances commonly observed during withdrawal. Chronic drug use can lead to adaptive changes in the brain's serotonin system. Abrupt cessation of drug intake during withdrawal may result in decreased serotonin levels. Serotonin dysregulation is often associated with symptoms of depression and dysphoria during drug withdrawal. Altered serotonin function can contribute to increased anxiety and irritability during drug withdrawal. Serotonin is involved in the regulation of sleep, and disruptions in serotonin function during withdrawal can contribute to sleep disturbances. Serotonin's role in mood regulation is interconnected with drug craving during withdrawal, potentially increasing the risk of relapse. Changes in its levels can contribute to symptoms of anhedonia, the inability to experience pleasure, during drug withdrawal. Serotonin is involved in regulating emotional states, and its dysregulation during withdrawal contributes to the overall negative affective experience.

Serotonin is involved in the regulation of gastrointestinal function, and alterations in serotonin levels during drug withdrawal can contribute to gastrointestinal symptoms such as nausea and diarrhea (Thompson & Lummis, 2007). Serotonin is associated with the regulation of appetite, and changes in serotonin levels during drug withdrawal can contribute to appetite changes and weight fluctuations. Gastrointestinal symptoms during drug withdrawal are influenced by various neurotransmitter systems, including serotonin. Serotonin is a key regulator of gastrointestinal function, and alterations in its levels can contribute to symptoms such as nausea, vomiting, and diarrhea. Serotonin is involved in the regulation of nausea and vomiting. Changes in serotonin levels during drug withdrawal can contribute to these gastrointestinal symptoms. Alterations in serotonin levels can impact gut motility and contribute to diarrhea during drug withdrawal. Changes in serotonin signaling may contribute to alterations in gut smooth muscle activity, leading to abdominal pain and cramps during withdrawal. Serotonin is implicated in the regulation of appetite. Alterations in serotonin function during drug withdrawal can contribute to appetite changes, including decreased or increased appetite. Serotonin is a key modulator of gastrointestinal motility. Changes in serotonin levels during drug withdrawal can influence the pace of gut transit (Crowell & Wessinger,

2007).Gastrointestinal symptoms during withdrawal, including vomiting and diarrhea, can contribute to dehydration and electrolyte imbalances. Understanding the role of serotonin in gastrointestinal symptoms during drug withdrawal is essential for developing targeted interventions to alleviate these symptoms. The interactions between serotonin and other neurotransmitter systems contribute to the complexity of the gastrointestinal effects observed during withdrawal from various substances of abuse. Drug craving and relapse also involve serotonin dysregulation, increasing the risk of relapse (Kosten & George, 2002).

Serotonin plays a crucial role in drug craving and relapse, influencing various aspects of the addiction cycle. Dysregulation of serotonin neurotransmission during withdrawal and abstinence can contribute to the intense desire for the drug and increase the risk of relapse. Serotonin is involved in the modulation of craving, affecting the subjective desire for drugs during withdrawal and abstinence. Alterations in serotonin levels can influence mood and contribute to drug craving as individuals may seek substances to alleviate negative affective states. Serotonin interacts with dopamine, another neurotransmitter involved in reward pathways, and these interactions play a role in drug craving (Di Giovanni & De Deurwaerdère, 2016). Specific serotonin receptors, such as the 5HT-1B receptor, have been implicated in the modulation of drug-seeking behavior and craving. Serotonin is involved in the response to drug-related cues, contributing to cue-induced craving and the likelihood of relapse.

Medications that influence serotonin, such as selective serotonin reuptake inhibitors (SSRIs), have been investigated for their potential in reducing drug craving. Stress-induced drug craving, a significant factor in relapse, involves serotonin pathways and their interaction with the stress response (Fox & Sinha, 2014). Understanding the role of serotonin in drug craving and relapse is critical for developing targeted pharmacotherapies and interventions aimed at reducing the risk of relapse during addiction treatment. The interactions between serotonin and other neurotransmitter systems contribute to the complexity of craving and relapse processes. Serotonin is implicated in mood regulation, and alterations in serotonin function during withdrawal can contribute to symptoms of depression and anhedonia (Hensler, 2003). It's important to note that the role of serotonin in drug withdrawal can vary depending on the specific drug of abuse and individual differences. Additionally, interactions with other neurotransmitter systems, such as the dopamine and noradrenaline systems, also contribute to the complex neurobiology of drug withdrawal. Ongoing research continues to deepen our understanding of these processes. Drug-induced depression and anhedonia can be associated with alterations in serotonin neurotransmission. Various substances of abuse can impact serotonin levels, leading to changes in mood and pleasure-seeking behaviors. Altered serotonin function is implicated in mood disorders, including drug-induced depression.

Drug-induced changes in serotonin levels may contribute to depressive symptoms. Serotonin is involved in the regulation of pleasure and reward. Dysregulation of serotonin function can contribute to anhedonia, the inability to experience pleasure. Serotonin plays a complex role in drug-induced anhedonia, which refers to the diminished ability to experience pleasure or a reduced interest in normally rewarding activities. Anhedonia is a common symptom observed in various psychiatric disorders, including those related to substance use. Serotonin is involved in the regulation of reward processing in the brain. Changes in serotonin levels can impact the brain's ability to perceive and respond to rewarding stimuli. Serotonin interacts with dopamine, another neurotransmitter associated with reward and pleasure. Disruptions in serotonin function can influence the balance between serotonin and dopamine signaling.

Serotonin is implicated in the regulation of hedonic tone, which is the level of pleasure or joy experienced. Dysregulation of serotonin may contribute to a blunted hedonic response observed in anhedonia (Der-Avakian & Markou, 2012). Abuse of different substances can impact serotonin levels and signaling pathways. Chronic drug use may lead to adaptations in serotonin function that contribute to anhedonic symptoms. Opioids, for example, can influence serotonin transmission. The interplay between opioids and serotonin pathways may contribute to anhedonia observed in opioid use. During drug withdrawal, especially from substances that impact serotonin function, individuals may experience anhedonic symptoms as a part of the withdrawal syndrome. Antidepressant medications that target serotonin, such as selective serotonin reuptake inhibitors (SSRIs), are sometimes used in the treatment of anhedonia associated with depression, including substance-induced depression. Understanding the role of serotonin in drug-induced anhedonia is essential for developing targeted interventions to address this symptom, particularly in the context of substance use disorders. The interactions between serotonin and other neurotransmitter systems contribute to the complexity of anhedonic states observed in individuals with a history of substance abuse.

Substance abuse can lead to mood disorders, including depression. The impact on serotonin levels is one of the contributing factors. Different drugs can affect serotonin receptors, influencing mood and emotional states. For example, MDMA (ecstasy) affects serotonin release and uptake. Opioid use can impact serotonin function, potentially contributing to mood disturbances and anhedonia. Some individuals with substance use disorders may experience comorbid depression. Antidepressants targeting serotonin, such as SSRIs, are used in the treatment 9 Spijker & Bijl, 2001). Drug withdrawal, especially from substances that affect serotonin levels, can lead to depressive symptoms as serotonin levels readjust. The interplay between serotonin and drug-induced depression and anhedonia is crucial for developing effective interventions and treatments for individuals experiencing mood disturbances in the context of substance use. The complexity of these interactions requires a comprehensive approach to both addiction and mental health treatment.

Serotonin and co-occurring disorders: Serotonin dysregulation is often implicated in the development and exacerbation of co-occurring mental health disorders in the context of drug abuse. Substance use disorders frequently co-occur with various psychiatric conditions, and serotonin, as a neurotransmitter, plays a crucial role in the neurobiological mechanisms underlying these comorbidities. Substance abuse, particularly with drugs that affect serotonin levels, can contribute to the development of depressive disorders. Dysregulation of serotonin neurotransmission is often observed in individuals with depression (Trivedi & Greer, 2014). Depression is a complex and debilitating mental health disorder characterized by persistent feelings of sadness, hopelessness, and a lack of interest or pleasure in activities. The neurobiological underpinnings of depression involve alterations in various neurotransmitter systems, with serotonin playing a central role. Serotonin, also known as the "feel-good" neurotransmitter, is involved in the regulation of mood, sleep, appetite, and overall emotional well-being. In the context of depression, there is a longstanding theory known as the serotonin hypothesis, suggesting that imbalances in serotonin levels contribute to the development and severity of depressive symptoms. Research has shown that individuals with depression often exhibit changes in serotonin neurotransmission. Specifically, there may be a deficiency of serotonin or dysfunction in the receptors that serotonin binds to. This serotonin imbalance is believed to disrupt the intricate neural circuits involved in mood regulation, leading to the characteristic symptoms of depression. Antidepressant medications, such as selective serotonin reuptake inhibitors (SSRIs) and serotonin-norepinephrine reuptake inhibitors (SNRIs), are commonly prescribed to address serotonin deficiencies in the brain. These medications work by increasing te availability of serotonin in the synaptic cleft, enhancing its binding to receptors and promoting mood stabilization.

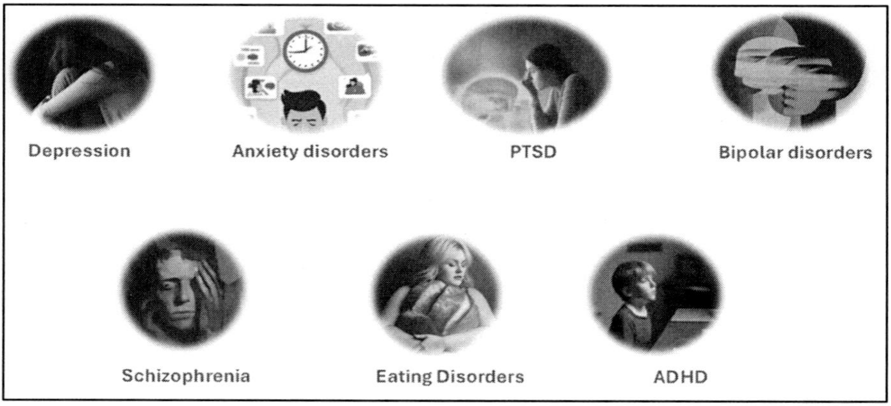

Serotonin dysregulation and co-occurring disorders in substance abuse

The relationship between depression and serotonin is not a simple cause-and-effect scenario. While serotonin imbalances are associated with depression, other factors, including genetic predisposition, environmental stressors, and individual differences in brain chemistry, also contribute to the development of depressive disorders. Understanding the role of serotonin in depression has led to the development of targeted pharmacotherapies, and ongoing research continues to refine our understanding of the intricate interplay between serotonin and other neurotransmitter systems in the context of depression. The multifaceted nature of depression underscores the importance of personalized and comprehensive approaches to treatment that address the unique neurobiological and psychosocial factors contributing to individual's experience of depression.

Drug abuse can lead to heightened anxiety levels. Serotonin is implicated in anxiety regulation, and disruptions in serotonin pathways may contribute to anxiety disorders (Graeff & Del-Ben, 2008). Anxiety disorders encompass a spectrum of mental health conditions characterized by excessive worry, fear, and apprehension. Serotonin, a neurotransmitter, plays a crucial role in the regulation of mood and emotional states, and its involvement in anxiety disorders is a topic of considerable research and clinical interest. The intricate relationship between serotonin and anxiety involves the modulation of neural circuits responsible for emotional processing. Serotonin acts as a key neurotransmitter in these circuits, influencing the balance between excitatory and inhibitory signals within the brain. Disruptions in serotonin levels or receptor functioning have been implicated in the pathophysiology of various anxiety disorders. Studies have shown that alterations in serotonin neurotransmission are associated with heightened anxiety states. Serotonin receptors, particularly those of the 5HT-1A subtype, are involved in the regulation of anxiety-related behaviors. Changes in the sensitivity or availability of these receptors may contribute to the development and maintenance of anxiety disorders.

Selective serotonin reuptake inhibitors (SSRIs) and serotonin-norepinephrine reuptake inhibitors (SNRIs) are commonly prescribed medications for the treatment of anxiety disorders. These drugs increase the concentration of serotonin in the synaptic cleft, enhancing its effects and promoting a more balanced neurotransmitter environment. The role of serotonin in anxiety extends beyond its direct influence on mood. Serotonin is also involved in the regulation of other physiological processes, such as sleep, appetite, and arousal, which are interconnected with anxiety symptoms. Dysregulation of serotonin in these areas may contribute to the diverse manifestations of anxiety disorders. While serotonin is a central player in anxiety disorders, it is important to recognize that anxiety is a complex condition influenced by a combination of genetic, environmental, and psychological factors. The interaction between serotonin and other neurotransmitter systems, such as gamma-aminobutyric acid (GABA) and norepinephrine, further contributes to the complexity of anxiety's neurobiology. The comprehensive nature of anxiety necessitates a holistic approach that considers individual differences and addresses the multifaceted factors contributing to the disorder.

Individuals with a history of substance abuse, especially with drugs affecting serotonin, may be at an increased risk of developing Post-Traumatic Stress Disorder (PTSD). Serotonin alterations are associated with the pathophysiology of PTSD (Price & Mello, 2020). Post-Traumatic Stress Disorder (PTSD) is a mental health condition that can develop in individuals who have experienced or witnessed a traumatic event. Serotonin, a neurotransmitter, is implicated in the neurobiology of PTSD, influencing various aspects of the disorder. Studies suggest that individuals with PTSD may exhibit alterations in serotonin neurotransmission. Changes in serotonin receptor sensitivity and availability have been observed in regions of the brain associated with emotional regulation. 5HT-1A serotonin receptors have been implicated in the modulation of fear responses and anxiety. Serotonin is involved in the regulation of hippocampal function, a brain region crucial for memory and emotion processing. Dysregulation of serotonin in the hippocampus may contribute to difficulties in trauma memory processing in PTSD (Jacobsen & Mork, 2006).

Selective serotonin reuptake inhibitors (SSRIs) are commonly used in the treatment of PTSD. These medications increase serotonin levels in the synaptic cleft, potentially alleviating symptoms of hyperarousal and intrusive thoughts. Genetic factors, including variations in the serotonin transporter gene, have been studied in relation to PTSD susceptibility. Certain genetic variants may influence serotonin reuptake and contribute to vulnerability to trauma-related conditions. Serotonin is involved in fear extinction processes, which are impaired in individuals with PTSD. Understanding the role of serotonin in fear extinction is crucial for developing targeted interventions. Understanding the role of serotonin in

PTSD is a complex and evolving area of research. While serotonin dysregulation is implicated in certain aspects of PTSD, the disorder's neurobiology involves intricate interactions with other neurotransmitter systems, genetics, and environmental factors. The integration of these factors is crucial for a comprehensive understanding of PTSD and the development of targeted therapeutic approaches. Co-occurrence of bipolar disorder and substance use is common. Serotonin dysregulation is implicated in both conditions, and drugs of abuse can impact mood regulation (Lee et al., 2022). The relationship between addiction and bipolar disorder involves complex interactions with neurotransmitters, including serotonin. Both conditions are characterized by dysregulation in mood and reward systems, and serotonin plays a crucial role in modulating these processes. Here's an overview of the connections between addiction, bipolar disorder, and serotonin, along with relevant references:

Bipolar disorder is associated with dysregulation in various neurotransmitter systems, including serotonin. Changes in serotonin levels are implicated in the mood swings observed in individuals with bipolar disorder (Lee et al., 2022). Serotonin is involved in mood stabilization, and alterations in serotonin levels are linked to the shifts between depressive and manic states in bipolar disorder. Individuals with bipolar disorder have higher rates of comorbid substance use disorders. Drugs of abuse, including those impacting serotonin, may be used to self-medicate or exacerbate mood symptoms. Substance abuse, particularly stimulants, can impact serotonin pathways. The interplay between substance use and serotonin dysregulation may contribute to the complexity of bipolar disorder symptoms. Mood stabilizers commonly prescribed for bipolar disorder, such as lithium, are believed to influence serotonin levels. These medications aim to stabilize mood by modulating neurotransmitter activity (Baldessarini & Tondo, 2019). Genetic variations in serotonin receptors have been investigated in relation to bipolar disorder susceptibility. These variations may contribute to individual differences in treatment response and symptom presentation.

Impulsivity is a common feature in bipolar disorder and is associated with serotonin dysfunction. Substance use as a form of self-medication may be influenced by impulsive behaviors in individuals with bipolar disorder. Understanding the interplay between bipolar disorder, addiction, and serotonin is crucial for developing effective treatment strategies. It involves considering the impact of both conditions on serotonin pathways, the potential use of substances to cope with mood symptoms, and the role of serotonin in the pharmacological management of bipolar disorder.

Substance use disorders are prevalent among individuals with schizophrenia. Serotonin alterations are implicated in the cognitive and affective symptoms of schizophrenia (Meltzer & Huang, 2008). The relationship between drug addiction, schizophrenia, and serotonin involves complex interactions within the brain's neurotransmitter systems. Serotonin dysregulation has been implicated in both substance abuse disorders and schizophrenia, and understanding these connections is crucial for developing comprehensive treatment approaches. Schizophrenia is associated with alterations in serotonin neurotransmission, particularly involving the 5-HT2A receptor. Dysregulation of serotonin pathways is thought to contribute to cognitive and affective symptoms in schizophrenia. Serotonin is involved in cognitive processes, and alterations in serotonin levels may contribute to cognitive deficits observed in schizophrenia. Cognitive impairment is a key feature of the disorder. Serotonin interacts with the mesolimbic dopamine pathway, which is implicated in reward processing and addiction. Dysregulation in this pathway may contribute to both schizophrenia and drug addiction.

Individuals with schizophrenia have a higher risk of comorbid substance use disorders. Substance abuse, including drugs affecting serotonin, may be an attempt to self-medicate or cope with symptoms. Serotonin dysregulation is associated with impulsivity, a trait linked to both substance use disorders and schizophrenia. Impulsivity may contribute to drug-seeking behavior and the development of addiction (Perry & Carroll, 2008). Antipsychotic medications, often prescribed for schizophrenia, influence serotonin receptors. These medications aim to modulate neurotransmitter activity, including serotonin, to alleviate symptoms. Shared neurobiological factors, including alterations in serotonin signaling, contribute to the overlap between substance use disorders and schizophrenia. Understanding these common pathways is essential for targeted interventions. Understanding the intricate interplay between serotonin, drug addiction, and schizophrenia is vital for developing effective interventions that address the complex needs of individuals with comorbid conditions. The shared neurobiological mechanisms may offer potential targets for novel therapeutic approaches. Certain drugs of abuse, including those affecting serotonin, may contribute to the development or exacerbation of eating disorders. Serotonin dysregulation is implicated in the neurobiology of eating disorders (Kaye et al., 2009). Eating disorders, such as anorexia nervosa and bulimia nervosa, are associated with alterations in serotonin neurotransmission. Dysregulation of serotonin pathways is thought to contribute to disturbances in mood, appetite regulation, and impulse control seen in these disorders. Serotonin plays a crucial role in the regulation of appetite and satiety. Dysregulation of serotonin signaling may contribute to abnormal eating behaviors observed in eating disorders. Individuals with eating disorders often have comorbid substance use disorders.

Substance abuse, including drugs affecting serotonin, may be used to cope with the emotional distress associated with eating disorders (Brewerton, & Dennis, 2014). Impulsivity is a trait associated with both eating disorders and substance use disorders. Serotonin dysregulation may contribute to impulsivity, influencing disordered eating patterns and substance abuse. Shared neurobiological factors, including alterations in serotonin signaling, contribute to the overlap between substance use disorders and eating disorders. Understanding these common pathways is essential for targeted interventions. Serotonin is involved in emotional regulation, and dysregulation of serotonin pathways may contribute to the emotional distress associated with both substance use and eating disorders. Understanding the intricate interplay between serotonin, drug abuse, and eating disorders is vital for developing effective interventions that address the complex needs of individuals with comorbid conditions. The shared neurobiological mechanisms may offer potential targets for novel therapeutic approaches.

Attention-Deficit/Hyperactivity Disorder (ADHD) and serotonin alterations may play a role in both ADHD and substance abuse. Understanding the intricate relationship between serotonin and drug abuse-induced co-occurring mental health disorders is crucial for developing comprehensive treatment strategies that address both substance use and psychiatric symptoms. The interactions between serotonin and other neurotransmitter systems contribute to the complexity of these comorbid conditions. The relationship between drug abuse, ADHD, and serotonin involves complex interactions within the brain's neurotransmitter systems. Serotonin dysregulation has been implicated in both ADHD and substance use disorders, and understanding these connections is crucial for developing comprehensive treatment approaches. ADHD is associated with alterations in serotonin neurotransmission, particularly involving the 5-HT1A receptor. Dysregulation of serotonin pathways is thought to contribute to attentional and impulse control deficits observed in ADHD (Zepf & Wöckel, 2016). Individuals with ADHD are at an increased risk of developing substance use disorders. Serotonin dysregulation may contribute to impulsive behaviors and a higher susceptibility to substance abuse in individuals with ADHD. Impulsivity is a core symptom of ADHD, and serotonin dysregulation is associated with impulsivity.

The interaction between serotonin and other neurotransmitter systems contributes to the impulsive behaviors seen in ADHD. Medications commonly used to treat ADHD, such as methylphenidate and amphetamines, primarily affect dopamine levels. However, the indirect impact on serotonin systems may contribute to the medications' therapeutic effects. Genetic variations in serotonin-related genes have been studied in relation to ADHD susceptibility. These variations may contribute to individual differences in serotonin function and ADHD risk. Serotonin is involved in executive function processes, which are often impaired in individuals with ADHD. Dysregulation of serotonin may contribute to difficulties in attention, planning, and self-control. Shared neurobiological factors, including alterations in serotonin signaling, contribute to the overlap between ADHD and substance use disorders. Understanding these common pathways is essential for targeted interventions. Intricate interplay between serotonin, drug abuse, and ADHD is vital for developing effective interventions that address the complex needs of individuals with comorbid conditions. The shared neurobiological mechanisms may offer potential targets for novel therapeutic approaches.

Genetic variations related to serotonin receptors and transporters in the context of drug abuse: Genetic variations in serotonin receptors and transporters play a significant role in the context of drug addiction. These variations can influence an individual's susceptibility to addiction, response to drugs, and risk of developing substance use disorders. Polymorphisms in serotonin receptors, especially the 5HT-2A and 5HT-2C receptors, have been linked to susceptibility to drug addiction. These variations can impact the reward pathway and the reinforcing effects of drugs (Sáiz et al., 2008). Genetic variations in serotonin receptors can influence an individual's susceptibility to addiction, response to drugs, and risk of developing substance use disorders. The serotonin transporter-linked polymorphic region (5HTTLPR) in the serotonin transporter gene (SLC6A4) influences serotonin reuptake. Variations in 5HTTLPR have been associated with susceptibility to substance use disorders (Kreek et al., 2005). Polymorphisms in the 5HT-1A receptor gene (HTR1A) have been linked to substance abuse, including alcohol dependence and vulnerability to addiction (Pattanaik et al., 2022).

The serotonin receptor 2A gene (HTR2A) has been implicated in various psychiatric disorders, and variations in this receptor may influence susceptibility to addiction. Polymorphisms in the serotonin receptor 2C gene (HTR2C) have been associated with substance abuse, including cocaine and alcohol dependence (Lee et al., 2005). Variations in the serotonin receptor 3A gene (HTR3A) have been linked to nicotine dependence, indicating a potential role in the addictive properties of tobacco (Ursini et al., 2011). Polymorphisms in the serotonin receptor 1B gene (HTR1B) have been associated with cocaine addiction, suggesting a role in the vulnerability to stimulant abuse. Genetic variations in the serotonin receptor 4 gene (HTR4) have been implicated in alcohol dependence, suggesting a potential role in the modulation of alcohol-related behaviors (Wang et al., 2004). Understanding the impact of serotonin receptor variations provides insights into the genetic factors contributing to individual differences in susceptibility to drug abuse and addiction. It's important to note that addiction is a complex and multifactorial disorder influenced by a combination of genetic, environmental, and behavioral factors.

The serotonin transporter gene (SLC6A4) encodes the serotonin transporter protein, which regulates serotonin reuptake. Genetic variations in this gene, such as the 5-HTTLPR polymorphism, have been associated with vulnerability to substance abuse. Genetic variations in the SLC6A4 gene have been implicated in alcohol dependence, with studies suggesting associations between certain alleles and the risk of alcohol-related disorders (Kim et al., 2008). Studies have explored the relationship between the 5-HTTLPR polymorphism and opioid dependence, revealing potential associations between certain genotypes and susceptibility to opioid abuse (Glatt et al., 2006). Genetic variations in the serotonin transporter gene have been investigated in the context of nicotine dependence, suggesting a potential role in the development of tobacco addiction (Munafo et al., 2004). Understanding the role of SLC6A4 gene variations provides valuable insights into the genetic factors contributing to individual differences in susceptibility to drug abuse and addiction. However, it's crucial to acknowledge the complexity of addiction, influenced by a combination of genetic, environmental, and behavioral factors.

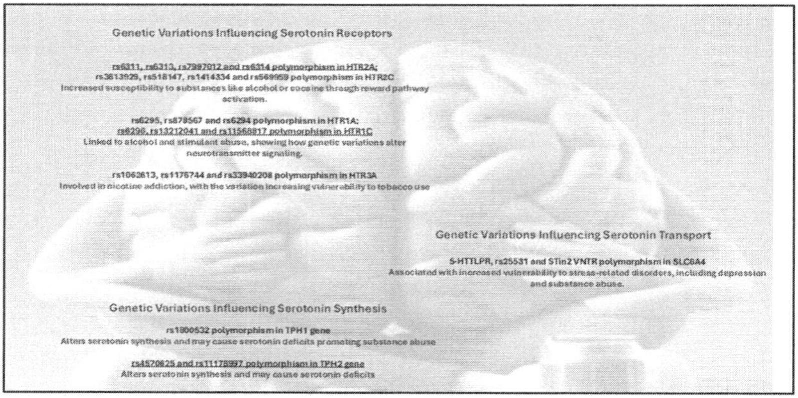

Genetic variations related to serotonin receptors and transporters in the context of drug abuse

Tryptophan hydroxylase is an enzyme involved in serotonin synthesis. Genetic variations in the TPH gene have been implicated in the susceptibility to drug addiction by influencing serotonin levels (Zill et al., 2007). Tryptophan hydroxylase (TPH) is an enzyme that plays a crucial role in the synthesis of serotonin, a neurotransmitter involved in mood regulation and various physiological functions. Variations in TPH genes can impact serotonin production and have been studied in the context of drug abuse. Polymorphisms in the TPH1 gene, which encodes the tryptophan hydroxylase 1 enzyme, have been investigated in relation to substance abuse, including alcohol dependence. TPH2, another isoform of tryptophan hydroxylase primarily found in the brain, has been implicated in the susceptibility to substance use disorders, including alcohol dependence and heroin addiction (Huang & Shyur, 2012).

Specific polymorphisms in the TPH1 gene have been associated with alcohol dependence, suggesting a role in the regulation of serotonin synthesis in the periphery (Kim et al., 2008). Genetic variations in TPH2 have been investigated in relation to opioid dependence, indicating potential links between serotonin synthesis in the brain and susceptibility to opioid abuse (Glatt et al., 2006). Variations in the TPH1 gene have been studied in relation to nicotine dependence, suggesting a potential role in the modulation of serotonin levels and the addictive properties of tobacco. Genetic variations in TPH genes provides insights into the biological mechanisms underlying serotonin synthesis and its potential role in the vulnerability to drug abuse. It's important to note that genetic factors are just one aspect of the complex interplay influencing substance use disorders, with environmental and behavioral factors also playing significant roles. Gene-environment interactions, such as variations in serotonin receptors interacting with stress or trauma, contribute to the risk of substance abuse and addiction. Understanding the genetic variations related to serotonin receptors and transporters provides insights into the biological underpinnings of drug addiction. However, it's important to note that addiction is a complex and multifactorial condition influenced by both genetic and environmental factors. The interaction between serotonin receptor variations and environmental factors plays a crucial role in the susceptibility to drug abuse and addiction. Environmental influences can modulate the impact of genetic variations on the risk of developing substance use disorders. The serotonin transporter-linked polymorphic region (5-HTTLPR) interacts with stressful life events to influence the risk of substance abuse. Individuals with specific 5-HTTLPR genotypes may be more vulnerable to the impact of stressors (Enoch et al., 2010). Various serotonin receptor polymorphisms, including those in HTR2A and HTR2C, may interact with environmental factors, such as childhood adversity, to influence the risk of developing substance use disorders (Nelson et al.,

2009). The serotonin receptor 2A gene (HTR2A) may interact with childhood maltreatment to influence the risk of substance abuse, particularly in individuals who experienced early-life stress (Nelson et al., 2009). Stressful life events may interact with variations in the tryptophan hydroxylase 2 gene (TPH2) to influence susceptibility to substance abuse and addiction (Nilsson et al., 2011). Interactions between genetic variations in serotonin receptors, such as HTR3A, and environmental factors may contribute to the risk of cocaine dependence (Han et al., 2015). The interaction between serotonin receptor polymorphisms and environmental factors, such as peer substance use, may contribute to the development of substance abuse behaviors. Understanding gene-environment interactions provides a more comprehensive view of the factors contributing to drug abuse and addiction. It emphasizes the need to consider both genetic and environmental influences to develop effective prevention and intervention strategies.

Therapeutic targeting of serotonin for drug abuse: Therapeutic targeting of serotonin receptors for drug abuse involves developing medications that modulate the activity of these receptors to reduce addictive behaviors. The goal is to influence the serotonin system, which plays a crucial role in mood regulation, reward processing, and impulse control. Drugs targeting the serotonin 5-HT3 receptor, such as ondansetron, have been explored for their potential in reducing alcohol consumption. 5-HT3 receptor antagonists may modulate the rewarding effects of alcohol (Johnson et al., 2003). Psilocybin, a classic hallucinogen that acts as a serotonin 5-HT2A receptor agonist, has shown promise in the treatment of substance use disorders, including addiction to nicotine and alcohol (Bogenschutz et al., 2015).

Buspirone, a partial agonist of the serotonin 5-HT1A receptor, has been investigated for its potential in reducing alcohol consumption and craving. Medications that increase serotonin synthesis by providing precursor molecules, such as tryptophan or 5-hydroxytryptophan (5-HTP), have been explored for their potential in reducing alcohol and drug cravings. SSRIs, such as fluoxetine and sertraline, which increase serotonin levels by inhibiting its reuptake, have been studied for their potential in treating co-occurring depression and substance use disorders (Addolorato et al., 2007). Medications that target both serotonin and norepinephrine reuptake, such as venlafaxine, have been investigated for their potential in treating comorbid depression and substance use disorders (Nunes et al., 2008). These examples illustrate the diverse approaches to therapeutic targeting of serotonin receptors for drug abuse, highlighting the complexity of serotonin's role in addiction and the potential for pharmacological interventions to address this complex issue. It's important to note that research in this field is ongoing, and individual responses to medications may vary.

CHAPTER 8

COMORBIDITY OF STRESS, DEPRESSION, AND DRUG ADDICTION

"Addiction is not a choice that anybody makes; it's a response to emotional pain. When people are in distress, they will do anything to relieve it—even if it means self-destruction."
~ Dr. Gabor Maté

It is interesting to know how stress and depression often go hand-in-hand with addiction. It's about the extra challenges people face when dealing with these together. We should consider how tough it is, but also how strong people can be in facing these battles. This chapter explains how the nexus of stress, depression, and drug addiction forms a complex interplay that underscores the intricate relationship between mental health and substance use disorders, shaping a landscape where these conditions frequently coexist. Examining the comorbidity of stress, depression, and drug addiction reveals a multifaceted dynamic, where the intertwining threads of emotional well-being and substance misuse contribute to a challenging terrain for individuals grappling with overlapping mental health concerns and addictive behaviors.

Stress is a complex and multifaceted concept that encompasses a range of physiological and psychological responses to external or internal challenges, known as stressors. It involves the body's adaptive response to perceived threats or demands, often referred to as the "fight-or-flight" response. Stress can be acute or chronic and may have both positive (eustress) and negative (distress) effects on an individual's well-being. Stress can be defined as a state of physiological and psychological arousal in response to a perceived threat or demand, leading to a complex set of adaptive reactions aimed at coping with or avoiding the stressor. Stress activates the body's neuroendocrine system, leading to the release of stress hormones such as cortisol and adrenaline, which prepare the body for a rapid response to the stressor (Chrousos, 2009). Stress involves cognitive and emotional responses to the perception of a stressor, including appraisals, coping strategies, and the subjective experience of distress. Eustress refers to positive stress that can enhance performance and motivation, while distress refers to negative stress associated with harm or threat. Stress involves both the physiological and psychological dimensions, as well as individual differences in how people perceive and respond to stressors. The referenced works provide foundational insights into the historical and contemporary understanding of stress.

Depression is a mental health disorder characterized by persistent feelings of sadness, hopelessness, and a lack of interest or pleasure in daily activities. It can affect how a person thinks, feels, and manages daily activities. Depression is a serious condition that can significantly impact one's quality of life, and it often requires professional intervention for effective treatment. Depression is a mood disorder marked by persistent feelings of sadness, hopelessness, and a lack of interest or pleasure in activities. It affects how a person thinks, feels, and functions on a daily basis. Key features of depression include persistent low mood or irritability, loss of interest or pleasure in activities once enjoyed, changes in appetite or weight, sleep disturbances, fatigue or loss of energy, feelings of worthlessness or excessive guilt, difficulty concentrating or making decisions and thoughts of death or suicide (National Institute of Mental Health, 2021). Depression is associated with alterations in neurotransmitter function, neuroendocrine regulation, and neuroplasticity (Duman et al., 2016).

Environmental stressors, trauma, and interpersonal difficulties can contribute to the development and exacerbation of depression. Drepression involves recognizing its multifaceted nature, considering both biological and psychosocial factors. Professional assessment and treatment are crucial for individuals experiencing depression. The referenced works provide foundational knowledge on the definition, features, and contributing factors of depression. The interrelationship between stress, depression, and drug abuse is a complex and multifaceted phenomenon. Each of these factors can influence and exacerbate the others, creating a cycle that poses significant challenges for individuals. Chronic stress can contribute to the development of both depression and substance abuse (Sinha, 2008). Chronic stress has been identified as a significant risk factor for the development of both depression and substance abuse. The relationship between chronic stress, depression, and substance abuse is complex and bidirectional, with each factor influencing and reinforcing the others. Prolonged exposure to chronic stressors, such as financial difficulties, work-related stress, or interpersonal conflicts, can dysregulate the body's stress response systems. Chronic activation of the stress response can lead to changes in the brain, particularly in areas associated with mood regulation, such as the hippocampus and prefrontal cortex. Over time, these changes may contribute to the development of depressive symptoms. Individuals experiencing chronic stress may turn to substances (such as alcohol or drugs) as a way to cope with the emotional distress and escape from negative feelings. Substance abuse can initially provide a sense of relief or pleasure, creating a potential for the development of a substance use disorder and it can further contribute to stress and exacerbate mental health issues. The relationship between chronic stress, depression, and substance abuse is often bidirectional, with each factor influencing and reinforcing the others. For example, substance abuse can worsen the effects of chronic stress, leading to a cycle of dependence and increased vulnerability to mental health issues.

Individuals experiencing stress and depression may turn to drug abuse as a way of self-medicating to alleviate emotional pain. Individuals experiencing stress and depression may turn to drug abuse as a way of self-medicating. Self-medication hypothesis suggests that individuals experiencing stress and depression may turn to drug abuse as a means of coping with or alleviating their emotional distress. This hypothesis proposes that substances such as drugs or alcohol are used as a form of self-treatment to manage the symptoms of psychological distress. Individuals facing stressors or experiencing symptoms of depression may seek relief from their emotional pain by using substances that temporarily alter mood or consciousness (Brady & Sinha, 2005). Drug abuse may provide a temporary sense of relief from feelings of sadness, anxiety, or stress, creating a perceived escape from emotional difficulties. Individuals may self-medicate with various substances, including alcohol, prescription medications, or illicit drugs, depending on their availability and personal preferences. Substance use may interact with the brain's reward system and neurotransmitter pathways, providing a temporary sense of pleasure or relief from negative emotions. While initially providing a sense of relief, self-medication with substances can lead to the development of substance use disorders, creating a cycle of dependence. Recognizing the interplay between stress, depression, and substance abuse, an integrated treatment approach that addresses both mental health and substance use is often essential for effective intervention (Mueser et al., 2003). Understanding of the complex relationship between stress, depression, and substance abuse is crucial for developing effective prevention and intervention strategies that address the underlying causes of these interconnected issues.

Stress and depression can affect the same neural circuits involved in addiction, contributing to a heightened vulnerability to substance abuse (Koob & Le Moal, 2008). The interplay of stress, depression, and drug abuse involves intricate neurobiological mechanisms that impact the brain's structure and function. Understanding these mechanisms is essential for comprehending the complex relationships among these phenomena. Chronic stress can lead to dysregulation of the Hypothalamic-Pituitary-Adrenal (HPA) Axis, resulting in increased release of stress hormones, particularly cortisol. Dysregulation of the HPA axis has been associated with both depression and substance abuse (Pariante & Lightman, 2008). Dysregulation of neurotransmitter systems, including serotonin, dopamine, and norepinephrine, is implicated in both depression and substance abuse. Substance abuse can directly impact these systems, leading to alterations in mood and reward processing. Chronic stress and depression have been associated with structural changes in the brain, particularly in areas such as the hippocampus and prefrontal cortex. Substance abuse can further impact neuroplasticity, affecting brain structure and function (Koob & Volkow, 2016). The mesolimbic dopamine system, associated with reward processing, is implicated in both depression and drug abuse. Substance abuse can lead to dysregulation of this system, contributing to the reinforcing effects of drugs. Chronic stress and substance abuse can induce epigenetic modifications, influencing gene expression patterns that may contribute to long-term changes in behavior and mood. These neurobiological mechanisms involved in the interplay of stress, depression, and drug abuse cover an active area of research. These mechanisms are complex and interconnected, involving various brain regions, neurotransmitter systems, and molecular pathways. Advances in neuroscience contribute to a more comprehensive understanding of how these factors interact and may inform the development of targeted interventions for individuals experiencing co-occurring stress, depression, and substance abuse.

Substance abuse can exacerbate stress and depression, creating a bidirectional relationship (Swendsen et al., 2010). The relationship between substance abuse and stress/depression is often bidirectional, meaning that each can contribute to and exacerbate the other. This bidirectional relationship is complex and involves various psychological, neurobiological, and social factors. Individuals may initially turn to substances as a way to cope with stress or alleviate symptoms of depression. Neurobiological changes in the brain take over, affecting areas associated with mood regulation and stress response. These changes may contribute to the persistence or exacerbation of depressive symptoms. Substance abuse can lead to a cycle of dependence, withdrawal, and cravings, which can increase stress and contribute to the onset or worsening of depressive symptoms. Substance abuse can have detrimental psychosocial consequences, such as strained relationships, financial difficulties, and legal problems, which can contribute to stress and exacerbate depressive symptoms. Addressing both substance abuse and mental health issues concurrently is often necessary for successful treatment. Integrated treatment approaches that target both conditions are associated with better outcomes (Mueser et al., 2003). Addressing the bidirectional relationship between substance abuse, stress, and depression is crucial for developing effective prevention and intervention strategies. This often involves a comprehensive and integrated approach that considers biological, psychological, and social factors. The co-occurrence of stress, depression, and substance abuse complicates treatment strategies, requiring an integrated approach.

Comprehensive prevention efforts should address the interconnected nature of stress, depression, and substance abuse. Understanding and addressing the interrelationship between stress, depression, and drug abuse requires a holistic approach that considers biological, psychological, and social factors. Research in this area continues to evolve, and staying informed about the latest literature is essential for effective intervention and treatment. Preventing the coexistence of stress, depression, and drug abuse involves a multi-faceted approach that addresses various factors contributing to these interconnected issues. Promoting the awareness about the relationship between stress, depression, and substance abuse is necessary to provide education on healthy coping mechanisms and the risks associated with self-medication. Implementing mental health promotion programs in schools, workplaces, and communities is crucial. Encouragement of open discussions about mental health to reduce stigma is needed. Stress management programs are required which could teach effective coping strategies, including mindfulness, relaxation techniques, and time management skills.

Resources must be provided to the individuals for identifying and managing stressors in their lives. Implementation of early intervention programs is required to identify and address mental health concerns before they escalate. Accessible mental health services in schools, workplaces, and community settings must be provided. Substance abuse prevention programs must be developed and implemented to focus on building resilience, decision-making skills, and refusal skills. Awareness of the risks of substance abuse and the potential impact on mental health must be created. Healthy lifestyles that include regular exercise, balanced nutrition, and sufficient sleep, all of which contribute to mental well-being would be helpful along with the activities that reduce stress and enhance overall health.

Implementation of workplace mental health programs that address stressors in the work environment would encourage a supportive workplace culture, flexible work arrangements, and access to mental health resources. Integrate mental health screening and assessment tools into healthcare settings to identify individuals at risk along with ensuring that healthcare providers are trained to recognize and address co-occurring issues. Integrated treatment approaches must be developed that address both mental health and substance abuse simultaneously. Collaboration between mental health professionals and substance abuse treatment providers must be ensured. Communities must be engaged in prevention efforts, involving schools, healthcare providers, law enforcement, and community organizations. This would create a supportive environment that discourages substance abuse and encourages mental health awareness. Preventing the coexistence of stress, depression, and drug abuse requires a comprehensive and collaborative effort across various sectors, including education, healthcare, community, and policy. Tailoring prevention strategies to specific populations and addressing the underlying determinants of mental health can contribute to more effective and sustainable prevention efforts.

The Stress-Drug Addiction Connection: There is an intricate relationship between stress and substance abuse and stress can act as a potent trigger for the initiation and escalation of substance abuse. Stress is a ubiquitous aspect of human life and has been identified as a significant factor contributing to the initiation and maintenance of substance use (Sinha, 2008). Physiological Mechanisms such as activation of the hypothalamic-pituitary-adrenal (HPA) axis and the release of stress hormones such as cortisol play important role in mediating stress response (Koob & Kreek, 2007). Chronic stress can dysregulate this system, leading to alterations in neural circuits associated with reward and motivation, potentially increasing susceptibility to substance use (Koob & Le Moal, 2008). Both drug abuse and the stress response are associated with the activation of the hypothalamic-pituitary-adrenal (HPA) axis. The HPA axis is a crucial component of the body's neuroendocrine system, playing a central role in the body's response to stress and the regulation of various physiological processes.

In the context of stress, when an individual encounters a stressor, the hypothalamus releases corticotropin-releasing hormone (CRH), which stimulates the pituitary gland to release adrenocorticotropic hormone (ACTH). ACTH, in turn, signals the adrenal glands to produce and release cortisol, a stress hormone. This cascade of events is known as the HPA axis activation and is designed to mobilize the body's resources to cope with stress. Similarly, drug abuse can also activate the HPA axis. Many substances of abuse, including drugs like cocaine and opioids, can stimulate the release of stress hormones such as cortisol. This activation is thought to contribute to the reinforcing effects of drugs and may play a role in the development of addiction. The parallel involvement of the HPA axis in both stress response and drug abuse suggests a potential overlap in the physiological mechanisms underlying these phenomena. Chronic activation of the HPA axis, whether due to prolonged stress or substance abuse, can lead to dysregulation and contribute to various health issues, including mental health disorders and addiction. Understanding the shared neurobiological pathways involving the HPA axis is crucial for developing comprehensive strategies to address both stress-related disorders and substance abuse.

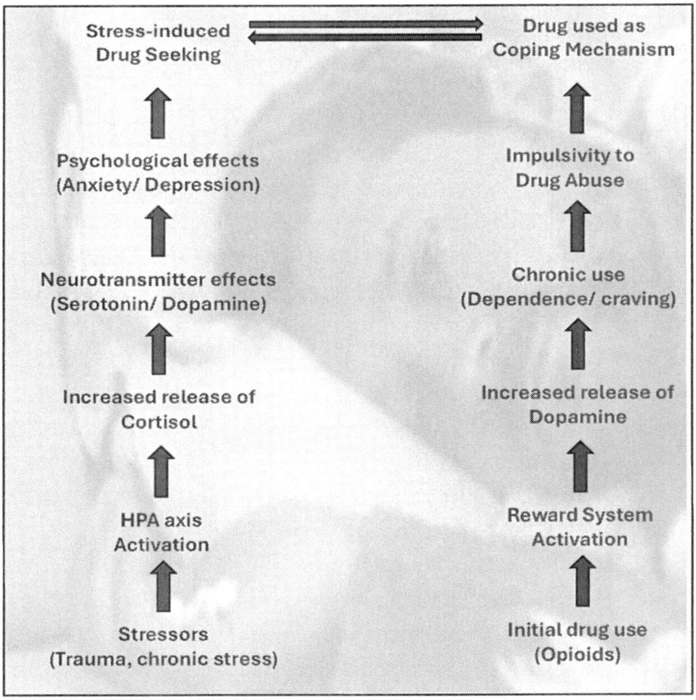

Stress-drug addiction connection

Psychological distress, often stemming from chronic stress, is a key contributor to substance use disorders (Sinha, 2001). Individuals may turn to substances as a coping mechanism to alleviate negative emotions or escape from stressors, creating a cycle of dependence (Sinha, 2008). The relationship between drug abuse and stress often involves psychological distress as a mediator. Psychological distress refers to emotional suffering, anxiety, or other negative emotional states that can result from various life stressors or internal conflicts. In the context of drug abuse and stress, psychological distress can play a significant role in mediating the connection between the two. Individuals experiencing stress may turn to substances as a coping mechanism to alleviate psychological distress. Drugs may provide a temporary escape or relief from emotional pain or discomfort associated with stress. Psychological distress can drive individuals to self-medicate with drugs as a means of managing emotional pain. The use of substances may be an attempt to regulate mood or cope with overwhelming feelings of anxiety or depression triggered by stressors.

The use of drugs to cope with psychological distress can contribute to a cycle of dependence. As individuals experience temporary relief through substance use, they may become reliant on drugs to manage ongoing stress, leading to a potential escalation of substance abuse. Psychological distress can impair decision-making abilities, making individuals more susceptible to engaging in risky behaviors, including drug abuse. Stress-induced alterations in cognitive function may contribute to poor judgment regarding substance use. Dual Vulnerability: Some individuals may be particularly vulnerable to both stress and psychological distress, creating a dual vulnerability that increases the likelihood of drug abuse. The interplay between stress, distress, and substance use can create a complex and reinforcing cycle. Understanding the mediating role of psychological distress in the relationship between drug abuse and stress is crucial for developing effective prevention and intervention strategies. Addressing psychological distress through therapeutic interventions, stress management techniques, and mental health support can be integral in breaking the cycle and reducing the risk of substance abuse in individuals experiencing stress-related psychological challenges. Behavioral pathways play important role in mediating influence of stress on decision-making and impulse control, making individuals more prone to risky behaviors, including substance use (Nock et al., 2017). Understanding these behavioral pathways is crucial for developing targeted interventions to break the stress-substance use cycle. Behavioral pathways play a crucial role in mediating the relationship between drug abuse and stress. Individuals experiencing stress may engage in maladaptive coping behaviors, such as drug use, to alleviate emotional discomfort or escape from stressors. Drug abuse can be a form of self-medication, where individuals use substances to cope with negative emotions or stress-induced psychological distress. Stress has been linked to increased impulsivity, which can contribute to risky behaviors, including drug experimentation and abuse. Individuals under stress may be more inclined to engage in risk-taking behaviors, such as experimenting with drugs, as a way to seek novelty or escape stressors temporarily. Chronic stress can impair cognitive function, affecting decision-making processes.

This impairment may lead individuals to make choices that increase the risk of drug abuse. Stress may diminish an individual's ability to delay gratification, making them more prone to seeking immediate relief through drug use. Stress can contribute to social withdrawal, leading individuals to isolate themselves. In this isolation, individuals may be more susceptible to engaging in drug abuse without the moderating influence of social connections. Stressful situations can increase vulnerability to peer pressure, with individuals turning to substance use as a way to fit in or gain social support. Drug use might be reinforced by the immediate positive effects experienced during stressful situations, creating a cycle of positive reinforcement that can contribute to continued substance abuse. Drug use may also serve as a means of negative reinforcement, helping individuals escape or avoid the aversive feelings associated with stress. Stress can contribute to the development of habits, including habitual drug use, as individuals seek routine and predictability in response to stressors. Understanding these behavioral pathways is critical for developing targeted interventions that address the specific factors linking stress and drug abuse. Interventions may include stress management strategies, cognitive-behavioral therapy, and programs aimed at enhancing coping skills to reduce the reliance on substances as a means of managing stress.

Gene-environment interactions play a significant role in mediating the relationship between drug abuse and stress. These interactions involve the interplay between genetic factors and environmental influences, shaping an individual's vulnerability or resilience to substance abuse in the context of stress. Genetic predispositions can interact with environmental stressors, amplifying the risk of substance use (Uhart & Wand, 2009). Research exploring gene-environment interactions provides valuable insights into individual differences in vulnerability to stress-induced substance abuse. Genetic factors can contribute to an individual's susceptibility to stress-related disorders and substance abuse. Certain genetic variations may increase the risk of both conditions. Drug abuse and stress are polygenic, involving multiple genes. The combination of specific genetic variants may heighten the risk or resilience to these conditions. Genetic variations in genes related to the dopaminergic system, which is involved in reward processing, can influence an individual's response to stress and susceptibility to drug abuse. Genes related to the serotonergic system may modulate mood and stress responses, impacting an individual's vulnerability to stress-induced drug-seeking behavior.

Variations in genes associated with the HPA axis, which regulates the stress response, can influence an individual's ability to cope with stress and, consequently, their susceptibility to drug abuse. Genetic variations in CRH-related genes may affect stress sensitivity and contribute to the development of substance use disorders. Stressful experiences can induce epigenetic modifications that alter gene expression patterns. Epigenetic changes may contribute to long-term changes in neural circuits related to reward and stress response, impacting susceptibility to drug abuse. Epigenetic modifications acquired during stress exposure may be passed on to future generations, potentially influencing the heritability of vulnerability to drug abuse. Individuals with certain genetic predispositions may actively seek out environments that expose them to stressors or increase the likelihood of drug availability, creating a correlation between their genes and environment.

Genetic factors in parents may influence both their own substance use and the environment in which their children are raised, contributing to a shared genetic-environmental risk. Understanding the intricate interplay between genetics and environmental stressors is crucial for tailoring prevention and intervention strategies. Personalized approaches that consider an individual's genetic background and environmental context can lead to more effective strategies for mitigating the risk of drug abuse in the presence of stress. Stress management techniques, cognitive-behavioral therapy, and pharmacological approaches could be implemented to mitigate the impact of stress on substance use (Nakao et al., 2021). Additionally, preventive strategies, including early intervention programs and resilience-building initiatives could also be explored. Reducing the risk of drug abuse in the presence of stress involves implementing a combination of preventive strategies, coping mechanisms, and support systems. Encourage the adoption of healthy coping mechanisms to manage stress, such as regular exercise, mindfulness, meditation, deep breathing exercises, and hobbies. These activities can help individuals cope with stress in a positive and constructive manner. Foster strong social connections and support networks. Having a reliable support system can provide emotional assistance during challenging times, reducing the inclination to turn to substances for solace. Encourage participation in activities that promote resilience, such as engaging in positive social interactions, building problem-solving skills, and developing a sense of purpose and meaning in life.

Provide education on the risks associated with substance abuse, especially in the context of stress. Increasing awareness about the negative consequences of drug abuse can empower individuals to make informed decisions. Offer stress management programs and workshops in schools, workplaces, and communities. These programs can teach effective stress reduction techniques and coping strategies to help individuals navigate stressful situations. Implement early intervention programs to identify and support individuals who may be at risk of drug abuse due to stress. Early detection and intervention can prevent the escalation of substance use. Improve accessibility to mental health services, including counseling and therapy. Providing mental health support can assist individuals in addressing the root causes of stress and developing healthier coping mechanisms. Establish and promote drug-free workplace policies that emphasize the importance of maintaining a healthy and substance-free work environment. This can contribute to a culture that discourages drug abuse. Provide parents with resources and educational materials on recognizing signs of stress in children and teens. Encouraging open communication and fostering a supportive home environment can be protective against substance abuse. Identify and address underlying issues contributing to stress, such as trauma, mental health disorders, or family conflicts. Treating these root causes can reduce the vulnerability to drug abuse. Engage community resources, such as local organizations, support groups, and community centers, to provide additional avenues of support for individuals facing stressors. Encourage positive peer influences and environments. Positive social interactions can contribute to a sense of belonging and reduce the likelihood of turning to substances for social connection. Monitor the use of prescription medications, especially those with abuse potential. Healthcare providers should educate patients on proper medication use and monitor for signs of misuse. By implementing a comprehensive and multi-faceted approach that addresses both individual and environmental factors, it is possible to decrease the risk of drug abuse in the presence of stress. Prevention efforts should be tailored to the specific needs of individuals and communities, recognizing the diverse factors that contribute to the complex relationship between stress and substance abuse. By synthesizing evidence from diverse studies, this review illuminates the multifaceted relationship between stress and substance use. Recognizing stress as a trigger for substance abuse is crucial for developing effective prevention and intervention strategies to address this public health concern.

The Depression-Drug Addiction Connection: The connection between depression and drug addiction is complex and multifaceted. Individuals experiencing depression may be at an increased risk of developing substance use disorders, and conversely, drug addiction can contribute to or exacerbate depressive symptoms. Depression can act as a motivator for drug abuse. Individuals with depression may turn to drugs as a form of self-medication to alleviate the emotional pain and distress associated with depressive symptoms. Substance use may provide temporary relief from feelings of sadness, hopelessness, and anxiety, reinforcing the association between drug use and mood regulation. Depression can serve as a motivator for drug addiction in several ways, as individuals may turn to substances as a means of coping with the emotional pain and distress associated with depressive symptoms. Individuals with depression often experience intense emotional pain, including feelings of sadness, hopelessness, and anxiety. Some may turn to drugs as a form of self-medication, seeking relief from these distressing emotions. Drugs can provide a quick and immediate escape from the overwhelming emotions associated with depression. The rapid onset of pleasurable sensations can offer a temporary reprieve from emotional suffering (Danek et al., 2023). Drug use may become a maladaptive coping mechanism for individuals with depression. In an attempt to manage and alleviate emotional distress, individuals may resort to substances, creating a reliance on drugs for emotional regulation.

The relief provided by drugs creates a negative reinforcement loop. Individuals learn that drug use is an effective way to escape or numb themselves from the negative emotions associated with depression, reinforcing the behavior. Depression can dampen the brain's reward system, making individuals more prone to seeking pleasure and reward. Drugs, by stimulating the reward pathways, become a compelling means of experiencing pleasure for those with depressive symptoms. Individuals with depression may use drugs in an attempt to experience a sense of normalcy or escape the emotional numbness that can accompany depressive states. Substances may be perceived as a way to temporarily lift the emotional burden. Drug use can be associated with social contexts where individuals find a sense of community or connection. For those experiencing depression and feelings of isolation, the social aspect of drug use may be a motivating factor (Leung et al., 2023). Depression often coexists with life stressors and challenges. Drugs may provide an escape from the pressures of reality, allowing individuals to temporarily disconnect from their problems. Depression can impair cognitive functions, including decision-making and impulse control. Impaired judgment may lead individuals to engage in drug use without fully considering the long-term consequences. As the negative emotions associated with depression persist, individuals may find themselves caught in a cycle of dependence, continually relying on drugs to cope with emotional pain and stress.

The co-occurrence of depression and addiction is associated with increased vulnerability. The presence of one condition may exacerbate the severity of the other, creating a complex interplay that reinforces the motivation for drug use. The motivation to use drugs as a coping mechanism for depression may pose challenges in seeking appropriate mental health treatment. Individuals may be less inclined to pursue therapeutic interventions when substances offer perceived immediate relief. Addressing the interplay between depression and drug addiction requires a comprehensive and integrated approach that includes mental health support, substance abuse treatment, and strategies for building healthier coping mechanisms. Recognizing and addressing the underlying factors contributing to both depression and addiction is essential for effective intervention and recovery.

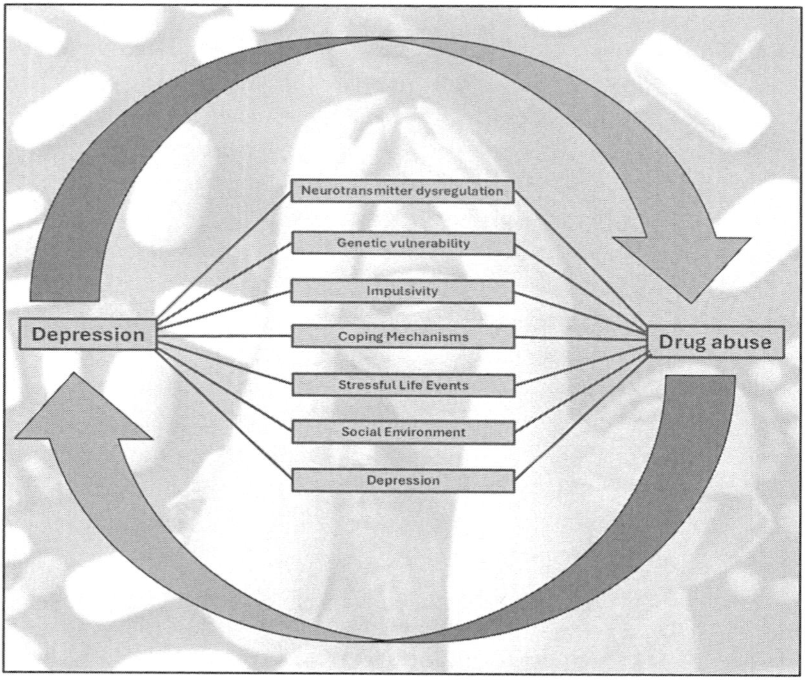

Depression-drug addiction connection

Neurobiological Changes mediating depression and drug addiction simultaneously involve neurotransmitter systems, such as the dopamine and serotonin pathways. Chronic drug use can alter these systems, contributing to the development and persistence of depressive symptoms. The neurobiological changes that mediate the connection between depression and drug addiction involve complex interactions within the brain's reward system, stress response pathways, and neurotransmitter systems. Reduced activity in the mesolimbic dopamine pathway, leading to decreased sensitivity to natural rewards and anhedonia (loss of pleasure). Drugs of abuse, including stimulants and opioids, increase dopamine release in the nucleus accumbens, creating a sense of euphoria and reinforcing drug-seeking behavior (Urban et al., 2023). Serotonin dysregulation is implicated in depressive disorders, contributing to mood disturbances. Some drugs, such as MDMA and hallucinogens, directly impact serotonin receptors, affecting mood and emotions. Reduced neuroplasticity, structural changes in the hippocampus, and alterations in the prefrontal cortex. Chronic drug use can lead to structural changes, affecting synaptic plasticity and connectivity, particularly in regions associated with reward and decision-making. Dysregulation of endorphins, contributing to decreased natural rewards and increased susceptibility to negative emotions.

Opioid drugs directly interact with the endorphin system, producing analgesic and euphoric effects. Alterations in the glutamatergic system may impact synaptic plasticity and connectivity. Drugs like ketamine and alcohol influence glutamate receptors, affecting mood and cognitive function, and may contribute to addictive processes. Changes in the endocannabinoid system are implicated in mood disorders. Cannabis, which acts on cannabinoid receptors, is associated with alterations in reward processing and addictive behaviors. Dysregulation of the GABAergic system may contribute to altered emotional regulation.

Drugs such as benzodiazepines, which enhance GABAergic activity, can have reinforcing effects and may be abused. Increased microglial activation and inflammation are observed in depressive states (Assadi et al., 2023). Chronic drug use can induce neuroinflammation, potentially contributing to the maintenance of addictive behaviors. Altered gene expression and epigenetic modifications may influence susceptibility to depression. Epigenetic changes induced by chronic drug use can contribute to the persistence of addictive behaviors. Understanding these neurobiological changes helps elucidate the shared mechanisms between depression and drug addiction. It's important to note that the relationship is bidirectional, with each condition influencing and exacerbating the other. Integrated approaches addressing both mental health and substance use are crucial for effective treatment and recovery. Bidirectional influence of depression and drug abuse exists. Depression can increase susceptibility to drug addiction by creating a vulnerability to the rewarding effects of substances.

Individuals with depression may seek the pleasurable sensations induced by drugs. On the other hand, drug addiction can exacerbate depressive symptoms through neurobiological changes, withdrawal effects, and the impact of substance use on one's overall well-being (Radhakrishnan et al., 2023). Indeed, there is a bidirectional relationship between depression and drug addiction. Each condition can increase susceptibility to the other, forming a complex interplay that presents unique challenges for individuals affected. Here's an exploration of how depression can increase susceptibility to drug addiction, and vice versa. Individuals experiencing depression may turn to drugs as a form of self-medication to alleviate emotional pain and distress.

The desire for relief from depressive symptoms can drive the initiation and maintenance of substance use. Depression often involves anhedonia, a reduced ability to experience pleasure from normally enjoyable activities. In an attempt to counter anhedonic feelings, individuals may seek the euphoria or pleasure induced by drugs, leading to an increased susceptibility to addiction. The emotional toll of depression can make individuals more vulnerable to maladaptive coping mechanisms. Drugs may be used to cope with stress, anxiety, or feelings of hopelessness, contributing to the development of addictive behaviors. Drugs may be perceived as a means of escaping from overwhelming negative emotions associated with depression. The desire to escape emotional pain can drive the use of substances, escalating the risk of addiction (Abu Al-Khair et al., 2023). Depression can lead to social withdrawal and isolation. Individuals may turn to drugs as a way to cope with loneliness and a lack of social support, further increasing susceptibility to addiction. Chronic drug use can lead to neurobiological changes that impact mood regulation and contribute to the development of depressive symptoms.

The dysregulation of neurotransmitter systems may persist even during periods of abstinence, increasing vulnerability to depression. The cycle of drug addiction often involves periods of withdrawal and intense craving. These withdrawal symptoms and cravings can contribute to the development or exacerbation of depressive symptoms, creating a reciprocal relationship. Substance abuse can dysregulate the stress response system, including the hypothalamic-pituitary-adrenal (HPA) axis. This dysregulation may contribute to chronic stress and increase susceptibility to depressive disorders. The social consequences of addiction, such as strained relationships, legal issues, and occupational challenges, can contribute to feelings of despair and hopelessness, increasing the risk of depression. The negative impact of drug addiction on various aspects of life, including physical health, financial stability, and overall functioning, can contribute to a sense of despair and contribute to the development of depressive symptoms (van Namen et al., 2023).

Both depression and addiction have genetic components. Individuals with a family history of either condition may be at an increased risk for developing both disorders. Childhood adversity, trauma, or abuse can increase the risk of both depression and substance use disorders, creating a shared vulnerability. Individuals with impaired coping skills may be more susceptible to both depression and addiction. The lack of effective coping mechanisms can contribute to the reliance on substances as a maladaptive coping strategy. The co-occurrence of depression and addiction can create a reinforcing loop, where one condition exacerbates the other. For example, depressive symptoms may lead to increased drug use, which, in turn, worsens depressive symptoms, creating a cycle that is challenging to break. Recognizing and addressing this bidirectional relationship is crucial for comprehensive treatment. Integrated interventions that target both mental health and substance use components are often necessary for effective recovery. Additionally, early intervention and prevention efforts can help mitigate the risk of this reciprocal relationship.

Common risk factors potentiating both depression and substance use disorders simultaneously include genetic factors, environmental stressors, trauma, chronic stress, or adverse life events, can contribute to the development of both depression and drug addiction. The comorbidity of depression and drug addiction is influenced by a range of common risk factors that contribute to the co-occurrence of these conditions. Understanding these shared risk factors is crucial for prevention, early intervention, and comprehensive treatment. Individuals with a family history of either depression or substance use disorders may have a genetic predisposition to both conditions, increasing the likelihood of comorbidity. Exposure to adverse childhood experiences, such as abuse, neglect, or trauma, is a significant risk factor for both depression and the development of substance use disorders later in life. Imbalances in neurotransmitter systems, such as serotonin and dopamine, can contribute to both depressive disorders and the vulnerability to substance abuse. Individuals who struggle with coping skills, whether due to environmental stressors or innate factors, may turn to substances as a maladaptive coping mechanism for managing emotional distress associated with depression.

Isolation, loneliness, or a lack of social support can contribute to both depression and the initiation or continuation of substance use as a way to cope or find a sense of connection. Conditions such as generalized anxiety disorder or post-traumatic stress disorder (PTSD) commonly co-occur with depression and may also increase the risk of substance use. Persistent exposure to chronic stressors, such as financial difficulties, relationship issues, or work-related stress, can contribute to the development of both depression and substance use disorders. Deficits in executive functions, such as decision-making and impulse control, can be associated with both depression and an increased susceptibility to drug addiction. Associations with peers who engage in substance use or have mental health challenges can contribute to the development of both depression and drug addiction (Merians et al., 2023). Individuals with a history of either substance use treatment or mental health treatment may be at an increased risk for the development of the other condition. Research suggests that the relationship between depression and substance use may vary by gender. For example, females may be more prone to depression, while males may be more prone to certain types of substance use. Easy access to alcohol or drugs in the environment may contribute to the initiation and continuation of substance use among individuals with depression.

Individuals with higher levels of impulsivity may be at an increased risk for both depression and drug addiction, as impulsivity is a common trait associated with both conditions. Individuals with chronic medical conditions that impact physical health and well-being may be more susceptible to depression and may turn to substances as a coping mechanism (Pautrat et al., 2022). Individuals facing economic hardship or limited educational opportunities may experience heightened stress, contributing to both depression and drug addiction. The stigma associated with mental health disorders and substance use may create additional challenges for individuals seeking help, potentially leading to the co-occurrence of both conditions. Limited access to mental health or substance use treatment services may prevent individuals from receiving timely and appropriate care for either condition. Certain personality disorders, such as borderline personality disorder, are associated with an increased risk of both depression and substance use disorders. It's important to note that the relationship between depression and drug addiction is complex and varies among individuals. These risk factors interact in unique ways, contributing to the heterogeneity observed in the co-occurrence of these conditions. Comprehensive and integrated approaches that address both mental health and substance use are essential for effective prevention and treatment strategies.

Changes in brain structure and function mediate chronic drug use and depression and affect regions involved in mood regulation, reward processing, and decision-making (Verovnik et al., 2023). Both conditions can impair cognitive function, influencing an individual's ability to cope with stress, regulate emotions, and make informed decisions. Changes in brain structure and function play a significant role in mediating the relationship between depression and drug addiction. Both conditions can influence various regions of the brain involved in emotional regulation, reward processing, decision-making, and stress response. Reduced volume and activity in the prefrontal cortex, impacting cognitive functions such as decision-making, impulse control, and emotional regulation. Chronic drug use, especially substances like cocaine and methamphetamine, can lead to structural changes in the prefrontal cortex, contributing to impaired executive functions and increased impulsivity.

Altered activity in the nucleus accumbens, a key region in the brain's reward system, may contribute to anhedonia and reduced responsiveness to pleasurable stimuli. Drugs of abuse, by directly influencing the release of dopamine in the nucleus accumbens, reinforce addictive behaviors and create a heightened sensitivity to drug-related cues. Changes in the amygdala, involved in processing emotions and stress responses, are associated with heightened emotional reactivity in depression. The amygdala plays a crucial role in associative learning related to drug reward and cues (Zhu et al., 2023). Changes in amygdala function contribute to drug craving and relapse. Reduced hippocampal volume is often observed in depression, affecting memory function and stress regulation. Chronic drug use, particularly substances like alcohol and opioids, can lead to structural changes in the hippocampus, impacting memory and learning processes. Dysregulation of the hypothalamus may contribute to disruptions in the HPA axis, leading to abnormal stress responses. Substance abuse can also affect the HPA axis, exacerbating stress-related responses and potentially maintaining addictive behaviors.

Changes in the cingulate cortex are associated with emotional processing and regulation. The cingulate cortex is implicated in drug craving and the processing of rewarding stimuli, contributing to the reinforcing effects of drugs. Altered striatal function is linked to motivational and reward processing deficits in depression. The striatum, particularly the dorsal striatum, is involved in habit formation and plays a role in the development of compulsive drug-seeking behavior. Changes in the vmPFC are associated with altered emotional regulation and decision-making. The vmPFC is involved in inhibitory control and is implicated in the inability to resist drug cravings and impulses in addiction. Serotonergic neurons in the dorsal raphe nucleus are involved in mood regulation. Drugs like MDMA and hallucinogens can impact serotonin release, influencing mood and emotions. Reduced neuroplasticity may limit the brain's ability to adapt and recover from stress (Wilson et al., 2023).

Neuroplastic changes induced by chronic drug use can contribute to the persistence of addictive behaviors and cravings. Changes in white matter integrity, affecting connectivity between brain regions, are observed in depression. Disruptions in white matter structure can be associated with cognitive deficits and impaired decision-making in individuals with substance use disorders. Altered connectivity within the default mode network (DMN) is implicated in ruminative thinking and self-referential thoughts. Changes in DMN connectivity are associated with altered self-awareness and may contribute to the reinforcing effects of drug use. Understanding these changes in brain structure and function provides insights into the shared neural mechanisms of depression and drug addiction. The bidirectional relationship between these conditions involves a complex interplay of genetic, environmental, and neurobiological factors. Integrated treatments that address both mental health and substance use components are essential for effective intervention and recovery.

Negative reinforcement loop is created in individuals with depression may use drugs to escape negative emotions, creating a negative reinforcement loop where the temporary relief provided by substances reinforces continued drug use. The negative reinforcement loop involving depression and drug addiction represents a cycle where individuals engage in drug use as a way to alleviate the negative symptoms associated with depression. This loop reinforces both conditions, creating a challenging cycle to break. Individuals experiencing symptoms of depression, such as persistent sadness, hopelessness, or anhedonia, may seek relief from these negative emotions (May et al., 2023). In an attempt to cope with the emotional pain and distress, individuals may turn to drugs as a means of self-medication. Substance use often provides immediate relief and a sense of euphoria. The rapid onset of pleasurable sensations creates a powerful incentive for continued drug use. The use of drugs temporarily alleviates the negative emotions associated with depression. This escape provides a sense of relief and may contribute to a perceived improvement in mood. The relief provided by drugs is short-lived, and as the effects wear off, the negative symptoms of depression return. This sets the stage for a cycle of repeated drug use to manage depressive symptoms. Individuals learn to associate drug use with the alleviation of depressive symptoms. This learned association reinforces the use of drugs as a primary means of emotional regulation.

Over time, the efficacy of the drug in alleviating depressive symptoms may diminish due to tolerance, leading individuals to escalate their drug use in an attempt to achieve the same level of relief. Escalating drug use can lead to negative consequences, including health problems, impaired functioning, strained relationships, and legal issues. Chronic drug use can dysregulate the stress response system, exacerbating stress responses in the body. Increased stress and the negative consequences of drug use contribute to the worsening of depressive symptoms, creating a cycle of escalating distress. The negative reinforcement loop perpetuates a cyclical pattern of drug use as individuals repeatedly turn to substances to cope with depressive symptoms. As the negative reinforcement loop continues, individuals may develop a dependence on drugs, leading to the development of addiction. The negative reinforcement loop reflects maladaptive coping mechanisms (Reich et al., 2023). Individuals may rely on drugs instead of developing healthier coping skills to manage stress and emotional distress. The reliance on drugs as a coping mechanism may create barriers to seeking mental health treatment. Individuals may be resistant to addressing the root causes of depression and addiction. Over time, cognitive and behavioral patterns become ingrained, reinforcing the association between drug use and relief from depressive symptoms. Breaking the negative reinforcement loop requires comprehensive intervention that addresses both the underlying depressive symptoms and the addictive behaviors. Integrated treatment approaches, including psychotherapy, pharmacotherapy, and support for developing healthier coping mechanisms, are essential for disrupting the cycle and promoting recovery. Additionally, addressing the social, environmental, and psychological factors contributing to the loop is crucial for sustained positive outcomes.

Drug dependence can lead to withdrawal symptoms, which, when experienced alongside depressive symptoms, may increase the risk of relapse (Sørensen et al., 2023). The craving for drugs and the compulsive use associated with addiction can persist even during periods of depression, contributing to a cycle of dependence. The co-occurrence of depression and drug addiction can complicate treatment. Addressing both conditions simultaneously is often necessary for effective recovery. Comorbid depression and addiction are associated with increased severity of both conditions and may require a comprehensive treatment approach, including therapy, medication, and support. Depression can impede treatment outcomes for substance use disorders, and vice versa. Comprehensive treatment that addresses both conditions is essential for achieving long-term recovery. Both depression and addiction can contribute to social isolation, creating a reinforcing cycle where individuals may use substances to cope with loneliness and depressive feelings. Understanding the depression-drug addiction connection is crucial for developing integrated and tailored interventions. Treatment approaches should address the unique challenges presented by comorbid depression and addiction, offering holistic support for emotional well-being and recovery. Integrated therapies, medication management, and ongoing psychosocial support are key components of effective treatment for individuals facing both depression and substance use disorders.

Common neurobiological pathways mediating comorbidity of stress, depression, and drug addiction: Stress, depression, and drug addiction are complex phenomena with overlapping neurobiological pathways. Understanding the commonalities can help shed light on why these conditions often co-occur and how they influence each other. It's important to note that the neurobiology of these conditions is still an active area of research, and our understanding continues to evolve. The HPA axis plays a central role in the body's response to stress. It involves the release of corticotropin-releasing hormone (CRH) from the hypothalamus, which stimulates the release of adrenocorticotropic hormone (ACTH) from the pituitary gland, leading to the release of cortisol from the adrenal glands. Chronic stress can dysregulate the HPA axis, leading to sustained high levels of cortisol. Dysregulation of the HPA axis is often observed in individuals with depression and is implicated in the development of drug addiction.

Monoamine neurotransmitters, including serotonin, norepinephrine, and dopamine, play a crucial role in the comorbidity of stress, depression, and drug addiction. The dysregulation of these neurotransmitter systems is a common thread in the neurobiology of these conditions. Serotonin, also known as 5-hydroxytryptamine (5-HT), is a neurotransmitter that plays a significant role in the comorbidity of stress, depression, and drug addiction. Chronic stress can lead to alterations in the serotonergic system. Stressful experiences may influence the synthesis, release, and reuptake of serotonin, contributing to changes in mood and emotional regulation (McEwen, 2005). Dysregulation of the serotonergic system is a common feature in depression. Lower levels of serotonin or alterations in serotonin receptor sensitivity are associated with the development and maintenance of depressive symptoms (Nestler et al., 2002). Serotonin is involved in the regulation of mood and reward, and its dysregulation is implicated in drug addiction. Drugs that affect serotonin levels, such as MDMA (ecstasy) and hallucinogens, can have reinforcing effects and contribute to addictive behaviors (Howell &

Cunningham, 2015). Chronic stress and depression can sensitize the brain to the effects of drugs, influencing the vulnerability to addiction. This cross-sensitization involves changes in monoamine neurotransmission, including serotonin (Sinha, 2008). Antidepressant medications that target the serotonergic system, such as SSRIs and SNRIs, are commonly used to treat both depression and certain anxiety disorders (Cipriani et al., 2018). These medications increase the availability of serotonin in the synaptic cleft. Understanding the role of serotonin in these conditions is an ongoing area of research, and these references provide insights into the complex interplay of serotonin in the neurobiology of stress, depression, and drug addiction.

Dysregulation of the noradrenergic system is associated with symptoms of anxiety and depression. Stress can lead to increased release of norepinephrine, contributing to the mood-related symptoms of depression. Norepinephrine is also involved in the brain's reward system. Stimulant drugs, such as cocaine and amphetamines, increase norepinephrine levels, contributing to their addictive properties. Chronic stress activates the sympathetic nervous system, leading to the release of norepinephrine. Dysregulation of the noradrenergic system is associated with the physiological and psychological responses to stress (Goldstein, 2010) as well as in the pathophysiology of depression. Increased noradrenergic activity is associated with symptoms such as anxiety, hyperarousal, and mood disturbances (Nestler et al., 2002). Noradrenaline is also involved in the brain's reward system. Stimulant drugs, such as cocaine and amphetamines, increase norepinephrine levels, contributing to the rewarding effects and addictive properties of these substances (Weinshenker & Schroeder, 2007).

Chronic stress and depression can sensitize the brain to the effects of drugs, including those that impact the noradrenergic system. This cross-sensitization contributes to the bidirectional relationship between stress, depression, and drug addiction (Russo & Nestler, 2013). Antidepressant medications, such as selective serotonin-norepinephrine reuptake inhibitors (SNRIs), modulate the levels of both serotonin and norepinephrine. By increasing the availability of these neurotransmitters, these medications alleviate depressive symptoms (Fava et al., 2006). Understanding the role of noradrenaline in stress, depression, and drug addiction is critical for developing targeted interventions and medications that address the shared neurobiological pathways in these conditions. These references provide further insights into the complex interactions involving noradrenaline.

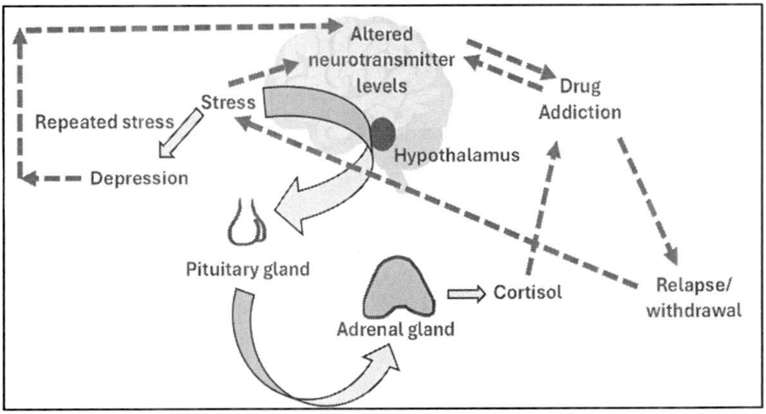

Common neurobiological pathways mediating comorbidity of stress, depression, and drug addiction

The dysregulation of the dopaminergic system is implicated in the reward circuitry of the brain and is associated with symptoms of anhedonia (loss of pleasure) in depression. Chronic stress can affect dopamine release and receptor sensitivity in brain regions involved in motivation and reward. Chronic stress can influence the dopaminergic system, affecting dopamine release and receptor sensitivity in brain regions associated with motivation and reward. Dysregulation of the dopaminergic system is also implicated in depressive disorders, particularly in the mesolimbic and mesocortical pathways. Changes in dopamine function contribute to symptoms such as anhedonia and motivational deficits (Nestler et al., 202).

Dopamine is a key player in the brain's reward system. Many drugs of abuse, including cocaine, amphetamines, and opioids, directly or indirectly increase dopamine levels, contributing to the reinforcing effects and addictive properties of these substances (Wise & Koob, 2014). Chronic stress and depression can sensitize the brain to the effects of drugs, influencing the vulnerability to addiction. This cross-sensitization involves changes in dopaminergic neurotransmission (Sinha, 2008). Some antidepressant medications indirectly affect dopamine levels by influencing other neurotransmitter systems. Tricyclic antidepressants, for example, can impact dopamine reuptake (Blier & Mansari, 2013). Understanding the role of dopamine in these conditions is crucial for developing targeted interventions. These references provide insights into the complex interplay of dopamine in the neurobiology of stress, depression, and drug addiction.

Comorbidity and cross-sensitization of stress, depression and drug abuse coexist. Chronic stress can sensitize the brain to the effects of drugs and increase vulnerability to addiction. This phenomenon is known as cross-sensitization and involves changes in monoamine neurotransmission. The interaction between stress, depression, and drug addiction is bidirectional. Substance abuse can lead to alterations in monoamine systems that contribute to mood disorders, and pre-existing mood disorders can increase susceptibility to drug addiction. Comorbidity refers to the simultaneous presence of two or more medical conditions in an individual, and cross-sensitization refers to the phenomenon where exposure to one factor sensitizes an individual to the effects of another. In the context of stress, depression, and drug abuse, there is a complex interplay involving comorbidity and cross-sensitization. Chronic stress is a well-established risk factor for the development of depression. Prolonged exposure to stressors can dysregulate the neurobiological systems involved in mood regulation, leading to the onset of depressive symptoms (Hammen, 2005).

Comorbidity between depression and substance use disorders is highly prevelant. Individuals with depression may turn to substances as a form of self-medication, attempting to alleviate their depressive symptoms. Conversely, substance abuse can contribute to the development or exacerbation of depressive disorders (Swendsen et al., 2010). Stressful life events can contribute to the initiation and maintenance of substance abuse. The interaction between stress and drug abuse involves the dysregulation of stress-responsive systems, such as the hypothalamic-pituitary-adrenal (HPA) axis, and changes in reward circuitry. Chronic exposure to stress can sensitize individuals to the reinforcing effects of drugs, making them more susceptible to substance abuse and addiction. This cross-sensitization involves neuroadaptive changes in the brain's reward circuitry (Lu & Wang,

2008). Individuals with a history of depression may be more vulnerable to the reinforcing effects of drugs, and exposure to substances can, in turn, exacerbate depressive symptoms. This bidirectional relationship involves changes in neurotransmitter systems, including serotonin, dopamine, and norepinephrine. Understanding the comorbidity and cross-sensitization between stress, depression, and drug abuse is crucial for developing comprehensive interventions that address the complex interactions between these conditions. The references provided offer insights into the scientific literature supporting these concepts.

Many antidepressant medications, such as selective serotonin reuptake inhibitors (SSRIs) and serotonin-norepinephrine reuptake inhibitors (SNRIs), work by increasing the availability of serotonin and/or norepinephrine in the synaptic cleft. These medications are commonly used to treat both depression and certain anxiety disorders, highlighting the shared involvement of monoamines in these conditions. Understanding the intricate interplay of monoamine neurotransmitters in stress, depression, and drug addiction is essential for developing effective therapeutic interventions that target these common neurobiological pathways. However, it's important to note that the relationship is complex, and other neurotransmitter systems and molecular pathways also contribute to the overall neurobiology of these conditions.

BDNF is a key neurotrophin involved in neuronal growth, survival, and synaptic plasticity. Stress and depression are associated with reduced levels of BDNF, particularly in brain regions involved in mood regulation such as the hippocampus. Drug addiction can also influence BDNF levels, and alterations in BDNF expression are observed in brain regions implicated in addiction. Chronic stress can influence BDNF levels in the brain. Stressful experiences may lead to a decrease in BDNF expression, particularly in brain regions involved in mood regulation and cognition (Duman & Monteggia, 2006). Altered BDNF levels are associated with depression. Reduced BDNF expression in the hippocampus and other brain regions has been observed in individuals with depressive disorders (Sen et al, 2006). Substance abuse and addiction can also impact BDNF levels. Chronic drug exposure may lead to changes in BDNF expression in brain regions associated with reward and addiction. Dysregulation of BDNF is suggested to contribute to the comorbidity between stress, depression, and drug abuse. Common neurobiological pathways involving BDNF alterations may underlie the interconnectedness of these conditions (Haile et al., 2014). Targeting BDNF and its signaling pathways is a potential therapeutic strategy for conditions involving comorbidity of stress, depression, and drug abuse. Some antidepressant and anti-addiction treatments may exert their effects, in part, through modulation of BDNF (Aurtry et al., .2014). Understanding the involvement of BDNF in the comorbidity of stress, depression, and drug abuse provides insights into potential targets for therapeutic interventions. It's important to note that research in this field is ongoing, and the mechanisms involved in BDNF-related comorbidity are complex and multifaceted.

Endogenous Opioid System, including endorphins and enkephalins, plays a role in stress modulation and reward processing. Dysregulation of this system is implicated in both depression and drug addiction. Opioid drugs, for example, directly target this system, leading to their addictive properties. The endogenous opioid system plays a significant role in the comorbidity of stress, depression, and drug abuse. This complex neurochemical system involves endorphins, enkephalins, and dynorphins, which are endogenous ligands that bind to opioid receptors in the brain. The interactions within the endogenous opioid system contribute to the regulation of mood, stress responses, and reward processes. The endogenous opioid system is involved in the modulation of stress responses. Stress can activate the release of endorphins, which bind to opioid receptors and play a role in dampening the perception of pain and stress (Bodnar, 2016). Dysregulation of the endogenous opioid system has been implicated in the pathophysiology of depression. Altered levels of endorphins and their receptors are observed in individuals with depressive disorders (Chartoff & Carlezon Jr, 2014). The endogenous opioid system is a key player in the brain's reward circuitry. Drugs of abuse, particularly opioids like heroin and prescription painkillers, mimic the effects of endorphins and activate the reward pathways, leading to the reinforcing effects of these substances (Koob & Le Moal, 2001).

Chronic stress and depression can influence the endogenous opioid system, altering the release and function of opioid peptides. This, in turn, can affect an individual's vulnerability to drug abuse, as opioids may be used to self-medicate or cope with stress and emotional distress (Ray & Hutchison, 2004). Understanding the role of the endogenous opioid system in the comorbidity of stress, depression, and drug abuse provides potential targets for therapeutic interventions. Medications that modulate the opioid system may be explored for the treatment of comorbid conditions (Lutz & Kieffer, 2013). The intricate interactions within the endogenous opioid system highlight its role in the interconnectedness of stress, depression, and drug abuse. Further research is essential to fully understand the specific mechanisms involved and to develop targeted interventions for individuals with comorbidities in these conditions.

Glutamatergic system is also involved in the comorbidity of stress, depression, and drug abuse. Glutamate is the primary excitatory neurotransmitter in the brain and is involved in synaptic plasticity. Alterations in glutamatergic transmission are implicated in the neurobiology of depression and drug addiction. Absolutely, the glutamatergic system, which primarily involves the neurotransmitter glutamate, plays a crucial role in the comorbidity of stress, depression, and drug abuse. Glutamate is the most abundant excitatory neurotransmitter in the central nervous system, and it interacts with several receptor types, including N-methyl-D-aspartate (NMDA) receptors, α-amino-3-hydroxy-5-methyl-4-isoxazolepropionic acid (AMPA) receptors, and kainate receptors. Chronic stress can lead to alterations in glutamate signaling. Stress activates the release of glutamate, particularly in brain regions associated with the stress response, such as the prefrontal cortex and the amygdala (Popoli et al., 2012). Dysregulation of the glutamatergic system is implicated in the pathophysiology of depression. Changes in glutamate release, receptor function, and synaptic plasticity contribute to altered mood states (Sanacora & Banasr, 2013). The glutamatergic system is involved in the neurobiological mechanisms of addiction. Glutamate transmission in the mesolimbic pathway, particularly in regions like the nucleus accumbens, is critical for the reinforcing effects of drugs of abuse (Kalivas & Volkow, 2005).

Chronic stress and depression can sensitize the glutamatergic system, influencing vulnerability to drug abuse. Conversely, drugs of abuse can affect glutamate transmission, contributing to the comorbidity between stress, depression, and addiction (Moussawi & Kalivas, 2010). Targeting the glutamatergic system has emerged as a promising avenue for the development of novel antidepressant and anti-addiction medications. Drugs that modulate glutamate release or receptor function are being investigated for their therapeutic potential (Sanacora et al., 2008). Exploring the interplay of the glutamatergic system in the comorbidity of stress, depression, and drug abuse is crucial for developing targeted interventions that address the shared neurobiological pathways in these conditions. Ongoing research in this field aims to identify novel therapeutic strategies for individuals with these complex comorbidities.

Inflammatory Pathways could be activated by chronic stress and neuroinflammation is associated with stress, depressive disorders and addiction. It's crucial to recognize that these pathways are interconnected, and alterations in one system can influence others. Additionally, genetic predispositions and environmental factors contribute to the complex interplay of these neurobiological mechanisms in stress, depression, and drug addiction. Advances in neuroscience continue to refine our understanding of these relationships. Stress activates the body's stress response system, including the release of stress hormones such as cortisol. Chronic stress can lead to dysregulation of the immune system, resulting in increased production of pro-inflammatory cytokines (Dantzer et al., 2008). Depression is associated with elevated levels of pro-inflammatory cytokines such as interleukin-1 (IL-1), interleukin-6 (IL-6), and tumor necrosis factor-alpha (TNF-α). This inflammation may contribute to the onset, severity, and persistence of depressive symptoms (Miller & Raison, 2016).

Substance abuse, including drugs like opioids and psychostimulants, can induce inflammation in the central nervous system. Inflammatory responses may contribute to the rewarding effects of drugs and the development of addiction. There is a bidirectional relationship between inflammation and the central nervous system. Inflammatory signals can impact neurotransmitter systems involved in mood regulation, stress responses, and reward pathways, influencing susceptibility to stress, depression, and drug abuse (Felger & Lotrich, 2013). Targeting inflammatory pathways has emerged as a potential therapeutic strategy for individuals with comorbid stress, depression, and drug abuse. Anti-inflammatory interventions may have beneficial effects on mood and substance use disorders. Role of inflammatory pathways in the interconnectedness of stress, depression, and drug abuse provides a framework for developing comprehensive interventions. However, it's essential to recognize that these relationships are multifaceted, and additional research is needed to fully understand the specific mechanisms and potential therapeutic targets involved in this complex interplay.

Neuroplasticity and Changes in Brain Structure in the comorbidity of stress, depression and drug abuse: The hippocampus is a critical brain region involved in learning, memory, and emotional regulation. It plays a significant role in the interconnectedness of stress, depression, and drug abuse. Chronic stress can lead to structural changes in the hippocampus, including a reduction in the volume of the hippocampal region. This phenomenon, known as hippocampal atrophy, is associated with impaired cognitive function and an increased risk of stress-related psychiatric disorders. Stress can also impact neurogenesis, the formation of new neurons, in the hippocampus. Chronic stress may suppress neurogenesis, and this has been linked to depressive-like behaviors (McEwen & Morrison, 2013). Individuals with depression often exhibit structural changes in the hippocampus, similar to those observed with chronic stress. Reduced hippocampal volume is a consistent finding in depression. Dysfunction in hippocampal function is associated with cognitive deficits and impairments in memory, which are common symptoms of depression (Campbell et al., 2004).

The hippocampus is crucial for learning and memory processes, including those associated with drug-related cues and rewards. Drug abuse can impact hippocampal function, contributing to the formation and maintenance of drug-associated memories (Castilla-Ortega et al., 2016). There is a bidirectional relationship between the hippocampus and stress, depression, and drug abuse. Chronic stress and depression can negatively impact the structure and function of the hippocampus, while alterations in the hippocampus may contribute to the vulnerability to stress and the development of depressive symptoms. The hippocampus is a region with high neuroplasticity, meaning it can adapt and change over time. Understanding the mechanisms of hippocampal plasticity is crucial for elucidating the interconnectedness of these conditions (Tanti & Belzung

2013). Therapeutic interventions that aim to enhance hippocampal neurogenesis or protect against stress-induced changes in the hippocampus are being explored for the treatment of depression and substance use disorders. Considering the role of the hippocampus in the interconnectedness of stress, depression, and drug abuse provides valuable insights into the shared neural mechanisms and potential targets for therapeutic interventions. However, it's important to note that research in this field is ongoing, and the relationships between these factors are complex and multifaceted.

The amygdala, a key region in the brain associated with emotional processing and responses, plays a significant role in the interconnectedness of stress, depression, and drug abuse. The amygdala is involved in the processing of emotionally salient stimuli, including those related to stress. It plays a central role in the initiation of the stress response by influencing the release of stress hormones, such as cortisol (McEwen, 2007). Altered amygdala function is often observed in individuals with depression, contributing to emotional dysregulation and heightened responses to negative stimuli. Hyperactivity in the amygdala is associated with the experience of negative affective states (Price & Drevets, 2012).

The amygdala is a crucial component of the brain's reward circuitry. It is involved in the processing of rewarding stimuli, including those associated with drugs of abuse. Drug-related cues can elicit amygdala activation, contributing to the reinforcement of drug-seeking behaviour (Koob & Volkow, 2010). There are bidirectional influences between the amygdala and stress, depression, and drug abuse. Chronic stress can lead to structural and functional changes in the amygdala, which may contribute to the development of depressive symptoms and an increased vulnerability to substance abuse. The amygdala exhibits neuroplasticity, and alterations in its structure and function can impact emotional responses and behavioral outcomes in the context of stress and drug abuse (Vyas et al., 2002). Therapeutic interventions that target the amygdala, such as cognitive-behavioral therapies, aim to modulate emotional responses and regulate stress. These interventions have been applied in the treatment of depression and substance use disorders. Medications that modulate amygdala function, such as certain antidepressants, are explored for their potential in managing both depressive symptoms and substance abuse (Etkin & Wager, 2007) Involvement of the amygdala in the interconnectedness of stress, depression, and drug abuse provides insights into shared neural mechanisms and potential targets for therapeutic interventions. However, it's crucial to recognize the complexity of these relationships, as multiple brain regions and circuits contribute to the overall neurobiology of these conditions.

Brain regions impacted.

Prefrontal cortex
Stress and Depression: Reduced volume and impaired decision-making.
Drug Abuse: Weakened executive control and impulse regulation.

Hippocampus:
Stress and Depression: Reduced neurogenesis and volume shrinkage, impacting memory and emotional regulation.
Drug Abuse: Damage to learning and memory processes.

Amygdala:
Stress: Hyperactivity, increased fear and anxiety.
Depression and Drug Abuse: Altered emotional responses.

Nucleus Accumbens (Reward System):
Stress and Depression: Diminished ability to process natural reward
Drug Abuse: Dysregulation of reward and pleasure pathways, overactivation with addictive substances.

Ventral Tegmental Area (VTA):
Stress, Depression, and Drug Abuse: Altered dopamine pathways related to reward and motivation.

Neuroplasticity Changes

Synaptic Changes in response to Stress, Depression and Addiction
Altered Connections: Disruption of normal synaptic plasticity, with excessive dopamine causing altered connections.

Dendritic Atrophy: Dendritic shrinking in the hippocampus and prefrontal cortex, leading to cognitive deficits.

Neurogenesis Impairment: Reduced neurogenesis in the hippocampus due to chronic stress and depression, and how drugs can further exacerbate this.

Structural Shrinkage: Structural shrinkage (e.g., reduced volume in the hippocampus and prefrontal cortex).

Neurochemical Impact

Dopamine, serotonin, and norepinephrine play important role in these conditions, and drug abuse, stress, and depression alter the balance and availability of these neurotransmitters.

Brain-derived Neurotrophic Factor (BDNF): Reduced BDNF levels impact neuroplasticity, especially in the hippocampus, and contribute to both mood disorders and addiction.

Neuroplasticity/ Changes in Brain Structure in the comorbidity of stress, depression and drug abuse

The prefrontal cortex (PFC) is a critical brain region that plays a key role in the interconnectedness of stress, depression, and drug abuse. Chronic stress can lead to impairments in the prefrontal cortex, particularly the dorsolateral prefrontal cortex (DLPFC), which is involved in executive functions such as decision-making, cognitive control, and emotional regulation. Stress-induced changes in the PFC may contribute to deficits in these functions (Arnsten, 2009). Individuals with depression often exhibit structural and functional alterations in the prefrontal cortex. Reduced gray matter volume and hypoactivity in regions such as the ventromedial prefrontal cortex

(VMPFC) are associated with depressive symptoms. Dysfunction in the prefrontal cortex is linked to cognitive deficits observed in depression, including difficulties in attention, memory, and decision-making (Price & Drevets, 2010). The prefrontal cortex, particularly the ventral prefrontal cortex (VPFC), is involved in inhibitory control and decision-making. Drug abuse can lead to impairments in PFC function, contributing to a loss of control over drug-seeking behavior. Substance use can affect the mesocorticolimbic pathway, involving the PFC, and influence reward processing. Changes in PFC function may contribute to the reinforcing effects of drugs (Goldstein & Volkow, 2011). There are reciprocal connections between the prefrontal cortex and limbic structures, such as the amygdala, which are involved in emotional processing. Dysregulation in these circuits may contribute to the interconnectedness of stress, depression, and drug abuse.

The prefrontal cortex exhibits neuroplasticity, and its function can be modulated by experiences such as stress and drug exposure. Understanding these plastic changes is crucial for unraveling the interconnected nature of these conditions (Sinha, 2008). Interventions that target the prefrontal cortex, such as cognitive-behavioral therapies, aim to enhance executive functions and emotional regulation. These approaches have been applied in the treatment of depression and substance use disorders. Medications that modulate PFC function, including certain antidepressants and anti-addiction medications, are explored for their potential in managing symptoms across these conditions (Naqvi & Bechara, A. 2009).

Altered reward processing is a crucial aspect of the interconnectedness of stress, depression, and drug abuse. Dysregulation in the brain's reward circuitry contributes to the development and maintenance of these conditions. Chronic stress can lead to a devaluation of natural rewards. The brain's response to pleasurable stimuli may be blunted, contributing to anhedonia (loss of interest or pleasure) – a common symptom in stress-related disorders. Conversely, chronic stress can sensitize the brain's reward circuitry to the reinforcing effects of drugs. Stress may increase vulnerability to drug abuse by enhancing the rewarding properties of substances (Ménard & Quirion, 2012). Individuals with depression often exhibit dysfunction in the brain's reward circuit, particularly in regions such as the nucleus accumbens and ventral tegmental area. This dysfunction contributes to reduced sensitivity to rewards and anhedonia. Depressed individuals may experience a reduced ability to derive pleasure from activities that were once rewarding, further contributing to the cycle of depression (Treadway & Zald, 2011).

Drugs of abuse can directly influence the brain's reward system, leading to intense feelings of pleasure and reinforcing drug-seeking behavior. Prolonged drug use induces neuroadaptations in the reward circuitry, leading to tolerance, dependence, and sensitization. These changes contribute to the cycle of addiction (Kalivas & O'Brien, 2008). There is evidence of cross-sensitization between stress, depression, and drug abuse. Chronic stress and depression can sensitize the brain's reward system, making individuals more susceptible to the reinforcing effects of drugs. Common neural pathways, including the mesolimbic dopamine system, are implicated in the processing of rewards, and alterations in these pathways contribute to the interconnected nature of these conditions (Russo, & Nestler, 2013)

Therapeutic approaches that focus on restoring healthy reward processing, such as behavioral activation therapy, are used in the treatment of depression. Medications targeting the reward circuitry, including antidepressants and anti-addiction medications, are explored for their potential to normalize reward processing in the context of stress and substance use disorders (Vrieze et al., 2013). Altered reward processing is a crucial aspect of the interconnectedness of stress, depression, and drug abuse. Dysregulation in the brain's reward circuitry contributes to the development and maintenance of these conditions. Implications for memory and emotional processing in the comorbidity of stress, depression and drug abuse has profound implications. Acute stress can enhance the encoding of emotionally salient information, leading to stronger memories for stress-related events. Chronic stress, however, can impair memory retrieval, particularly in tasks requiring cognitive flexibility and declarative memory processes. Depression is often associated with deficits in episodic memory, impacting the ability to remember personal experiences and events. Individuals with depression may exhibit a bias toward recalling negative memories over positive ones, contributing to the maintenance of depressive symptoms. Substance abuse, especially in the context of addiction, is linked to the formation of strong memories associated with drug use and drug-related cues. Prolonged substance abuse, particularly with drugs like alcohol and opioids, can lead to cognitive impairments affecting various memory domains. Chronic stress and depression can impact memory processes, creating vulnerability to substance abuse. Conversely, substance abuse can further disrupt memory and exacerbate the cognitive impact of stress and depression. Shared neural circuits, including the hippocampus and amygdala, play a crucial role in memory formation and emotional processing, forming a link between stress, depression, and substance abuse (Joëls, 2009; Sandi, 2011; MacQueen & Frodl, 2011; Bora et al., 2012;).

Cognitive interventions that focus on memory enhancement and cognitive remediation may be incorporated into treatment plans to address cognitive deficits associated with stress, depression, or substance abuse. Stress can lead to heightened emotional reactivity, making individuals more responsive to emotional stimuli. The amygdala plays a key role in this process. Chronic stress may impair emotional regulation, contributing to mood disorders and increasing vulnerability to substance abuse as individuals seek relief from emotional distress. Depression is associated with emotional blunting, where individuals may experience a reduction in the intensity of both positive and negative emotions. Changes in the processing of emotional stimuli in the amygdala and prefrontal cortex contribute to altered emotional reactivity in individuals with depression. When abused, drugs can induce intense and euphoric emotional states, contributing to the reinforcing effects of substances.

Chronic drug use can lead to emotional dysregulation, where individuals may experience mood swings, irritability, and difficulties in managing emotions. The amygdala, prefrontal cortex, and limbic system, which are involved in emotional processing, are common substrates that contribute to the interconnectedness of stress, depression, and drug abuse. Emotional processing influences and is influenced by stress, depression, and substance abuse in a bidirectional manner, forming a complex interplay. Interventions that target emotion regulation strategies, such as dialectical behavior therapy (DBT) or mindfulness-based approaches, are used in the treatment of conditions involving emotional dysregulation, including certain mood disorders and substance use disorders (Disner et al., 2011; Siegle et al., 2007; Koob & Volkow, 2016; Everitt & Robbins, 2016). Certain medications, such as antidepressants and mood stabilizers, may be used to modulate emotional processing in the treatment of depression and co-occurring substance use disorders.

In conclusion, the interconnected nature of stress, depression, and drug abuse reflects a complex interplay of biological, psychological, and environmental factors. These conditions are not isolated entities but are intricately linked through shared neurobiological pathways, behavioral patterns, and environmental influences. Stress, depression, and drug abuse share common neurobiological pathways, including the involvement of neurotransmitters (e.g., serotonin, dopamine, norepinephrine) and neural circuits (e.g., amygdala, prefrontal cortex, hippocampus). These shared pathways contribute to the cross-sensitization and bidirectional influences observed in these conditions. Stress, depression, and drug abuse exert profound effects on memory and emotional processing. Chronic stress can modulate memory formation and retrieval, while depression is associated with episodic memory deficits and emotional blunting. Drug abuse, in turn, shapes the formation of drug-related memories and induces emotional dysregulation.

The relationships between stress, depression, and drug abuse are reciprocal. Chronic stress and depressive symptoms can increase vulnerability to substance abuse, and substance abuse can exacerbate stress and depressive symptoms. This bidirectional influence contributes to the persistence and chronicity of these conditions. Genetic, environmental, and developmental factors contribute to shared vulnerabilities for stress-related disorders, depression, and substance use disorders. Early life experiences, trauma, and genetic predispositions can amplify the risk for the development of these interconnected conditions. Integrated treatment approaches that address the holistic nature of these conditions are crucial. Therapeutic interventions should consider the bidirectional influences and shared neural substrates, employing a combination of psychotherapy, pharmacotherapy, and psychosocial support. Given the heterogeneity of individuals experiencing these interconnected conditions, a one-size-fits-all approach may not be effective. Tailored, individualized treatment plans that consider the unique biological, psychological, and social factors of each person are essential for successful outcomes. Prevention efforts should target common risk factors and focus on building resilience against stressors. Early intervention and education can play a vital role in preventing the escalation from stress and depression to substance abuse, breaking the cycle before it becomes entrenched. Further research is needed to unravel the intricate mechanisms underlying the interconnectedness of stress, depression, and drug abuse. Advances in neuroscience, genetics, and behavioral science can provide valuable insights, opening new avenues for more effective prevention and treatment strategies.

CHAPTER 9

ANIMAL MODELS OF DRUG ADDICTION

"An over-indulgence of anything, even something as pure as water, can intoxicate."
~ Criss Jami

Excessive consumption or engagement in any behavior, even those considered benign or essential, can lead to harmful consequences. The abuse or overuse of substances, whether they are initially perceived as harmless or even beneficial, can result in intoxication or negative outcomes. This chapter helps explore the intricate landscape of drug addiction begins with the utilization of animal models, provides insights into the neurobiological and behavioral aspects of substance use disorders. In the quest to unravel the complexities of drug addiction, researchers turn to animal models as essential frameworks, allowing the study of behavioral, genetic, and neurochemical aspects to better understand the mechanisms underlying addictive behaviors.

Animal models of drug addiction play a crucial role in understanding the neurobiological, behavioral, and environmental factors that contribute to substance abuse. These models provide valuable insights into the mechanisms underlying addiction, facilitate the development of potential treatments, and aid in the identification of risk factors. Animal models help researchers study the neurobiological and behavioral changes associated with drug addiction, shedding light on the underlying mechanisms. These models are instrumental in the preclinical evaluation of potential pharmacotherapies for addiction treatment.

Preclinical drug development: Animal models play a crucial role in preclinical drug development for various diseases, including drug addiction.

These models allow researchers to investigate the safety, efficacy, and potential side effects of new medications before they are tested in human clinical trials. Animal models help identify and validate potential drug targets by elucidating the neurobiological mechanisms involved in addiction. Animal models allow researchers to assess the effectiveness of potential medications in altering drug-seeking behavior, relapse, and other relevant endpoints (Kalivas & Volkow, 2005; Venniro et al., 2016). Animal models help assess the absorption, distribution, metabolism, and excretion of potential drugs, as well as their pharmacodynamic effects. Using these animal models potential adverse effects and toxicity of candidate drugs could be identified, ensuring safety before progressing to human trials (Pugsley, 2008). Animal models help determine the optimal dosage range for a potential drug, ensuring therapeutic efficacy without excessive side effects.

Animal models help elucidate the specific mechanisms through which a drug exerts its effects, providing insights into the pharmacology of potential medications (Nestler, 2014). Animal models contribute to the validation of therapeutic targets by demonstrating whether interventions at specific points in the addiction process lead to desired outcomes (Neisewander & Cheung, 2019). Animal models allow researchers to assess the potential of novel treatment modalities, such as gene therapies or neuromodulation techniques, in the context of addiction (Thanos et al., 2001). Findings from animal models help inform the design of human clinical trials, improving the likelihood of success in translating preclinical research to effective treatments (Littman & Williams, 2005). While recognizing the importance of animal models, ethical considerations, such as the refinement, reduction, and replacement of animal use (the 3Rs), are critical to ensure humane treatment. Animal models provide a critical bridge between basic research and clinical applications in drug addiction. They enable a systematic and ethical approach to preclinical drug development, laying the groundwork for the advancement of effective treatments for substance use disorders.

Types of animal models: Various types of animal models are utilized in scientific research to study different aspects of drug addiction. Each model is designed to mimic certain features of human addiction, allowing researchers to investigate the neurobiological, behavioral, and environmental factors involved.

a. Self-administration models: Animals are trained to self-administer drugs, reflecting the voluntary drug-taking behavior observed in humans. Self-administration models are a class of animal models widely used in addiction research to study voluntary drug-taking behavior, reinforcement mechanisms, and the development of addiction-like behaviors. These models involve 'operant conditioning' which refers to training animals to self-administer drugs, providing insights into the neurobiological and behavioral aspects of addiction. Animals learn to perform specific operant responses (e.g., pressing a lever) to receive drug infusions. Animals may have continuous access to the drug (free-access) or restricted access during specific sessions (limited-access). Animals must make a response (e.g., lever press) to receive a drug infusion, establishing a contingent relationship between behavior and drug delivery. The stages of self-administration models include, acquisition (animals learn to associate a specific response with drug delivery), maintenance (animals continue to self-administer the drug under stable conditions) and (extinction: the drug is no longer available following the operant response, leading to a decrease in drug-seeking behavior) and reinstatement (factors such as drug priming or exposure to drug-associated cues can reinstate drug-seeking behavior after extinction). Self-administration models elucidate the involvement of brain reward pathways, particularly the mesolimbic dopamine system (Volkow & Fowler, 2000).

Long-term changes in neurotransmitter systems, receptor expression, and synaptic plasticity are studied in this animal model. It could be tailored for various substances, including psychostimulants, opioids, alcohol, and cannabinoids. It also investigates how prior exposure to one drug influences the response to another and could also be helpful in studying the impact of different drug doses on self-administration behavior. Fixed or progressive ratio schedules influence the effort required for drug access. The role of environmental cues and context in drug-seeking behavior could also be studied. This model has translational relevance and face validity as it mimics key features of human drug-taking behavior, enhancing the translational relevance of findings. Successful pharmacotherapies identified in self-administration models may progress to clinical trials. Challenges associated with this animal model include species differences as responses may vary between species, emphasizing the need for cautious interpretation. Self-administration models capture certain aspects but may not fully replicate the complexity of human addiction. This model could facilitate successful modulation of drug self-administration can suggest potential medications for addiction treatment and evaluates the abuse potential of novel compounds (Everitt & Robbins, 2005). Self-administration models provide a valuable tool for understanding the behavioral and neurobiological underpinnings of addiction, offering insights into the development, maintenance, and potential treatment of substance use disorders.

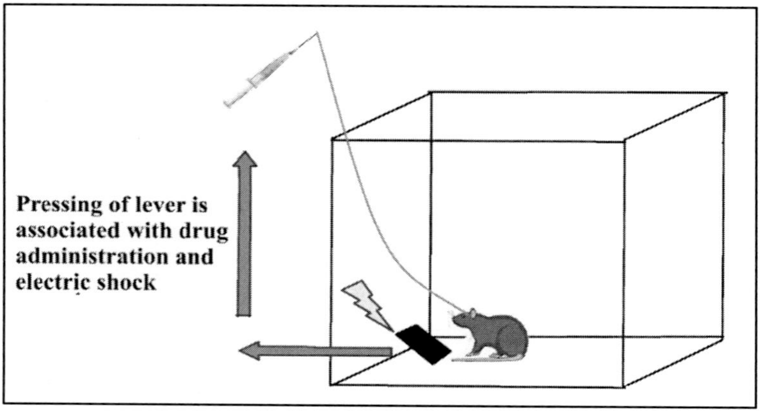

Animal model of drug self-administration

b. Conditioned place preference (CPP): The Conditioned Place Preference (CPP) paradigm is a widely used animal model in addiction research, providing insights into the rewarding properties of drugs of abuse and the neural circuits involved in associative learning (Tzschentke, 2007). This model is based on the principle of classical conditioning. CPP animal model involves classical conditioning where animals learn to associate the rewarding effects of a drug with a particular environment. The experimental procedure involves three distinct phases: (i) Pre-conditioning phase: animals are exposed to two distinct environments, often with different sensory cues such as color / texture. Baseline preference for each environment is determined by measuring the time spent in each compartment. (ii) Conditioning phase:

animals receive drug administration in one of the environments (paired with the drug's effects) and vehicle administration (no drug) in the other environment. Pairing creates an association between the drug's rewarding effects and the environmental cues. (iii) Post-conditioning phase: animals are once again given free access to both environments without drug administration. Changes in the time spent in drug-paired vs. non-drug-paired environments are assessed.

An increase in the time spent in the drug-paired environment indicates the development of a conditioned place preference, suggesting that the drug has rewarding or reinforcing properties. The mesolimbic dopamine system, particularly the nucleus accumbens, is implicated in the rewarding effects observed in CPP.

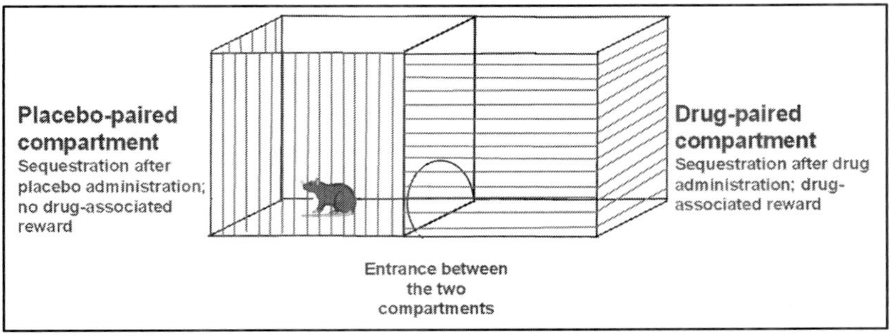

Conditioned place preference

CPP models the associative learning processes underlying drug reward. It evaluates the rewarding properties of various drugs of abuse and if combined with repeated drug exposure, CPP can be used to study the development of behavioral sensitization. The dose and timing of drug administration during conditioning influence the magnitude of CPP. Sensitivity to CPP may also vary among different strains and individual animals. The specific context and cues associated with CPP may not fully capture the complexity of drug use in humans. Responses in rodents may not precisely translate to human drug-taking behavior (Bardo & Bevins, 2000; Cunningham et al., 2006). The CPP animal model provides a valuable tool for assessing the rewarding properties of drugs and understanding the associative learning processes associated with drug addiction. It complements other animal models, contributing to a comprehensive understanding of the neurobiology of addiction.

c. Extinction and Reinstatement Models: The extinction and reinstatement models are experimental paradigms used in animal research to investigate the processes of drug-seeking behavior, extinction, and the potential for relapse. These models are particularly relevant for understanding the dynamics of addiction and evaluating interventions aimed at preventing relapse. Animals learn to extinguish drug-seeking behavior, and reinstatement tests assess factors triggering relapse (Shaham et al., 2003). Animals are trained to self-administer a drug until a stable baseline of drug-seeking behavior is established. The drug is then withheld, and the animal undergoes sessions where responding no longer results in drug delivery. Over time, the animal learns that the previously drug-paired response is no longer followed by drug reinforcement. Decrease in Drug-Seeking Behavior: Extinction training results in a gradual reduction or extinction of drug-seeking behavior. Involves neural circuits associated with inhibitory learning, including the prefrontal cortex and the amygdala. Challenges include the potential for the reappearance of drug-seeking behavior after a period of abstinence (Peters & Kalivas, 2006; Caprioli & Venniro, 2020).

In reinstatement model of drug addiction, after extinction training, a relapse (reinstatement) is triggered by exposing animals to specific stimuli or conditions. Reinstatement can be induced by drug priming, exposure to drug-associated cues, stressors, or other factors. Reinstatement results in the rapid resurgence of drug-seeking behavior. This model is considered a relapse model, as it simulates the vulnerability to return to drug-seeking after a period of abstinence. It involves neural circuits associated with drug reward, stress response, and associative learning, including the mesolimbic dopamine system and the amygdala. It covers three types of reinstatements i.e., 'drug-primed reinstatement' observed following administration of a small dose of the drug of abuse, 'cue-induced reinstatement' expressed post exposure to drug-associated cues or contexts and 'stress-induced reinstatement' expressed post exposure to stressors or aversive stimuli. The reinstatement model captures certain aspects of relapse but may not fully replicate the complexity of human relapse (Epstein et al., 2006).

There are combined extinction-reinstatement models. Integration involves sequential phases i.e., combining extinction and reinstatement procedures to study the transition from drug-seeking to extinction and then relapse. It can therefore give deep insight into behavioral dynamics and captures the dynamic processes of extinction learning, maintenance, and factors contributing to relapse. It could have immense research applications in the evaluation of pharmacological interventions and could be highly beneficial in testing the effectiveness of pharmacological or behavioral interventions in preventing or attenuating relapse (Bossert et al., 2006; Grimm et al., 2001). These models collectively provide valuable insights into the behavioral and neurobiological mechanisms underlying addiction, extinction learning, and relapse. They contribute to the development and evaluation of interventions aimed at preventing or mitigating relapse in individuals recovering from substance use disorders.

d. Withdrawal Models: Withdrawal models in drug addiction research are designed to simulate the physiological and behavioral changes that occur when an individual abruptly stops or reduces the intake of a drug after prolonged use. These models are crucial for understanding the neurobiological mechanisms underlying withdrawal symptoms, which can contribute to the maintenance of drug dependence. Morphine withdrawal model, there is an abrupt cessation of chronic morphine administration. Withdrawal symptoms include hyperalgesia, piloerection, increased anxiety-like behavior, diarrhea, and other symptoms. Opioid withdrawal model involves endogenous opioid system and adaptations in neurotransmitter systems (Koob & Le Moal, 2008). In alcohol withdrawal model there is abrupt cessation of chronic alcohol exposure and withdrawal symptoms include symptoms like tremors, seizures, anxiety, dysregulation of autonomic functions, and potential delirium tremens. There is kindling model in which repeated withdrawal episodes lead to increased severity of withdrawal symptoms with each subsequent episode (Heilig et al., 2010). The nicotine withdrawal model exhibits cessation of chronic nicotine administration with withdrawal symptoms like irritability, anxiety, increased appetite, cognitive deficits, and craving for nicotine. Neurobiological mechanisms include involvement of nicotinic acetylcholine receptors and neurotransmitter systems (Jackson et al., 2015). Benzodiazepine withdrawal model involves abrupt cessation of chronic benzodiazepine administration. Withdrawal symptoms of anxiety, insomnia, increased sensitivity to stimuli, and potential seizures are exhibited by rats. GABAergic system and adaptations in neurotransmitter systems mediate the neurochemical changes exhibited in this model (Stephens & King, 2009). Withdrawal models provide valuable insights into the neurobiological and behavioral changes associated with the discontinuation of various drugs. These models are instrumental in understanding the processes of dependence, withdrawal, and relapse, contributing to the development of effective treatment strategies for substance use disorders.

e. Genetic Models: Animal genetic models of drug addiction play a crucial role in understanding the genetic factors that contribute to the susceptibility, development, and maintenance of substance use disorders. These models involve selectively breeding animals with specific genetic traits or manipulating specific genes to investigate their role in addiction-related behaviors. High- and low-responder lines are the selective breeding based on the animals' response to a drug challenge. Animals showing a high response to a drug challenge (e.g., locomotor activity or preference) are bred together to create a high-responder line, while low responders are bred together to create a low-responder line. These lines help identify genes associated with the intensity of drug responses and vulnerability to addiction. Alcohol-preferring (P) and non-preferring (NP) rat lines are the selective breeding based on the animals' preference for alcohol. P rats show a strong preference for alcohol compared to NP rats, which do not exhibit a strong preference. P and NP rats are used to study genetic factors influencing alcohol consumption, withdrawal, and addiction-related behaviors. Animal models such as selective breeding for cocaine sensitivity also are used which include selective breeding based on the animals' sensitivity to the effects of cocaine. Animals that are more sensitive to the locomotor-stimulating effects of cocaine are bred together to create a line with high cocaine sensitivity (Roy et al., 2023).

Dopamine receptor knock out mice model helps identify genes associated with individual differences in response to cocaine and susceptibility to addiction. Dopamine receptor knock out mice involve genetic manipulation to create mice lacking specific dopamine receptor subtypes (e.g., D1 or D2 receptors). These could help in studying the role of specific dopamine receptors in reward-related behaviors and addiction. They also provide insights into the neurobiological mechanisms involving dopamine receptors in addiction-related processes. Mu-Opioid Receptor Knockout Mice Genetic manipulation to create mice lacking mu-opioid receptors. It helps in investigating the role of mu-opioid receptors in the rewarding effects of opioids and susceptibility to opioid addiction. It helps elucidate the contribution of mu-opioid receptors to opioid-induced behaviors.

CRF (Corticotropin-Releasing Factor) overexpression is a genetic manipulation to overexpress crf, a stress-related neuropeptide. It facilitates the study of the impact of heightened stress response on addiction-related behaviors. CRF overexpression models help understand the role of stress in addiction vulnerability. Neuropeptide Y (NPY) overexpression can also be used as genetic manipulation to overexpress neuropeptide Y, a peptide with anxiolytic and anti-stress effects. Investigating the role of NPY in modulating stress responses and addiction-related behaviors could help understand the mechanisms better. NPY overexpression models contribute to understanding the protective effects of NPY against stress-induced relapse. These genetic models allow researchers to dissect the contributions of specific genes and molecular pathways to addiction-related behaviors (Corder et al., 2020). By combining genetic approaches with behavioral, neurobiological, and pharmacological studies, scientists can gain insights into the complex interplay between genetics and environmental factors in the development of substance use disorders.

f. Stress-Induced Models: Stress-induced animal models of drug addiction are designed to investigate how stressors contribute to the initiation, maintenance, and relapse of drug-seeking behavior. These models are valuable for understanding the complex interactions between stress and substance use and for elucidating the neurobiological mechanisms involved. In chronic mild stress (CMS) model, animals are exposed to a series of mild, unpredictable stressors over an extended period. It induces anhedonia (reduced responsiveness to rewards), changes in exploratory behavior, and alterations in sucrose consumption. It mimics chronic stressors that individuals may face in daily life and provides insight into how chronic stress influences susceptibility to drug addiction. In social defeat stress model animals are exposed to repeated social defeat experiences, where it is subjected to aggressive encounters with a dominant conspecific. This results in social avoidance, heightened anxiety-like behavior, and altered reward sensitivity. Social defeat stress can increase vulnerability to drug self-administration and relapse, reflecting the impact of social stressors on addictive behaviors. Restraint stress model includes animals which are physically restrained for a specific duration, inducing psychological stress. It elicits increased corticosterone levels, anxiety-like behavior, and alterations in neurotransmitter systems. Restraint stress can lead to increased drug self-administration and reinstatement of drug-seeking behavior, demonstrating its role in addiction vulnerability (Logrip et al., 2012). Footshock stress model involves exposing animals to mild electric foot shocks. Behavioral effects induce stress-related responses, such as increased corticosterone levels and anxiety-like behaviors. It can also enhance drug self-administration and reinstatement of drug-seeking, modeling stress-induced relapse. Animals experience intermittent footshocks, creating a more unpredictable and severe stress paradigm. it produces a greater impact on anxiety-like behaviors and HPA axis activation. This model is particularly useful for studying stress-induced escalation of drug use and reinstatement of drug-seeking behavior.

Chronic social stress model involves exposing animals to prolonged social instability or conflict. It also leads to social avoidance, altered neuroendocrine function, and changes in reward-related behaviors. Chronic social stress can increase vulnerability to drug self-administration and promote the escalation of drug intake. These stress-induced animal models contribute to our understanding of the intricate relationship between stress and drug addiction. They help identify neurobiological mechanisms involved in stress-induced changes in behavior and provide a platform for testing potential interventions aimed at mitigating the impact of stress on addiction vulnerability and relapse.

g. Social Models: Animal social models of drug addiction involve studying the influence of social interactions, social hierarchy, and social environments on drug-related behaviors. These models aim to understand how social factors contribute to the development, maintenance, and relapse of substance use disorders. Social facilitation and peer influence models involve exposure of animals to conspecifics (members of the same species), and their drug-related behaviors are observed. It helps in studying how the presence of other animals influences drug self-administration, drug preference, and drug-seeking behavior. It mimics social situations where individuals are influenced by the drug-related behaviors of their peers (Strickland, Acuff, 2023). Social defeat stress model involves exposing an animal to social defeat experiences, where it is subjected to aggressive encounters with a dominant conspecific. Behavioral effects include social avoidance, heightened anxiety-like behavior, and alterations in reward sensitivity. It can influence susceptibility to drug self-administration and relapse, reflecting the impact of social stressors on addictive behaviors (Pantoja-Urbán et al., 2024).

Social learning models include learning of animals about drug-related behaviors through observation of conspecifics and also investigating how social learning contributes to the acquisition and expression of drug-seeking behaviors. It reflects the role of observational learning in the development of drug preferences and drug-related behaviors (Zhang et al., 2023). Social isolation models involve housing of animals in isolation or limited social environments. Behavioral effects include changes in stress-related behaviors, anxiety, and alterations in neurotransmitter systems. In relevance to addiction, social isolation can impact vulnerability to drug addiction, reflecting the importance of social factors in mental health (Powell & Swerdlow, 2023). Dominance hierarchy models involve housing animals in groups with established dominance hierarchies and studying how social status and dominance influence drug self-administration and access to drugs. It mimics social structures where access to drugs may be influenced by social dominance (Jozifkova et al., 2022). Conditioned place preference (CPP) with social interaction model combines the CPP paradigm with the presence of a conspecific during drug conditioning and helps in investigating how the association between drug effects and social interaction influences reward-related behaviors. In relevance to addiction, it reflects the impact of social context on the rewarding properties of drugs (Jozifkova et al., 2022). Social stress models involve exposing animals to social stressors, such as aggressive encounters or social instability. It induces changes in stress-related behaviors and may influence drug-related behaviors. It examines the impact of social stress on susceptibility to drug addiction and relapse. These social models contribute to our understanding of the social determinants of drug addiction. They help uncover the complex interactions between social factors, environmental influences, and neurobiological mechanisms involved in substance use disorders. Additionally, these models provide insights into potential social interventions for preventing and treating drug addiction.

h. Adolescent Models: Adolescent models of drug addiction involve studying the effects of drug exposure during the adolescent period on subsequent drug-related behaviors. Adolescence is a critical developmental stage characterized by ongoing neurobiological changes, including synaptic pruning, myelination, and alterations in neurotransmitter systems. Exposure to drugs during this period can have lasting effects on brain structure and function, influencing vulnerability to addiction. Adolescent drug exposure models involve exposure of animals to drugs during adolescence, and the long-term effects on drug-related behaviors are assessed in adulthood. This involves investigating how adolescent drug exposure influences drug self-administration, reward sensitivity, and susceptibility to addiction later in life. It mimics the vulnerability of human adolescents to the long-term effects of drug exposure during a critical period of brain development (Maldonado et al., 2023).

Adolescent social models make it feasible to study the impact of social interactions during adolescence on subsequent drug-related behaviors. It helps in investigating how peer influence, social learning, and social stress during adolescence contribute to drug-seeking behaviors in adulthood and reflects the importance of social factors during adolescence in shaping susceptibility to drug addiction (Renner et al., 2023). Adolescent stress models involve exposing animals to stressors during adolescence and assessing the impact on drug-related behaviors. This helps in studying how stress during adolescence influences vulnerability to drug addiction and stress-induced relapse. It facilitates examining the role of stress during a critical developmental period in shaping the neurobiology of addiction (Deng et al., 2023).

Adolescent brain development models help in investigating the impact of drug exposure on the developing adolescent brain and assessing changes in brain structure, neurotransmitter systems, and synaptic plasticity following adolescent drug exposure. These animal models facilitate us in understanding that how drugs may alter the developing neural circuitry, leading to increased susceptibility to addiction (Ray et al., 2023). Adolescent impulsivity models assess impulsive behavior during adolescence and its association with drug-related behaviors in adulthood and could be used for investigating the link between adolescent impulsivity and the development of addiction-like behaviors. This impulsive behavior during adolescence is associated with an increased risk of substance use disorders in adulthood (Cajiao-Manrique et al., 2023). Adolescent sensitization models examine the development of behavioral sensitization to drugs during adolescence and assess the persistence of drug sensitization and its impact on subsequent drug-related behaviors. Behavioral sensitization is associated with an increased vulnerability to addiction-like behaviors (Buthmann et al., 2023). These adolescent models contribute to our understanding of the unique vulnerabilities and sensitivities of the adolescent brain to drugs of abuse. They help identify critical periods during development when exposure to drugs may have lasting effects on behavior and neurobiology, ultimately influencing the susceptibility to drug addiction in adulthood. Studying these models provides insights into potential intervention strategies aimed at preventing or mitigating the long-term consequences of adolescent drug exposure.

i. Transgenic Models: Transgenic models of drug addiction involve genetically modifying animals to express or lack specific genes related to addiction-related processes. These models are essential for elucidating the molecular and genetic mechanisms underlying drug dependence and addictive behaviors. ΔFosB overexpression models involve overexpression of transcription factor ΔFosB implicated in addiction. Overexpression models aim to understand its role in drug-induced neuroplasticity (Nestler, 2015). CREB (cAMP response element-binding protein) is involved in long-term neuronal changes associated with drug addiction. CREB overexpression or knockdown models involve modifying expression of CREB to provide insights into addiction mechanisms (Carlezon et al., 2005).

Dopamine receptor knockout models involve genetic manipulation of dopamine receptors (e.g., d1 or d2 receptors) to investigate their role in reward and addiction (Bello et al., 2011). Opioid Receptor knockout models investigate the role of opioid receptors (e.g., mu-opioid receptors) in addiction-related behaviors (Contet et al., 2010). Neuropeptide Y (NPY) overexpression models facilitate examining the effects of overexpressing neuropeptide Y, which has anti-stress and anxiolytic properties (Thorsell et al., 2000). Calcium/Calmodulin-Dependent Protein Kinase II (CaMKII) overexpression models investigate the role of CaMKII, a key enzyme in synaptic plasticity, in drug addiction (Jia et al., 2021). These transgenic models provide valuable insights into the molecular and genetic basis of drug addiction. Researchers use these models to explore specific gene functions, signaling pathways, and neuroadaptations associated with drug dependence, helping to identify potential targets for therapeutic interventions in addiction treatment. These animal models collectively provide a comprehensive approach to studying the multifaceted nature of drug addiction, allowing researchers to explore different aspects of the disorder and develop potential interventions.

Neurobiological Insights: Animal model studies have been instrumental in providing neurobiological insights into addictive behaviors, shedding light on the underlying mechanisms of substance abuse and dependence. Animal models have demonstrated the central role of the dopaminergic system, particularly the mesolimbic pathway, in mediating the rewarding effects of drugs and the development of addictive behaviors (Wise, 2004). Animal models have revealed neuroadaptations and synaptic plasticity in response to chronic drug exposure, contributing to the transition from casual drug use to compulsive drug-seeking behavior (Kalivas & O'Brien, 2008). Animal models, including Pavlovian conditioning paradigms, have demonstrated the role of environmental cues in eliciting drug-associated responses and triggering cravings. They also have delineated the neural circuits involved in drug craving and relapse, emphasizing the role of interconnected brain regions such as the prefrontal cortex, amygdala, and nucleus accumbens (Everitt & Robbins, 2016). Animal models have elucidated the complex interactions between stress, the hypothalamic-pituitary-adrenal (HPA) axis, and drug addiction, highlighting the role of stress in vulnerability to substance abuse (Sinha, 2008). Neurobiological basis of addictive behaviors, provide insights into the molecular, cellular, and circuit-level changes that drive substance abuse and dependence. Animal models allow for controlled experimentation, manipulations, and precise measurements, facilitating the discovery of potential targets for addiction treatment.

Dopaminergic system plays a significant role in addiction and animal model studies have significantly contributed to our understanding in this regard. Animal models, particularly rodents, have demonstrated that the mesolimbic dopaminergic pathway, connecting the ventral tegmental area (VTA) to the nucleus accumbens (NAc), plays a central role in mediating the rewarding effects of drugs and natural rewards (Wise, 2004). Animal models, including microdialysis studies, have shown that drugs of abuse increase dopamine release in the NAc, leading to enhanced dopaminergic signaling, which is associated with the reinforcing properties of addictive substances (Nestler, 2005). Animal models have demonstrated that repeated exposure to drugs induces neuroplastic changes in the dopaminergic system, leading to sensitization—a phenomenon where the response to the drug becomes amplified over time (Vezina & Leyton, 2009). Animal models, including studies using genetically modified mice, have helped elucidate the specific roles of dopamine receptor subtypes (D1 and D2 receptors) in addiction-related behaviors and neuroplasticity (Lobo & Nestler, 2011). Animal models have demonstrated the role of dopamine in conditioned responses and cue-induced craving, emphasizing the importance of associative learning processes in addiction (Flagel & Robinson, 2017). These insights from animal model studies highlight the intricate role of the dopaminergic system in addiction, providing a foundation for understanding the neurobiology of addictive behaviors and potential targets for therapeutic interventions.

The serotonergic system, centered around the neurotransmitter serotonin (5-hydroxytryptamine or 5-HT), plays a complex role in addiction. Animal model studies have contributed valuable insights into the involvement of the serotonergic system in addictive behaviors. Animal models have demonstrated that serotonin regulates reward circuitry, influencing the reinforcing effects of drugs. Serotonergic projections to the mesolimbic system, including the nucleus accumbens, modulate dopamine release and impact the perception of reward (Müller et al., 2007). Animal studies suggest that serotonin is involved in the regulation of impulsivity and compulsive drug-seeking behaviors. Dysregulation of the serotonergic system may contribute to the development of addiction-related traits (Dalley & Roiser, 2012).

Serotonin is implicated in stress response and coping mechanisms. Animal models show that alterations in the serotonergic system may influence an individual's susceptibility to stress-induced relapse and the use of drugs as a coping strategy (Lowry et al., 2005). Insights: Animal models have been used to explore the impact of serotonin on mood and affective states, with relevance to addiction. Dysregulation of the serotonergic system is associated with depressive-like states that may contribute to drug-seeking behavior (Müller & Homberg, 2015). Animal models have been crucial for testing pharmacotherapeutic interventions targeting the serotonergic system to mitigate addictive behaviors. Selective serotonin reuptake inhibitors (SSRIs) and other serotonergic drugs have been explored (Cunningham & Anastasio, 2014). These findings collectively underscore the multifaceted role of the serotonergic system in addiction, providing a basis for understanding the neurobiology of addictive behaviors and potential avenues for therapeutic interventions.

The noradrenergic system, involving the neurotransmitter norepinephrine (NE), plays a significant role in various aspects of addiction. Animal model studies have provided valuable insights into the involvement of the noradrenergic system in addictive behaviors. The noradrenergic system, particularly projections from the locus coeruleus (LC) to reward-related brain regions, modulates the processing of rewarding stimuli and contributes to addiction-related behaviors (Ventura & Alcaro, 2016). Animal models have been employed to investigate how the noradrenergic system contributes to stress-induced craving and relapse. Noradrenergic signaling is implicated in the interaction between stress and drug-seeking behavior (McReynolds et al., 2014). Animal models have provided insights into the noradrenergic system's involvement in withdrawal symptoms and negative affective states associated with drug cessation (Valentino & Van Bockstaele, 2008). Animal models have been used to explore the potential therapeutic effects of medications targeting the noradrenergic system in the treatment of addiction (Fu & Shen, 2018). Animal models have been instrumental in investigating the interactions between the noradrenergic system and other neurotransmitter systems, such as dopamine and serotonin, in the context of addiction (McElligott & Winder, 2009). These findings underscore the diverse roles of the noradrenergic system in addiction, ranging from reward processing to stress responses, withdrawal, and potential therapeutic interventions. Animal models have played a critical role in elucidating these neurobiological mechanisms.

The GABAergic system, centered around the neurotransmitter gamma-aminobutyric acid (GABA), plays a crucial role in the regulation of neural activity and is implicated in addiction. Animal model studies have provided valuable insights into the involvement of the GABAergic system in addictive behaviors. Animal models have demonstrated that the GABAergic system exerts inhibitory control over the mesolimbic dopamine system, influencing reward processing and addiction-related behavior. Animal models have been employed to investigate how the GABAergic system modulates incentive salience and cue-induced craving, influencing drug-seeking behavior. Animal models have provided insights into how the GABAergic system regulates withdrawal symptoms and the development of dependence on drugs of abuse (Chaudhri et al., 2007). Animal models have been employed to investigate the role of the GABAergic system in modulating stress responses, which can influence vulnerability to addiction (Roberto et al., 2012). Animal models have been utilized to explore the efficacy of GABAergic medications in the treatment of addiction, including medications that modulate GABA receptor (Kalluri et al., 2003). These findings highlight the intricate involvement of the GABAergic system in addiction and its potential as a target for pharmacological interventions in the treatment of substance use disorders. Animal models have been crucial in uncovering these neurobiological insights.

Behavioral Paradigms: Behavioral paradigms in animal models of drug addiction are experimental setups designed to mimic and study different aspects of substance abuse, dependence, and related behaviors. These paradigms help researchers understand the neurobiological and behavioral mechanisms underlying drug-seeking and drug-taking behaviors. These behavioral paradigms provide researchers with tools to investigate different aspects of drug addiction, from initial drug reinforcement to relapse and withdrawal. By using these paradigms, scientists can gain valuable insights into the neurobiology of addiction and identify potential targets for therapeutic interventions.

a. Operant conditioning: Operant conditioning is a key concept in the study of animal models of addiction, providing a framework for understanding how behavior is influenced by its consequences. In the context of addiction research, operant conditioning paradigms are widely used to investigate the development and maintenance of drug-seeking and drug-taking behaviors. Animals are trained to perform a specific response (e.g., pressing a lever) to receive a drug infusion. The delivery of the drug serves as a positive reinforcement, and animals learn to self-administer the drug. The main objective is to study the reinforcing properties of drugs, the motivation for drug intake, and the development of drug-seeking behavior.

Fixed-Ratio (FR) Schedules: Reinforcement is provided after a specific number of responses (e.g., every 10 lever presses). Different FR schedules (e.g., FR-1, FR-5) can be used to examine the effort required for obtaining a drug reward. It serves the purpose of investigating the response rates, the intensity of drug-seeking behavior, and the impact of effort on drug intake.

Variable-Ratio (VR) Schedules: Reinforcement is provided after an average number of responses, and the ratio requirement varies unpredictably. This schedule mimics intermittent drug availability to model patterns of drug intake that are variable and unpredictable, similar to real-world drug use.

Extinction and Reinstatement Models: After animals are trained to self-administer drugs, the drug-reinforced behavior is extinguished by withholding the drug. Reinstatement is then triggered by various factors (e.g., drug priming, stress) to assess relapse-like behavior. It is helpful in studying the persistence of drug-seeking behavior and factors contributing to relapse.

Cue-Induced Reinstatement Models: Animals are exposed to cues associated with drug administration after extinction, leading to the reinstatement of drug-seeking behavior. It studies the role of environmental cues in relapse and to understand the neural mechanisms underlying cue-induced drug-seeking behavior.

Progressive Ratio (PR) Schedules: The response requirement increases progressively following each reinforcement. This schedule assesses the maximum effort an animal is willing to exert for a drug reward to measure the motivation for drug intake and the breaking point at which the animal discontinues responding.

Fixed-Interval (FI) Schedules: Reinforcement is provided for the first response after a fixed time interval has elapsed (e.g., every 5 minutes). This schedule can be used to study temporal patterns of drug-seeking behavior to investigate the timing of drug-seeking behavior and the anticipation of drug availability.

These operant conditioning paradigms allow researchers to systematically investigate various aspects of drug-related behaviors, including the reinforcing effects of drugs, the impact of schedules of reinforcement, and the factors contributing to relapse. They provide valuable insights into the behavioral and neurobiological mechanisms underlying addiction.

b. Pavlovian conditioning: Pavlovian conditioning plays a significant role in drug addiction by establishing associations between environmental cues and the rewarding effects of drugs. This form of associative learning contributes to the development, maintenance, and relapse of addictive behaviors. Here are key aspects of Pavlovian conditioning in the context of drug addiction:

Cue-Drug Associations: Pavlovian conditioning involves pairing neutral stimuli (cues) with the administration of drugs. Over time, these cues become associated with the rewarding effects of drugs. The cues can elicit conditioned responses, such as craving and physiological changes, even in the absence of the drug.

Conditioned Place Preference (CPP): In CPP, animals learn to associate specific environments with drug administration. The environment itself becomes a conditioned stimulus that elicits a preference due to its association with the rewarding effects of drugs. CPP reflects the learned preference for contexts associated with drug reward and provides a model for studying environmental influences on drug-seeking behavior.

Cue-Induced Craving: Pavlovian cues associated with drug use can trigger craving, an intense desire for the drug. This craving is a conditioned response to the cues predicting drug availability. Cue-induced craving is a major factor in relapse, as exposure to drug-associated cues can lead individuals to seek and use drugs even after a period of abstinence.

Extinction and Reinstatement: After Pavlovian conditioning, if drug-associated cues are presented without the drug, extinction occurs. However, the presentation of these cues later can reinstate drug-seeking behavior. Reinstatement models mimic relapse situations, where exposure to drug-related cues can lead to the resurgence of drug-seeking behavior.

Pavlovian-to-Instrumental Transfer (PIT): Pavlovian cues can influence instrumental behaviors (e.g., lever-pressing for drugs) through PIT. The presentation of Pavlovian cues enhances drug-seeking behaviors. PIT reflects the impact of learned associations on goal-directed behaviors and helps understand how environmental cues influence instrumental drug-seeking actions.

Cue-Induced Reinstatement Models: Animals trained to self-administer drugs undergo extinction, and the presentation of drug-associated cues can reinstate drug-seeking behavior. This model mimics situations in which exposure to environmental cues triggers a relapse to drug-seeking and drug-taking behaviors.

Stress and Pavlovian Conditioning: Interaction: Stressful situations can interact with Pavlovian conditioning, exacerbating the impact of drug-associated cues on craving and relapse. Stress-induced relapse often involves the activation of Pavlovian conditioning processes in response to stressors.

Understanding the role of Pavlovian conditioning in drug addiction provides insights into the complex interplay between environmental cues, learned associations, and the motivational aspects of drug-seeking and drug-taking behaviors. This knowledge is crucial for developing effective therapeutic interventions aimed at preventing relapse and promoting long-term recovery.

c. Cue-induced reinstatement: Animals exhibit drug-seeking behavior in response to cues associated with drug use, modeling relapse triggers. Cue-induced reinstatement is a behavioral paradigm commonly used in preclinical models of drug addiction to study the relapse-like behavior triggered by exposure to drug-associated cues or contexts. This paradigm helps researchers understand how environmental cues, which have been previously paired with drug use, can reinstate drug-seeking behavior after a period of abstinence or extinction.

Experimental Setup involves training phase in which animals are initially trained to self-administer drugs in the presence of specific cues or within certain environmental contexts and extinction phase in which drug administration is discontinued, and animals undergo extinction training, during which responding for the drug-associated cues is no longer reinforced. The extinction phase aims to reduce the association between drug-associated cues and the rewarding effects of the drug. After extinction, animals are exposed to the drug-associated cues (e.g., visual, auditory, or olfactory stimuli) without receiving the drug. Reinstatement refers to the subsequent increase in drug-seeking behavior triggered by the presentation of these cues. Cue-induced reinstatement models are considered a preclinical representation of relapse in individuals with a history of drug addiction. Environmental cues play a significant role in relapse, and this model specifically addresses the impact of drug-associated cues. Cue-induced reinstatement involves neural circuits in the brain, including areas associated with reward, learning, and memory. Dopamine, glutamate, and other neurotransmitter systems are implicated in mediating the effects of cue-induced reinstatement. Cue-induced reinstatement models aim to capture aspects of cue-induced relapse observed in individuals recovering from addiction. Understanding the mechanisms underlying cue-induced reinstatement can inform the development of therapeutic interventions to prevent or mitigate relapse.

Animals may differ in their sensitivity to drug-associated cues, mirroring the variability in cue reactivity observed among individuals with substance use disorders. Factors influencing reinstatement include stress, mood, and other factors which can modulate the impact of cues on reinstatement. Researchers can use cue-induced reinstatement models to test the efficacy of pharmacological or behavioral interventions in preventing cue-triggered relapse. The model aids in identifying potential therapeutic targets for preventing relapse in human addiction. Cue-induced reinstatement is a valuable tool for investigating the neural and behavioral mechanisms involved in cue-triggered relapse, providing insights into the vulnerability of individuals in recovery from drug addiction and informing the development of relapse prevention strategies.

Neuroadaptations and Plasticity: Animal models facilitate investigating the neural plasticity underlying addiction, including changes in synaptic strength and connectivity. Studies in animals reveal alterations in brain structures, such as the prefrontal cortex and amygdala, associated with addiction. The study of neuroadaptations and plasticity in animal models of addiction involves investigating changes in the structure and function of neural circuits in response to chronic drug exposure. These adaptations are crucial for understanding the long-term effects of drugs on the brain and how they contribute to addictive behaviors. Brain samples isolated from these animal models could be examined for monitoring adaptive changes.

Electrophysiology: In vivo and in vitro electrophysiological recordings measure the electrical activity of neurons in specific brain regions. It could be utilized to assess changes in synaptic strength, long-term potentiation (LTP), and long-term depression (LTD) in circuits associated with addiction.

Neurochemistry: Neurotransmitter assays, microdialysis, and immunohistochemistry quantify changes in neurotransmitter levels and receptor expression and to examine alterations in dopamine, serotonin, glutamate, and other neurotransmitter systems associated with addiction.

Neuroimaging: Functional magnetic resonance imaging (fMRI), positron emission tomography (PET), and other imaging modalities visualize brain activity and structure. Mapping changes in brain regions could be explored and connectivity associated with addiction, providing a non-invasive perspective could be studied.

Molecular Biology: Polymerase chain reaction (PCR), Western blotting, and gene expression analysis reveal changes at the molecular level. Alterations in gene expression, transcription factors, and signaling pathways involved in addiction-related plasticity could be studied in detail.

Optogenetics: Using light to control genetically modified neurons expressing light-sensitive proteins, specific neural circuits could be manipulated to elucidate their role in addiction-related behaviors and plasticity.

Chemogenetics: Modifying neurons to respond to synthetic ligands for selectively activating or inhibiting specific neural circuits to study their involvement in addiction-related plasticity.

Behavioral Models: Leveraging various addiction-related behavioral paradigms, such as self-administration and conditioned place preference, linking observed behavioral changes to underlying neuroadaptations and plasticity.

Synaptic Plasticity Models: Studying changes in synaptic strength using electrophysiological approaches to investigate how chronic drug exposure alters synaptic plasticity in reward-related brain regions.

Longitudinal Studies: Following animals over extended periods after drug exposure for assessing the persistence and time course of neuroadaptations and plasticity associated with addiction.

Environmental Enrichment and Rehabilitative Interventions: Providing enriched environments or rehabilitative interventions for studying how positive environmental factors influence neuroplasticity and recovery from addiction-related changes.

By employing these techniques and approaches, researchers can gain insights into the molecular, cellular, and circuit-level changes that occur in the brain as a result of chronic drug exposure. Understanding these neuroadaptations is crucial for developing targeted interventions and treatments for addiction.

Pharmacological Intervention: Animal models contribute to the development and testing of medications targeting specific neurotransmitter systems or neural circuits involved in addiction.

Using animal models for drug development is a common and longstanding practice in the pharmaceutical and biomedical research fields. Animal models play a crucial role in the early stages of drug discovery and development, serving several important purposes. Animals, especially mammals, share many biological similarities with humans. Studying the effects of drugs in animals can provide valuable insights into how these drugs might behave in the human body. However, it's important to note that differences between species exist, and not all findings in animals can be directly extrapolated to humans. Animal models are used to assess the safety of potential drug candidates. This includes identifying potential toxic effects, understanding the drug's metabolism, and evaluating its potential impact on various organs and systems within the body (Kuhn et al., 2019). Researchers use animal models to determine whether a drug candidate has the desired therapeutic effects. This involves studying the drug's effectiveness in treating a specific disease or condition.

Animal studies help researchers understand how drugs are absorbed, distributed, metabolized, and excreted in the body (pharmacokinetics) and how they exert their effects (pharmacodynamics). This information is crucial for determining the appropriate dosage and administration of a drug in humans. Animal models are often used to replicate human diseases, allowing researchers to study the underlying mechanisms and test potential treatments. This is particularly important for conditions that cannot be easily studied in humans or for which human samples are limited. Regulatory agencies, such as the U.S. Food and Drug Administration (FDA) and the European Medicines Agency (EMA), typically require data from animal studies as part of the regulatory approval process for new drugs. While animal models are valuable tools in drug development, they also have limitations. Differences in biology between species and the inability to fully replicate human complexity can lead to disparities in drug responses (Teal et al., 2023). As a result, there is ongoing research into alternative methods, such as in vitro (cell-based) and computational models, to complement and, in some cases, replace the use of animals in drug development. These alternative approaches aim to enhance the predictive accuracy of preclinical testing and reduce reliance on animal models.

Challenges and Considerations: Using animal models for drug development is a common and longstanding practice in the pharmaceutical and biomedical research fields. Animal models play a crucial role in the early stages of drug discovery and development, serving several important purposes. Animals, especially mammals, share many biological similarities with humans. Studying the effects of drugs in animals can provide valuable insights into how these drugs might behave in the human body. However, it's important to note that differences between species exist, and not all findings in animals can be directly extrapolated to humans. Animal models are used to assess the safety of potential drug candidates. This includes identifying potential toxic effects, understanding the drug's metabolism, and evaluating its potential impact on various organs and systems within the body.

Researchers use animal models to determine whether a drug candidate has the desired therapeutic effects. This involves studying the drug's effectiveness in treating a specific disease or condition. Pharmacokinetics and Pharmacodynamics: Animal studies help researchers understand how drugs are absorbed, distributed, metabolized, and excreted in the body (pharmacokinetics) and how they exert their effects (pharmacodynamics). This information is crucial for determining the appropriate dosage and administration of a drug in humans. Animal models are often used to replicate human diseases, allowing researchers to study the underlying mechanisms and test potential treatments. This is particularly important for conditions that cannot be easily studied in humans or for which human samples are limited.

Regulatory agencies, such as the U.S. Food and Drug Administration (FDA) and the European Medicines Agency (EMA), typically require data from animal studies as part of the regulatory approval process for new drugs. While animal models are valuable tools in drug development, they also have limitations. Differences in biology between species and the inability to fully replicate human complexity can lead to disparities in drug responses. As a result, there is ongoing research into alternative methods, such as in vitro (cell-based) and computational models, to complement and, in some cases, replace the use of animals in drug development. These alternative approaches aim to enhance the predictive accuracy of preclinical testing and reduce reliance on animal models.

Ethical Considerations: The use of animal models in drug development raises various ethical considerations that researchers and institutions must carefully address. Balancing the potential benefits of advancing medical knowledge and developing new treatments with the welfare of animals is a complex and ongoing challenge. Ensuring the well-being of animals involved in research is a primary ethical concern. Researchers must provide appropriate housing, nutrition, veterinary care, and environmental enrichment to minimize stress and promote the overall welfare of animals. Ethical guidelines emphasize the importance of minimizing any pain, distress, or suffering experienced by animals during experiments. This involves using anesthesia, analgesia, and humane endpoints to reduce or eliminate discomfort.

The 3Rs framework—Replacement (finding alternatives to animal use), Reduction (minimizing the number of animals used), and Refinement (enhancing animal welfare and experimental techniques)—guides researchers in ethical animal experimentation. Researchers must provide a strong scientific justification for using animals in their studies. This includes demonstrating that the research question cannot be adequately addressed through alternative methods and that the potential benefits justify the use of animals. Ethical practices require transparency in reporting methodologies, procedures, and outcomes of animal studies. This helps the scientific community and the public assess the ethical rigor of the research. Most research institutions have an IACUC that reviews and approves animal research protocols. The committee assesses the ethical and scientific aspects of proposed studies, ensuring compliance with relevant regulations and guidelines. Researchers are encouraged to explore and use alternative methods that do not involve animals whenever possible. In vitro models, computational modeling, and other non-animal techniques are continually being developed to reduce reliance on animal experimentation.

Ethical decisions involve choosing the most appropriate species for a particular study and using the minimum number of animals necessary to obtain valid results. Selecting species that closely mimic human biology can enhance the relevance of the research. Ethical considerations should not end with protocol approval. Regular and ongoing ethical review ensures that researchers adhere to ethical standards throughout the duration of the study. Researchers and laboratory staff involved in animal research should receive proper education and training in ethical considerations, animal care, and experimental techniques. Engaging with the public and communicating the ethical framework of animal research is essential for maintaining public trust. Transparency in communication about the ethical considerations and benefits of animal research can help address concerns and misconceptions. Efforts are ongoing to refine and improve ethical standards in animal research, and researchers are encouraged to stay informed about the latest guidelines and best practices. Additionally, advancements in technology and alternative methods continue to offer opportunities to reduce and replace the use of animals in research while maintaining scientific rigor.

Future Directions: The future directions for using animal models in drug development involve addressing current limitations, incorporating technological advancements, and exploring alternative approaches. Researchers aim to improve the predictive validity of animal models by identifying and addressing species-specific differences in drug responses. This involves refining existing models and developing new ones that better mimic human physiology and disease. Advancements in technology, such as high-throughput screening, organoids, and microphysiological systems (organ-on-a-chip), offer opportunities to enhance the efficiency and accuracy of preclinical drug testing. These technologies provide more relevant in vitro models and reduce reliance on animal studies. The development of animal models that incorporate individualized or precision medicine aspects, considering genetic and environmental factors, can improve the understanding of variable drug responses among individuals. Humanized animal models, where specific human genes or tissues are introduced into animals, aim to better replicate human physiology and disease. These models can be particularly useful for studying diseases with a strong genetic component. Integrating big data and systems biology approaches allows researchers to analyze complex interactions within biological systems comprehensively. This can provide a more holistic understanding of drug effects and identify potential biomarkers.

Given the challenges in developing treatments for neurological and psychiatric disorders, there is a continued emphasis on refining animal models for conditions such as Alzheimer's disease, depression, and schizophrenia. This involves incorporating more relevant behavioral and cognitive endpoints. Ongoing efforts to refine and reduce the use of animals in research include the development and validation of alternative methods, such as in vitro models, computational modeling, and human-based assays. Researchers are working to enhance the translatability of findings from animal studies to human clinical outcomes. This involves a better understanding of the biological and physiological similarities and differences between species. Increased collaboration and data sharing among researchers and institutions can accelerate progress in drug development.

Peclinical data allows for a more comprehensive evaluation of potential drug candidates. The use of patient-derived cells, tissues, or organoids can provide more personalized and clinically relevant models for drug testing. This approach considers the heterogeneity of diseases and individual patient responses. Longitudinal studies in animal models can provide valuable insights into the chronic effects of drugs, including potential side effects and the development of tolerance or dependence. Continued collaboration between researchers, industry, and regulatory agencies is essential to establish and refine guidelines for the ethical use of animal models in drug development. Clear regulatory standards can facilitate the development and approval of novel treatments. As technology and scientific understanding advance, the future of using animal models in drug development will likely involve a combination of traditional approaches, innovative technologies, and a commitment to ethical and transparent research practices. Researchers are continually exploring ways to enhance the relevance, efficiency, and human predictability of preclinical studies while minimizing the use of animals when possible.

To complement these advancements, emerging technologies like artificial intelligence and machine learning are being leveraged to analyze complex datasets from both animal models and human studies, identifying predictive biomarkers that bridge the translational gap. The integration of multi-omics approaches—including genomics, proteomics, and metabolomics—into preclinical research allows for a more comprehensive understanding of disease mechanisms and drug responses across species. Advanced imaging techniques, such as high-resolution PET and fMRI, now enable researchers to track neurobiological changes in real-time, improving the correlation between animal model findings and human pathophysiology. Humanized mouse models, incorporating patient-derived xenografts or genetic modifications, are providing unprecedented opportunities to study disease progression and treatment responses in more clinically relevant systems. Concurrently, microfluidic organ-on-a-chip platforms are being refined to replicate complex human organ systems, offering ethical alternatives for preliminary drug screening while reducing reliance on animal testing. The development of sophisticated computational models that simulate disease progression and drug interactions is further enhancing the predictive value of preclinical research, allowing for more targeted and efficient animal studies when necessary.

International consortia are now establishing standardized protocols for animal research to improve reproducibility and data comparability across laboratories worldwide. Investment in open-source platforms for sharing both positive and negative preclinical results is helping to minimize redundant animal studies while accelerating therapeutic discovery. Ethical considerations remain paramount, with the implementation of the "3Rs" principle (Replacement, Reduction, Refinement) being continuously updated to reflect technological advancements and evolving societal values. These collective efforts are driving a paradigm shift toward more human-relevant, efficient, and ethically responsible approaches in neuroscience drug development. The ultimate goal remains to develop effective treatments for neurological and psychiatric disorders while progressively minimizing animal use through innovation and interdisciplinary collaboration. As these strategies converge, they promise to transform the landscape of preclinical research, making it more predictive, personalized, and aligned with both scientific rigor and ethical imperatives.

CHAPTER 10

PHARMACOTHERAPEUTIC APPROACHES TO TREAT DRUG ADDICTION

"Rising from the ashes, I am born again, powerful, exultant, majestic through all the pain."
~ Shannon Perry

The imagery of being "born again" signifies a profound and positive change, highlighting the individual's journey towards recovery and self-discovery. Despite enduring pain and hardship, there is a sense of newfound strength, celebration, and a majestic quality in the process of overcoming addiction. This chapter suggests that navigating the complex landscape of drug addiction requires a thorough exploration of pharmacotherapeutic approaches, where medications play a pivotal role in addressing the multifaceted challenges associated with substance use disorders. The realm of treating drug addiction unfolds through the lens of pharmacotherapy, unveiling diverse strategies and medications that aim to mitigate the physiological, psychological, and behavioral aspects inherent in the spectrum of addictive behaviors.

Treating drug addiction poses several challenges, reflecting the complex nature of substance use disorders and the diverse factors influencing addiction. Stigmatization of individuals with substance use disorders can hinder their willingness to seek help and contribute to a lack of understanding among healthcare providers and the general public. Stigma may result in delayed or inadequate treatment, perpetuating the cycle of addiction. There is often a shortage of treatment facilities, particularly in certain geographic areas, leading to long waiting lists and limited access to evidence-based interventions. Delayed treatment can exacerbate the severity of addiction, increase the risk of overdose, and impede recovery efforts. Many individuals with substance use disorders also have co-occurring mental health conditions such as depression, anxiety, or trauma. Treating both addiction and co-occurring disorders concurrently is complex but crucial for successful outcomes. Failure to address underlying mental health issues may contribute to relapse.

Addiction is often a chronic, relapsing condition with periods of remission and recurrence. Achieving sustained recovery is challenging, and relapses can occur even after successful treatment. A long-term and comprehensive approach is needed to manage the chronic nature of addiction. Individuals may use multiple substances simultaneously, complicating the treatment approach. Treating polydrug use requires a comprehensive understanding of the interactions between different substances and their effects on the individual's health and recovery. Some individuals may lack the motivation to engage in or adhere to treatment, particularly in the early stages. Motivational barriers can hinder the effectiveness of interventions. Building and sustaining motivation for treatment are ongoing challenges. While pharmacotherapy plays a crucial role in addiction treatment, not all substances have approved medications, and individual responses vary. Limited pharmacotherapy options may limit the effectiveness of medical interventions, leaving some individuals without targeted treatment options.

High rates of treatment dropout, whether due to personal reasons, lack of perceived effectiveness, or external factors, can impede treatment success. Incomplete treatment may result in suboptimal outcomes, and individuals may not fully benefit from the available interventions. Socioeconomic factors, such as poverty, lack of education, and unemployment, can pose barriers to accessing and completing treatment. Individuals facing these challenges may struggle to engage in treatment, and addressing underlying socioeconomic issues is often essential for successful recovery. The integration of behavioral therapies with medical treatments is not always seamless, and some treatment settings may lack a comprehensive, multidisciplinary approach. A holistic approach that combines behavioral, medical, and psychosocial interventions is essential for addressing the various dimensions of addiction. Addressing these challenges requires a multifaceted and collaborative approach involving healthcare professionals, policymakers, communities, and individuals affected by addiction. Continued research, increased access to evidence-based treatments, and destigmatization efforts are crucial components of a comprehensive strategy to improve drug addiction treatment outcomes.

Goals of Pharmacotherapy in Drug Addiction: Pharmacotherapy, the use of medications to treat drug addiction, is guided by several key goals aimed at addressing various aspects of the addiction cycle. Reduction of craving is targeted to minimize or eliminate the intense desire or urge to use drugs. Craving is a common trigger for relapse. Medications that target cravings help individuals resist the temptation to use substances. Prevention of relapse reduces the likelihood of a return to drug use after a period of abstinence. Relapse is a common challenge in addiction recovery. Pharmacotherapies aim to stabilize individuals, making sustained recovery more achievable. Alleviation of withdrawal symptoms to manage and alleviate the physical and psychological symptoms associated with drug withdrawal is pivotal. Withdrawal symptoms can be severe and contribute to relapse. Medications help individuals cope with the discomfort, facilitating the early stages of recovery.

Restoration of neurological functions and addressing neurobiological changes induced by chronic drug use and restore normal brain function. Prolonged drug use can alter neural circuits, affecting decision-making, impulse control, and stress response. Pharmacotherapies target these neural changes to support recovery. Maintenance of treatment engagement to encourage individuals to remain engaged in treatment over the long term must be accomplished. Long-term engagement is critical for sustained recovery. Medications that help manage cravings and prevent relapse contribute to treatment retention. Reduction of drug-related harm is required to minimize the negative health and social consequences associated with drug use. Beyond abstinence, reducing harm associated with drug use is an important goal, especially in cases where complete cessation may be challenging. Improvement of Psychosocial Functioning is needed to enhance an individual's overall well-being, including mental health, social functioning, and quality of life. Addiction often leads to disruptions in various aspects of life. Medications, in conjunction with behavioral therapies, contribute to comprehensive recovery.

Reduction of criminogenic behaviors is required to address behaviors related to criminal activities associated with drug use. Substance use disorders are often linked to criminal behavior. Effective pharmacotherapy can contribute to a reduction in drug-related criminal activities. Individualized Treatment strategies are needed to tailor pharmacotherapy to the individual's specific needs, considering factors such as co-occurring disorders, medical history, and treatment preferences. Individualized treatment approaches acknowledge the heterogeneity of addiction and the varying needs of different individuals. Promotion of abstinence to facilitate and support complete abstinence from illicit substances. Achieving and maintaining abstinence is a primary goal of addiction treatment, and medications play a crucial role in supporting individuals in this effort. These goals are often pursued in conjunction with behavioral therapies, counseling, and psychosocial interventions as part of a comprehensive treatment approach. The integration of pharmacotherapy with other evidence-based treatments enhances the effectiveness of addiction treatment programs, offering individuals a more comprehensive and tailored recovery experience.

a. Reduction of Craving: Craving, defined as an intense desire or urge to use drugs, plays a crucial role in the dynamics of drug addiction. Understanding the significance of craving is essential for comprehending the challenges individuals face during addiction and the development of effective treatment strategies. It is a multifaceted and dynamic aspect of drug addiction with profound implications for the initiation, maintenance, and recovery from substance use disorders. Recognizing the significance of craving informs the development of comprehensive and personalized treatment approaches aimed at addressing this critical aspect of addiction.

Pharmacotherapeutic approaches for opioid use disorder include methadone; a long-acting opioid agonist that helps stabilize individuals and reduce opioid cravings and buprenorphine; a partial opioid agonist that can alleviate cravings and withdrawal symptoms and naltrexone; opioid receptors blocker, reducing the reinforcing effects of opioids and cravings. For alcohol use disorder treatment options include drugs like acamprosate; modulates neurotransmitter systems, reducing alcohol cravings and promoting abstinence, naltrexone; reduces alcohol cravings by blocking opioid receptors and disulfiram; creates aversive reactions to alcohol consumption, discouraging use. Nicotine Replacement Therapies (NRT) deliver controlled amounts of nicotine to reduce withdrawal and cravings. Varenicline also Partially stimulates nicotine receptors, reducing withdrawal symptoms and cravings. Bupropion also alleviates nicotine cravings and withdrawal symptoms (Fiore et al., 2008; Anthenelli et al., 2016; Cahill et al., 2014).

Cocaine induced cravings could be attenuated by disulfiram which inhibits cocaine metabolism, leading to aversive effects and reduced cravings or by topiramate which modulates neurotransmitter systems, reducing cravings for cocaine (Pettinati et al., 2008; Johnson et al., 2007). For cannabis use disorder, cannabidiol; modulates the endocannabinoid system, potentially reducing cannabis cravings and sativex (nabiximols); showing potential for reducing cannabis use, are the treatment options (Freeman et al., 2019). Apart from therapeutic approaches, Cognitive-Behavioral Therapy (CBT) also addresses distorted thought patterns and helps individuals develop coping strategies to manage cravings. Techniques like mindfulness meditation can enhance awareness and reduce impulsive responses to cravings. Contingency management also provides tangible rewards for drug-free behaviors, reinforcing abstinence and reducing cravings (Drummond et al., 2000; Brewer et al., 2009; Petry, 2000).

Integrated approaches such as pharmacotherapy and behavioral interventions include combining medications and therapy by integrating pharmacotherapy with behavioral interventions often yields more significant reductions in cravings and enhances overall treatment outcomes. Synergistic effects address both the neurobiological and psychological aspects of craving concurrently can lead to synergistic effects in craving reduction. Lifestyle modifications and holistic approaches include physical activity such as regular exercise has been shown to positively impact mood and reduce cravings through various neurobiological mechanisms. Nutritional support via a balanced diet can contribute to overall well-being and may influence neurotransmitter systems related to cravings.

Stress reduction strategies, such as yoga or meditation, can mitigate triggers for cravings. Recognizing the individual variability in treatment response and addressing unique needs is crucial for effective craving reduction. Providing ongoing support and adjusting treatment plans based on the individual's progress and changing needs. The reduction of drug craving requires a comprehensive, individualized approach that addresses both the biological and psychological aspects of addiction ongoing research and the development of innovative interventions are essential for improving the efficacy of craving reduction strategies.

b. Reduction of Relapse: Relapse is a common challenge in the treatment of substance use disorders. Implementing effective strategies to reduce drug relapse involves a comprehensive approach that addresses biological, psychological, and social factors. Effective treatment for drug relapse involves a comprehensive, individualized approach that addresses various aspects of addiction. A comprehensive assessment is required for thorough evaluation of the individual's substance use history, including patterns, triggers, and co-occurring mental health issues. Assessment of the severity of addiction and the specific substances involved is also important. Any acute health issues or overdose symptoms should be addressed promptly, and medical intervention and stabilization should be provided as per need.

Medications should be considered based on the substance of abuse and must be tailored to the individual's needs and preferences. Dosage should also be adjusted accordingly, optimizing effectiveness. Behavioral interventions should be adapted, such as engaging individuals in evidence-based therapies such as Cognitive-Behavioral Therapy (CBT), contingency management, and Motivational Enhancement Therapy (MET). Focus should be on identifying and addressing maladaptive thought patterns and behaviors and effective relapse prevention strategies should be developed. Individualized treatment plans include development of personalized treatment plans that consider the unique needs, preferences, and circumstances of the individual. This treatment plan should be continuously reassessed and adjusted as per necessity. Addressing co-occurring mental health disorders through integrated treatment approaches to prevent relapse. Collaboration with mental health professionals is a must to ensure holistic care. Peer Support and counseling is equally important to encourage participation in support groups like Alcoholics Anonymous (AA) or Narcotics Anonymous (NA).

Family involvement is very important to prevent drug relapse in future. Family members must be involved in the treatment process and educated about addiction, relapse triggers, and coping strategies. Cognitive restructuring and coping skills assist individuals in recognizing and challenging negative thought patterns. Adaptive coping skills must be taught to manage stress, cravings, and emotional triggers. Continuous monitoring of progress and subsequent adjustment of treatment plans is necessary to monitor for signs of relapse, including changes in behavior or attendance. A comprehensive aftercare plan that includes ongoing outpatient treatment, counseling, and support group participation must be there. Transitional housing or sober living arrangements should also be considered, if necessary.

Technology-based interventions, such as mobile apps or teletherapy, to enhance support and provide tools for relapse prevention. Adoption of a healthy lifestyle, including regular exercise, proper nutrition, and sufficient sleep is required to promote overall well-being to enhance resilience against relapse. Positive support network to assist individuals in building and maintaining positive social connections is necessary to foster relationships with individuals who support recovery goals. Crisis intervention planning is necessary to develop a crisis intervention plan to address emergencies or intense cravings. It's essential to tailor interventions to everyone's unique circumstances and continually reassess and adjust the treatment plan based on their progress and needs.

c. Alleviation of drug Withdrawal: Alleviating drug withdrawal symptoms is a crucial aspect of the early stages of addiction treatment. It's important to note that treatment approaches may vary based on the specific substance of abuse, individual needs, and medical considerations. Management of withdrawal symptoms post opioid use disorder (OUD) could be done by FDA-approved medications methadone, buprenorphine, and naltrexone (Mattick et al., 2009). Benzodiazepines are used for the management of alcohol withdrawal symptoms (Mayo-Smith et al., 2004). Certain anticonvulsant medications, such as gabapentin or carbamazepine, may be used to manage withdrawal symptoms for substances like benzodiazepines (Soyka, 2017). Nicotine replacement therapy options include patches, gum, lozenges, nasal spray, or inhalers (Stead et al., 2012). Cognitive-Behavioral

Therapy (CBT) and contingency management are effective in addressing withdrawal and reducing the risk of relapse.

Counseling and motivational enhancement strategies can assist individuals in managing withdrawal symptoms associated with cannabis use. Non-addictive medications may be used to address specific withdrawal symptoms, such as nonsteroidal anti-inflammatory drugs (NSAIDs) for pain or antiemetics for nausea. Adequate nutrition and hydration support the body during withdrawal and promote overall well-being (Budney et al., 2003; Mars et al., 2014). Supervised medical detoxification in either inpatient or outpatient settings may be recommended based on the severity of withdrawal symptoms. Psychosocial support, including individual and group counseling, helps individuals cope with the emotional aspects of withdrawal. These interventions should be implemented within the context of a comprehensive treatment plan tailored to the individual's specific needs and circumstances. It's crucial to consult with healthcare professionals to determine the most appropriate and effective strategies for managing withdrawal symptoms based on the substance of abuse and the individual's overall health.

d. Restoration of Neurological Function: The restoration of neurological function after drug addiction is a complex process that involves various neuroadaptive changes in the brain. Recovery often depends on factors such as the type of substance used, duration of use, individual differences, and the presence of co-occurring conditions. While the brain has a remarkable capacity for recovery, some changes may persist. Neuroplasticity and structural changes in the brain play a crucial role in the process of recovery after drug addiction. Neuroplasticity refers to the brain's ability to reorganize itself by forming new neural connections throughout life. Structural changes involve alterations in the anatomy and architecture of the brain. Chronic drug use can lead to alterations in synaptic plasticity, affecting communication between neurons. During recovery, the brain undergoes synaptic rewiring to restore normal communication patterns. Drugs of abuse can impact dendritic spine density, affecting the connections between neurons. In recovery, there is evidence of restoration in dendritic spine density. Chronic drug use may suppress neurogenesis in the hippocampus, a region important for learning and memory. Abstinence from drugs has been associated with the restoration of hippocampal neurogenesis. Prolonged drug use can lead to changes in gray matter volume. Studies suggest partial recovery of gray matter volume during abstinence. Drug addiction can affect white matter integrity, disrupting communication between different brain regions. Abstinence may contribute to the restoration of white matter integrity. Chronic drug use may influence cortical thickness. Studies have shown evidence of cortical thickness changes during abstinence and recovery (Momenan et al., 2012).

The prefrontal cortex, involved in decision-making and impulse control, can undergo structural changes during addiction and recovery. Neuronal hypertrophy and atrophy are observed in different brain regions during addiction and recovery, reflecting dynamic changes in neural structure. Chronic drug use can lead to microglial activation and neuroinflammation. Restoration involves the resolution of neuroinflammatory processes. Epigenetic changes, including alterations in DNA methylation and histone acetylation, contribute to long-term structural modifications during addiction and recovery (Robison & Nestler, 2011; Nock et al., 2017). Understanding the restoration of neuroplasticity and structural changes after drug addiction provides valuable insights into the potential for recovery and the development of targeted interventions for individuals seeking to overcome addiction. Research in this field is ongoing, and a comprehensive approach to treatment may involve a combination of behavioral therapies, pharmacological interventions, and support services.

Dopaminergic system recovery plays a crucial role in reward, motivation, and reinforcement learning, and it is often affected by drug use. Chronic drug use can lead to dysregulation of dopamine receptors, affecting the balance of dopamine transmission. After drug withdrawal, there is evidence of receptor regulation as the brain attempts to restore normal functioning. Prolonged drug use, such as in the case of stimulants, can reduce dopamine transporter density. During withdrawal, there may be an increase in transporter availability as part of the recovery process. Chronic drug use can alter dopamine release and synthesis. After withdrawal, there may be attempts to restore normal dopamine release patterns. Dopamine D2/D3 receptor availability is often reduced in individuals with substance use disorders. During abstinence, there may be a gradual increase in receptor availability. The prefrontal cortex and striatum are integral to the dopaminergic reward system. After drug withdrawal, there may be efforts to restore prefrontal-striatal function (Nutt et al., 2015).

Drug withdrawal can impact both the mesolimbic (reward) and mesocortical (cognitive) pathways. Recovery involves a process of restoring balance in these pathways. Neurotrophic factors, such as brain-derived neurotrophic factor (BDNF), play a role in neuronal survival and function. The dopaminergic system may rely on neurotrophic support during recovery. Drug-associated cues can trigger dopamine release, contributing to cravings. Over time, cue-induced dopamine release may normalize during abstinence. Executive functions, including decision-making and impulse control, are modulated by dopamine. Recovery may involve the restoration of these cognitive processes. Glutamate, the primary excitatory neurotransmitter, modulates dopamine release. Changes in glutamatergic signaling may contribute to dopaminergic system recovery (Kalivas & Volkow, 2011).

Glutamatergic system restoration is an important aspect of neurological functions restoration. The glutamatergic system, which involves the neurotransmitter glutamate, plays a crucial role in various brain functions, including learning, memory, and synaptic plasticity. Drug use, especially substances of abuse, can have profound effects on the glutamatergic system. Chronic drug use, such as with substances like alcohol and opioids, can lead to alterations in N-methyl-D-aspartate (NMDA) receptor function. During withdrawal, there may be efforts to restore normal NMDA receptor activity. Changes in α-amino-3-hydroxy-5-methyl-4-isoxazolepropionic acid (AMPA) receptor function are associated with drug addiction. Recovery involves restoring AMPA receptor activity to regulate synaptic transmission. mGluRs play a modulatory role in glutamatergic signaling. Modulation of mGluR activity during withdrawal may contribute to restoring balance in glutamatergic transmission. Glutamate transporters regulate the extracellular concentration of glutamate. During withdrawal, there may be changes in the expression of these transporters to maintain glutamate homeostasis (Knackstedt et a., 2010). Emerging research suggests targeting specific glutamate receptor subtypes could offer novel therapeutic avenues for addiction treatment. Pharmacological agents that normalize metabotropic glutamate receptor (mGluR5) activity show promise in reducing craving and relapse behaviors.

Long-Term Potentiation (LTP) and Long-Term Depression (LTD) are forms of synaptic plasticity crucial for learning and memory. Drug withdrawal may involve the restoration of normal LTP and LTD mechanisms. Neurotrophic factors, such as brain-derived neurotrophic factor (BDNF), are involved in synaptic plasticity. During withdrawal, there may be efforts to restore BDNF signaling for synaptic function. Astrocytes play a role in glutamate homeostasis. Drug withdrawal may involve astrocytic contributions to the restoration of glutamatergic balance. The immediate early gene Homer1a is involved in synaptic plasticity. During withdrawal, changes in Homer1a expression may contribute to synaptic adaptations. Chronic drug use can affect dendritic spine density. Recovery may involve efforts to normalize dendritic spine density for proper synaptic connectivity. Glutamate serves as the primary excitatory neurotransmitter in the brain. The restoration of glutamate-mediated neurotransmission is a critical aspect of recovery (Kalivas & Volkow, 2005). Understanding the intricacies of glutamatergic system restoration after drug withdrawal is essential for developing targeted interventions to support recovery. Research in this field continues to uncover novel therapeutic strategies to address glutamate dysregulation associated with addiction.

Neurotransmitter receptor regulation is a complex process involving changes in the density, sensitivity, and function of receptors in response to alterations in neurotransmitter levels. After drug withdrawal, the brain undergoes adaptive changes to restore balance and function in neurotransmitter systems (Hyman et al., 2006). Chronic drug use often leads to dysregulation of dopamine receptors, particularly dopamine D2/D3 receptors. During drug withdrawal, there may be an attempt to restore normal dopamine receptor density and sensitivity. Opioid receptors, including mu, delta, and kappa receptors, can undergo changes in response to chronic opioid use. After withdrawal, there may be adaptations in opioid receptor expression. Chronic drug use, particularly substances like alcohol and cocaine, can affect glutamate receptor subtypes, such as N-methyl-D-aspartate (NMDA) and α-amino-3-hydroxy-5-methyl-4-isoxazolepropionic acid (AMPA) receptors. After withdrawal, there may be efforts to restore normal glutamate receptor function. Gamma-aminobutyric acid (GABA) receptors, particularly GABAA receptors, are modulated by chronic drug use. After withdrawal, there may be adaptations in GABAergic neurotransmission. Chronic drug use can influence serotonin receptor subtypes, including 5-HT1A and 5-HT2A receptors. After withdrawal, there may be changes in serotonin receptor expression and function. Nicotinic acetylcholine receptors are affected by chronic nicotine exposure. After smoking cessation, there may be adaptations in nicotinic receptor density and function (Changeux & Taly, 2008).

Chronic cannabis use can impact cannabinoid receptors (CB1 and CB2). After withdrawal, there may be changes in endocannabinoid signaling and receptor regulation. Chronic use of substances like cocaine and methamphetamine can affect adrenergic receptors. After withdrawal, there may be adaptations in adrenergic receptor density and responsiveness. Histamine receptors can be influenced by chronic drug use. After withdrawal, there may be changes in histamine receptor expression and sensitivity. Endogenous opioids, including endorphins and enkephalins, act on opioid receptors. Chronic drug use may impact the endogenous opioid system, and during withdrawal, there may be adaptations in endorphin and enkephalin receptor regulation (Bodnar, 2016). Understanding the changes in neurotransmitter receptor regulation after drug withdrawal is essential for developing effective treatments for substance use disorders. It highlights the dynamic nature of the brain's response to chronic drug exposure and the potential for targeted interventions to support recovery.

Cognitive function recovery after drug withdrawal is a dynamic process that involves adaptive changes in the brain's structure and function. Chronic drug use, depending on the type of substance and duration of use, can impact various cognitive functions, including memory, attention, executive function, and decision-making (Crews & Boettiger, 2009). Chronic drug use, such as with substances like alcohol and benzodiazepines, can lead to memory deficits. Abstinence from drugs allows for the gradual recovery of memory function. Studies have shown improvements in both short-term and long-term memory following drug withdrawal. Stimulant drugs, like amphetamines and cocaine, can affect attention and concentration. With abstinence, attention and concentration often improve. However, the timeline for recovery can vary based on factors such as the type of drug and the duration of use. Executive functions, including decision-making and impulse control, are often affected by drug use. Abstinence allows for improvements in executive function. Cognitive-behavioral therapy and other interventions can further enhance recovery in these areas (Verdejo-García et al., 2006).

Long-term abstinence may be associated with more significant recovery. Verbal and non-verbal reasoning abilities can be affected by substance use. Cognitive recovery in reasoning skills is often observed during abstinence. Individual differences and the presence of co-occurring conditions may influence the extent of recovery. Decision-making skills are impaired during drug use and withdrawal from substance abuse can impact decision-making abilities. Abstinence and participation in treatment programs can lead to improvements in decision-making skills over time. Substance use can also affect emotional regulation as it involves reward circuit. Abstinence and therapeutic interventions support the recovery of emotional regulation. Cognitive-behavioral therapy may be particularly effective in addressing emotional aspects of recovery. Structural changes in the brain, including alterations in gray and white matter, are associated with chronic drug use. Abstinence allows for neuroplasticity and structural changes that contribute to cognitive recovery. These changes may be observed in various brain regions (Goldstein & Volkow, 2011). It's important to note that individual responses to drug withdrawal and cognitive recovery can vary, and the extent of recovery may depend on factors such as the severity and duration of drug use, the presence of co-occurring conditions, and engagement in supportive interventions. The process of cognitive recovery is ongoing, and continued research contributes to a better understanding of the brain's resilience and adaptability.

Neurogenesis and hippocampal recovery after drug withdrawal is required for normal neorlogical functions retrieval. Neurogenesis refers to the generation of new neurons, and the hippocampus is a brain region particularly associated with learning, memory, and emotional regulation. Chronic drug use can impact neurogenesis and the structure of the hippocampus (Noonan et al., 2010). Several drugs of abuse, including alcohol, opioids, and stimulants, have been associated with a reduction in adult hippocampal neurogenesis. This reduction may contribute to cognitive impairments and emotional dysregulation observed in individuals with substance use disorders. Chronic drug use can lead to structural changes in the hippocampus, including alterations in dendritic morphology, synaptic plasticity, and reductions in the volume of the hippocampal region. Abstinence from drugs has been associated with a partial restoration of neurogenesis in the hippocampus. The extent of recovery may depend on factors such as the duration and severity of drug use (Volkow et al., 2004).

Longer periods of abstinence have been associated with more significant recovery of neurogenesis. This suggests that continued abstinence allows for a gradual restoration of hippocampal structure and function. Physical activity has been shown to enhance neurogenesis, and exercise during drug withdrawal may support the recovery of hippocampal function. Some antidepressant medications, such as selective serotonin reuptake inhibitors (SSRIs), have been shown to promote neurogenesis and may have potential benefits during drug withdrawal. Restoration of neurogenesis in the hippocampus may contribute to cognitive recovery during drug withdrawal, including improvements in learning and memory. Individual differences may influence the degree of recovery in neurogenesis and hippocampal structure. Genetic, environmental, and neurobiological factors can contribute to variability in recovery outcomes (Hill et al., 2015). Understanding the interplay between chronic drug use, neurogenesis, and hippocampal recovery is crucial for developing targeted interventions to support cognitive and emotional well-being during drug withdrawal. Continued research in this area aims to uncover novel therapeutic strategies that enhance neuroplasticity and promote recovery of hippocampal function.

White matter integrity restoration after drug withdrawal is a complex and dynamic process involving adaptive changes in the brain's structure and connectivity. Chronic drug use, particularly substances of abuse, can have detrimental effects on white matter, which consists of myelinated axons that facilitate communication between different brain regions (Monnig et al., 2013). Chronic drug use has been associated with disruptions in white matter integrity. Changes may include alterations in myelin structure, axonal damage, and compromised connectivity between brain regions. Different drugs may impact specific white matter tracts. For example, cocaine and methamphetamine use has been associated with changes in the integrity of the corpus callosum and frontal white matter tracts. After drug withdrawal, the brain undergoes adaptive changes, including neuroplasticity. This process involves the reorganization of neural networks and can contribute to the restoration of white matter integrity. The timeline for white matter integrity restoration can vary based on factors such as the type and duration of drug use, individual differences, and the presence of co-occurring conditions. Some recovery may occur relatively quickly, while other improvements may take more time (Bora & Zorlu, 2017).

Complete abstinence from drugs is a crucial factor in the recovery of white matter integrity. Supportive interventions, such as behavioral therapy, counseling, and rehabilitation programs, can contribute to overall recovery. Regular physical exercise and a healthy lifestyle have been associated with positive effects on white matter integrity. These factors may complement the recovery process after drug withdrawal. Advanced neuroimaging techniques, such as diffusion tensor imaging (DTI) and magnetic resonance imaging (MRI), allow researchers to assess white matter integrity and changes during recovery after drug withdrawal. Individual differences, including genetic factors and pre-existing vulnerabilities, can contribute to variability in the recovery of white matter integrity. Understanding these differences is crucial for personalized treatment approaches (Bjork et al., 2003). Understanding the process of white matter integrity restoration after drug withdrawal is essential for developing effective treatments for substance use disorders. Ongoing research continues to uncover the mechanisms underlying these changes and inform interventions that support recovery at the structural level of the brain.

While research has provided valuable insights into the neurological recovery process, it's important to note that individual responses to treatment can vary. Focus should be on understanding the foundation for investigating the complex mechanisms involved in the restoration of neurological function after drug addiction. Continued research in this field is critical for developing targeted interventions and optimizing outcomes for individuals in recovery.

Pharmacotherapeutic Interventions for Specific Substances: Pharmacotherapeutic interventions for substances of abuse involve the use of medications to treat addiction and related conditions. The choice of medication depends on the specific substance of abuse and the individual's needs. The field of addiction medicine is dynamic, and ongoing research may lead to the development of new medications and treatment approaches. The effectiveness of pharmacotherapeutic interventions can vary among individuals, and treatment plans should be tailored to each person's unique needs and circumstances. Additionally, individuals seeking treatment for substance use disorders should consult with healthcare professionals to determine the most appropriate and evidence-based interventions for their situation.

a. Opioids: Pharmacotherapeutic interventions for treating opioid abuse involve the use of medications to help individuals manage cravings, withdrawal symptoms, and achieve abstinence. Some commonly used medications include:

Methadone: Methadone is a long-acting opioid agonist that binds to the same receptors as opioids, reducing cravings and withdrawal symptoms.

Buprenorphine: Buprenorphine is a partial opioid agonist that can reduce cravings and withdrawal symptoms without producing the same level of euphoria as full agonists.

Naltrexone: Naltrexone is an opioid receptor antagonist that blocks the effects of opioids, reducing the rewarding effects and cravings.

Naloxone: Naloxone is an opioid receptor antagonist used for the emergency treatment of opioid overdoses.

Buprenorphine/Naloxone Combination: This combination product contains buprenorphine and naloxone. Buprenorphine helps with cravings and withdrawal, while naloxone discourages misuse by causing withdrawal symptoms if injected.

Methadone Maintenance Treatment (MMT): MMT involves the long-term use of methadone as a replacement for the opioid of abuse, helping to stabilize individuals and reduce illicit drug use.

Extended-Release Naltrexone: Extended-release naltrexone is administered monthly and helps prevent relapse by blocking opioid receptors.

These medications are often used as part of a comprehensive treatment approach that includes counseling, psychosocial support, and behavioral therapies (Mattick et al., 2009; Lee et al., 2016; Tanum et al., 2017). The choice of medication depends on individual factors, including the severity of addiction, medical history, and patient preferences. It's important to note that successful treatment often involves a combination of pharmacotherapy and psychosocial interventions tailored to the individual's needs. Regular medical monitoring and follow-up are critical components of opioid use disorder treatment.

Nicotine: Pharmacotherapeutic interventions for treating nicotine abuse primarily aim to assist individuals in quitting tobacco use by reducing cravings and withdrawal symptoms. The choice of medication should be tailored to the individual's preferences, medical history, and potential side effects. Combining pharmacotherapy with behavioral interventions, counseling, or support groups can enhance treatment outcomes. Nicotine replacement therapies are often used in a step-down approach, allowing individuals to gradually reduce their nicotine intake. Some commonly used medications include:

Nicotine Replacement Therapy (NRT): NRT provides controlled doses of nicotine to help reduce withdrawal symptoms and cravings, allowing individuals to gradually decrease their dependence. It is available in various forms, including patches, gum, lozenges, nasal spray, and inhalers.

Bupropion (Zyban): Bupropion is an antidepressant that also acts as a nicotine receptor antagonist, helping to reduce cravings and withdrawal symptoms.

Varenicline (Chantix): Varenicline is a partial nicotine receptor agonist, reducing withdrawal symptoms while also blocking the rewarding effects of nicotine if smoking occurs.

Combination Therapy: Combining different forms of NRT or combining NRT with medications like bupropion has been shown to enhance efficacy.

Cytisine: Cytisine is a partial agonist to the nicotinic acetylcholine receptor, helping to reduce withdrawal symptoms and cravings.

Clonidine: Clonidine, an alpha-2 adrenergic agonist, can help manage withdrawal symptoms associated with nicotine cessation.

It's essential for individuals seeking to quit smoking to consult with healthcare professionals to determine the most suitable pharmacotherapeutic interventions from the above mentioned ones (Stead et al., 2008; Cahill et al., 2016; Stead & Lancaster, 2012) for their situation. Additionally, ongoing support and follow-up are crucial components of successful smoking cessation programs.

Alcohol: Pharmacotherapeutic interventions for treating alcohol use disorder (AUD) include medications that target different aspects of the addiction, such as reducing cravings, blocking rewarding effects, or alleviating withdrawal symptoms. Some commonly used medications include:

Disulfiram: Disulfiram inhibits the enzyme acetaldehyde dehydrogenase, leading to an accumulation of acetaldehyde when alcohol is consumed. This results in unpleasant reactions, discouraging alcohol consumption.

Acamprosate: Acamprosate modulates glutamatergic neurotransmission and is thought to reduce symptoms of protracted withdrawal, helping to maintain abstinence.

Naltrexone: Naltrexone is an opioid receptor antagonist that reduces the rewarding effects of alcohol, helping to decrease cravings and the likelihood of relapse.

Topiramate: Topiramate is an antiepileptic medication that has been studied for its potential in reducing alcohol consumption.

Nalmefene: Nalmefene is an opioid receptor modulator that helps reduce alcohol consumption by reducing the reinforcing effects of alcohol.

Baclofen: Baclofen, a GABA-B receptor agonist, has been explored for its potential in reducing alcohol cravings.

The choice of medication from the above mentioned ones (Mann et al., 2004; Garbutt et al., 2005; Johnson et al., 2003; van den Brink et al., 2013) depends on factors such as the individual's medical history, severity of alcohol dependence, and treatment goals. Combining medications with behavioral therapies and counseling can enhance treatment outcomes. Close monitoring and follow-up with healthcare providers are important to assess the effectiveness and tolerability of the chosen medication. It's important for individuals with alcohol use disorder to consult with healthcare professionals for a comprehensive assessment and to determine the most appropriate pharmacotherapeutic interventions tailored to their needs. Additionally, ongoing support, counseling, and lifestyle changes are often integral components of successful treatment for alcohol abuse.

Cocaine: Cocaine use disorder (CUD) poses a notable public health concern without any approved medication from the Food and Drug Administration (FDA). Drug repurposing seeks economical alternatives by exploring new applications for already approved drugs. This study introduces a comprehensive approach to pinpoint FDA-approved drugs suitable for repurposing in the treatment of CUD. Some commonly used medications include:

Disulfiram: Disulfiram, while approved for alcohol use disorder, has been explored for its potential to reduce cocaine use by creating aversive reactions to cocaine ingestion.

Modafinil: Modafinil, a wakefulness-promoting agent, has been studied for its potential in reducing cocaine use and improving cognitive performance.

Topiramate: Topiramate, an antiepileptic medication, has been investigated for its potential in reducing cocaine use and promoting abstinence.

N-Acetylcysteine (NAC): NAC, an antioxidant and glutamate modulator, has shown promise in reducing cravings and improving treatment outcomes for cocaine dependence.

Dextroamphetamine: Mechanism of Action: Dextroamphetamine, a stimulant, has been investigated for its potential in reducing cocaine use by addressing attention and arousal deficits.

It's important to emphasize that the effectiveness of these medications for treating cocaine use disorder is still under investigation, and results from studies may vary (Carroll et al., 2001; Dackis et al., 2005; La Rowe et al., 2006; Grabowski et al,. 2001). Behavioral therapies and counseling remain crucial components of treatment for cocaine abuse. Individuals seeking help for cocaine use disorder should consult with healthcare professionals to explore the most appropriate and evidence-based interventions for their specific situation.

Cannabis: The primary approach to addressing cannabis use disorder typically involves behavioral interventions, counseling, and support. It's essential to note that the field of addiction treatment is dynamic, and research is ongoing to explore potential pharmacotherapeutic interventions. Some commonly used medications include:

N-Acetylcysteine (NAC): NAC, an antioxidant and glutamate modulator, has been studied for its potential in reducing cannabis use by affecting the endocannabinoid system.

Gabapentin: Gabapentin, an anticonvulsant, has been explored for its potential in reducing cannabis withdrawal symptoms and cravings.

Dronabinol: Dronabinol, a synthetic form of THC (tetrahydrocannabinol), has been investigated for its potential in reducing cannabis withdrawal symptoms.

Quetiapine: Quetiapine, an atypical antipsychotic, has been studied for its potential in reducing cannabis use and associated symptoms.

It's important to emphasize that the effectiveness of these medications for treating cannabis use disorder is still under investigation (Gray et al., 2012; Mason et al., 2012; Levin et al., 2013; Green et al., 2003), and results from studies may vary. Additionally, behavioral therapies and counseling are crucial components of treatment for cannabis use disorder. Individuals seeking help for cannabis use disorder should consult with healthcare professionals to explore the most appropriate and evidence-based interventions for their specific situation.

Adjunctive Medications and Supportive Therapies: The treatment of drug addiction often involves a combination of medications and supportive therapies to address both the physical and psychological aspects of substance use disorders, such as Behavioral therapies aim to modify attitudes and behaviors related to drug use, enhance life skills, and promote abstinence. Cognitive-Behavioral Therapy (CBT) helps individuals recognize and cope with triggers and cravings, develop coping strategies, and prevent relapse. Motivational Enhancement Therapy (MET) aims to enhance an individual's motivation to change by exploring and resolving ambivalence. Contingency Management (CM) provides tangible rewards for maintaining abstinence and achieving treatment goals. Community Reinforcement Approach and Family Training (CRAFT) involves involving the family in the treatment process and reinforcing non-drug-related behaviors. Mindfulness-Based Relapse Prevention (MBRP) combines mindfulness meditation with cognitive-behavioral relapse prevention strategies. These interventions are often used in combination, and treatment plans should be tailored to the individual's needs (Skinner et al., 2016; Chick et al., 2003). It's important to consult with healthcare professionals for personalized treatment recommendations based on the latest research and clinical guidelines.

a. Antidepressants: The use of antidepressants in the treatment of drug addiction is a complex and evolving area of research. Antidepressants may be prescribed to address co-occurring mood disorders, such as depression or anxiety, that often accompany substance use disorders. Additionally, some antidepressants have shown potential in directly influencing certain aspects of drug addiction. However, it's crucial to note that the efficacy of antidepressants in treating drug addiction can vary, and individual responses may differ.

Selective Serotonin Reuptake Inhibitors (SSRIs): SSRIs are commonly used to treat depression and anxiety by increasing serotonin levels in the brain.

Tricyclic Antidepressants (TCAs): TCAs, although less commonly prescribed today due to their side effect profile, have been investigated for their potential in treating substance use disorders.

Norepinephrine-Dopamine Reuptake Inhibitors (NDRIs): NDRIs, such as bupropion, have been studied for their potential in treating stimulant (e.g., cocaine) dependence.

Serotonin-Norepinephrine Reuptake Inhibitors (SNRIs): SNRIs, like venlafaxine, have been explored for their potential in reducing cocaine use.

Agomelatine: Agomelatine, a melatonergic antidepressant, has been investigated for its potential in reducing alcohol intake.

Mirtazapine: Mirtazapine, an atypical antidepressant, has been studied for its potential in reducing methamphetamine use.

While some studies suggest potential benefits of these antidepressants in treating drug addiction (Myrick et al., 2001; Poling et al., 2006; Levin et al., 2010; Leggio et al., 2012; Elkashef et al., 2008), the field is dynamic, and research is ongoing. Treatment decisions should be made based on a comprehensive assessment of an individual's specific needs and in consultation with healthcare professionals.

b. Anxiolytics: The use of anxiolytics, or anti-anxiety medications, in the treatment of drug addiction is often focused on managing anxiety symptoms that may co-occur with substance use disorders. Anxiety is a common comorbidity in individuals with addiction, and addressing anxiety symptoms can be an important aspect of comprehensive treatment.

Benzodiazepines: Benzodiazepines are a class of anxiolytic medications that enhance the effect of the neurotransmitter gamma-aminobutyric acid (GABA) in the brain.

Buspirone: Buspirone is a non-benzodiazepine anxiolytic that affects serotonin receptors and is sometimes used to manage anxiety symptoms.

Pregabalin: Pregabalin, an anticonvulsant, has been studied for its potential in reducing anxiety and cravings in individuals with substance use disorders.

Hydroxyzine: Hydroxyzine, an antihistamine with anxiolytic properties, has been used to manage anxiety symptoms in individuals with substance use disorders.

Gabapentin: Gabapentin, an anticonvulsant, has been studied for its potential in reducing anxiety and cravings in individuals with alcohol use disorder.

Clonidine: Clonidine, an alpha-2 adrenergic agonist, has been used to manage withdrawal symptoms and anxiety in individuals with substance use disorders.

The use of these anxiolytics in the context of drug addiction should be carefully considered (Martinotti et al., 2010; Mason et al., 2014), as some medications may have the potential for misuse or dependence. Treatment decisions should be made based on a thorough assessment of an individual's specific needs, and consultation with healthcare professionals is essential.

c. Cognitive-Behavioral Therapy (CBT): Cognitive-Behavioral Therapy (CBT) is a widely used and evidence-based therapeutic approach for the treatment of drug addiction. CBT focuses on identifying and modifying maladaptive thoughts, beliefs, and behaviors associated with substance use. It aims to help individuals develop coping skills, increase self-awareness, and prevent relapse. CBT is adapted for substance use disorders to address cognitive distortions, triggers for drug use, and the development of coping strategies. It emphasizes relapse prevention by identifying high-risk situations, developing coping skills, and enhancing self-efficacy to resist drug use. CBT is often integrated with the treatment of co-occurring mental health disorders, such as depression or anxiety, commonly associated with substance use (Back & Brady, 2008; Iqbal et al., 2019).

CBT is applied to address the challenges specific to opioid use disorder, including cravings, pain management, and medication adherence. It is also adapted to address the unique features of stimulant use disorders, focusing on cognitive restructuring and coping strategies (Carroll & Onken, 2005). CBT is tailored for adolescents, addressing developmental factors and peer influences in the context of substance use. It is also effective in treating individuals with dual diagnoses, addressing both substance use and co-occurring mental health disorders (Mueser et al., 2003). CBT is often part of comprehensive treatment programs for drug addiction and may be delivered in individual or group settings. It is adaptable to various substances of abuse and can be implemented in different stages of recovery.

d. Contingency Management: Contingency Management (CM) is a behavioral therapy approach that provides tangible incentives as rewards to reinforce positive behaviors such as abstinence from drug use. It is based on the principles of operant conditioning, where desired behaviors are strengthened by the systematic delivery of rewards. CM involves the systematic reinforcement of target behaviors, such as drug abstinence or adherence to treatment plans, through the provision of tangible rewards. CM typically uses a variety of incentives and rewards, such as vouchers, prizes, or privileges, to reinforce abstinence and positive behaviors. It has shown effectiveness in the treatment of opioid use disorder, particularly in improving retention in treatment and reducing opioid use. CM has been effective in reducing cocaine use and promoting abstinence in individuals with cocaine use disorder. CM can be combined with medications for substance use disorders, enhancing overall treatment outcomes. CM has been applied successfully in the treatment of stimulant use disorders, including methamphetamine and amphetamine use. Contingency management has been utilized to promote smoking cessation, providing incentives for abstinence from tobacco use (Stitzer & Petry, 2006; Prendergast et al., 2006; Petry et al., 2005; Higgins et al., 2000). Contingency management has demonstrated effectiveness across various substances of abuse and treatment settings. It is often used in conjunction with other therapeutic approaches to enhance treatment outcomes. The references provided offer more in-depth information on each aspect of contingency management in the treatment of drug addiction.

Novel and Experimental Approaches for the treatment of drug addiction: Novel and experimental approaches for the treatment of drug addiction are areas of active research. Researchers are exploring innovative strategies, including pharmacological, behavioral, and neurobiological interventions such as:

Neurofeedback: Neurofeedback is a therapeutic approach that involves providing individuals with real-time feedback about their brain activity, allowing them to learn how to self-regulate and optimize neural functioning. In the context of drug addiction, neurofeedback is being explored as a potential intervention to address underlying neural dysregulation associated with substance use disorders. (Meng et al., 2023).

Transcranial Magnetic Stimulation (TMS): Transcranial Magnetic Stimulation (TMS) is a non-invasive neurostimulation technique that uses magnetic fields to modulate neuronal activity in specific brain regions. It is being investigated for its potential in reducing cravings and promoting abstinence. It has been explored as a potential treatment for various psychiatric disorders, including drug addiction (Amerio et al., 2023).

Deep Brain Stimulation (DBS): Deep Brain Stimulation (DBS) is a neurosurgical procedure that involves implanting electrodes into specific brain regions particularly nucleus accumbens and delivering electrical impulses to modulate neural activity. While DBS has been primarily used for movement disorders, such as Parkinson's disease, it has also been explored as a potential treatment for drug addiction. (Shaheen et al., 2023).

Immunotherapy: Immunotherapy for the treatment of drug addiction involves the development of vaccines or antibodies that target drugs in the bloodstream, preventing them from reaching the brain and eliciting rewarding effects. This approach aims to reduce the reinforcing effects of drugs and decrease the likelihood of relapse (Hossain et al., 2023).

Psychedelic-Assisted Therapy: Psychedelic-assisted therapy involves the use of psychedelics, such as psilocybin (found in certain mushrooms) and MDMA (3,4-methylenedioxymethamphetamine), in conjunction with psychotherapy to facilitate therapeutic processes. This approach has gained attention for its potential in treating various mental health conditions, including substance use disorders. (Sharma et al., 2023)

Oxytocin Administration: Oxytocin, often referred to as the "bonding hormone," is a neuropeptide that plays a role in social bonding, trust, and emotional regulation. Some studies have explored the potential of oxytocin administration as a treatment for drug addiction. In general, oxytocin not only inhibits the rewarding effects of drugs during the binge phase of addiction but also diminishes stress reactions and social difficulties during withdrawal. Ultimately, it prevents the reinstatement of drug-related cues and stress-induced relapses (Mellentin et al., 2023).

Cannabinoid-Based Therapies:

Cannabinoid-based therapies have been explored for their potential in the treatment of drug addiction, with a focus on the endocannabinoid system and compounds derived from the cannabis plant. Results from placebo-controlled randomized controlled trials suggest that synthetic delta-9-tetrahydrocannabinol reduces withdrawal symptoms, although not cannabis use, in adults with daily cannabis use. Meanwhile, findings on formulations containing tetrahydrocannabinol combined with cannabidiol are varied. Initial evidence from two placebo-controlled randomized controlled trials in adults with cannabis abuse indicates that both fatty acid amide hydrolase inhibitors and cannabidiol may decrease cannabis use. Nevertheless, larger trials are necessary to bolster this evidence. Insights from studies in adults highlight cannabinoid-based treatments as a potential strategy that warrants exploration in youth with cannabis use disorder (Romer Thomsen et al., 2022). These novel and experimental approaches represent areas of ongoing research, and their effectiveness and safety are subjects of continued investigation. As the field advances, new findings and interventions may emerge. Always consult the latest scientific literature and healthcare professionals for the most up-to-date information on novel and experimental treatments for drug addiction.

Challenges and Considerations in the treatment of drug addiction: The treatment of drug addiction is a complex and multifaceted process, and various challenges and considerations impact the effectiveness of interventions. Stigma associated with addiction can hinder individuals from seeking treatment and receiving support. Discrimination may also affect the quality of care. Promoting public awareness, education, and destigmatization efforts are crucial to encourage individuals to seek help without fear of judgment. Many individuals face barriers such as geographical limitations, financial constraints, and lack of available treatment options. Expanding access to affordable and diverse treatment services, including telehealth options, can improve the reach and effectiveness of interventions. Individuals with substance use disorders often experience co-occurring mental health issues, complicating treatment. Integrated treatment approaches that address both substance use and mental health conditions concurrently are essential for comprehensive care.

One-size-fits-all approaches may not be effective, as individuals have unique factors influencing their addiction and recovery. Personalized treatment plans, considering factors such as age, gender, cultural background, and specific substance use patterns, can enhance treatment outcomes. Many individuals struggle with completing the full course of treatment, leading to relapse. Providing ongoing support, follow-up care, and addressing barriers to treatment adherence are crucial to sustaining recovery efforts. The neurobiological changes associated with addiction make relapse a common challenge. Ongoing research into the neurobiology of addiction can inform the development of targeted interventions and medications to prevent relapse. Some individuals may not respond adequately to existing treatments, highlighting the need for continued research and innovation. Investing in the development of new therapeutic approaches and medications can improve overall treatment efficacy.

Relapse is a common occurrence, and maintaining long-term abstinence can be challenging. Providing individuals with effective coping strategies, ongoing support, and relapse prevention education is essential to reducing the risk of relapse. Achieving a balance between behavioral and pharmacological interventions and ensuring their seamless integration can be challenging. Collaborative, multidisciplinary treatment teams can work together to provide comprehensive care that addresses both psychological and physiological aspects of addiction. Cultural differences can impact the effectiveness of treatment, and a lack of cultural competence may lead to disparities in care. Culturally sensitive treatment approaches that consider diverse backgrounds, beliefs, and values can enhance engagement and outcomes. Addressing these challenges and considerations requires a holistic and patient-centered approach, incorporating ongoing research, community support, and a commitment to reducing barriers to effective treatment.

a. Individual Variability in Treatment Response: Individual variability in treatment response is a crucial aspect in the treatment of drug addiction. The diverse responses among individuals undergoing addiction treatment can be influenced by various factors, including genetic, neurobiological, psychological, and environmental variables. Understanding and addressing this variability is essential for developing personalized and effective treatment approaches.

Genetic factors play a significant role in individual variability in the treatment response to drug addiction. The influence of genetic variations on treatment outcomes is a complex interplay of multiple genes, each contributing to the risk of addiction, treatment response, and susceptibility to relapse. Genetic variations can influence an individual's susceptibility to addiction and their response to treatment interventions. Genetic factors contribute to an individual's vulnerability to developing substance use disorders. Polymorphisms in drug metabolism enzymes can impact the rate at which drugs are metabolized, influencing treatment response. Genetic influences on neurotransmitter systems and neural pathways involved in addiction can affect treatment response. Genetic factors influence how individuals respond to pharmacological treatments for addiction. It can also influence an individual's likelihood of remaining in treatment and susceptibility to relapse. Genetic factors may interact with environmental influences, such as stress or trauma, affecting treatment outcomes. Understanding the genetic factors influencing treatment response allows for the development of more targeted and personalized interventions (Uhl & Grow, 2004). However, it's important to note that genetic factors are just one component of the complex interplay of influences contributing to addiction and treatment outcomes. Further research is needed to unravel the intricate relationship between genetics and treatment response fully.

Neurobiological Factors including brain structure and function, can impact how individuals respond to pharmacological and behavioral interventions. Neurobiological factors play a crucial role in individual variability in the treatment response to drug addiction. The complex interplay of brain structures, neurotransmitter systems, and neuroplasticity contributes to differences in how individuals experience and respond to addiction treatment. Dysregulation of the dopamine system, particularly in the mesolimbic pathway, is a common neurobiological feature of addiction (Urban et al., 2023). Neuroplastic changes in brain circuits involved in reward, motivation, and learning contribute to the development and maintenance of addiction.

Impaired functioning of the prefrontal cortex, involved in decision-making and impulse control, is associated with addiction. Changes in glutamate transmission, particularly within the cortico-striatal circuitry, contribute to addictive behaviors. The serotonin system influences mood and impulse control, and its dysregulation is implicated in addiction. The endocannabinoid system plays a role in reward processing and motivation, impacting responses to addictive substances. Dysregulation of the stress response system, particularly involving CRF, is associated with drug addiction and relapse (Cavanagh et al., 2022). Understanding individual differences in neurobiological factors is crucial for tailoring treatment approaches. Personalized interventions that consider the unique neurobiological profile of each individual may lead to more effective and targeted treatment strategies in the context of drug addiction.

Psychological factors significantly contribute to the variability in treatment response to drug addiction. Individual differences in cognitive processes, emotional regulation, motivation, and coping strategies play a crucial role in determining how individuals engage with and benefit from addiction treatment. Variability in an individual's motivation to change their addictive behaviors influences treatment engagement and outcomes. Differences in cognitive processes, such as impulsivity and decision-making abilities, contribute to variations in treatment response. Varied coping skills and stress management strategies impact an individual's ability to deal with triggers and stressors that may lead to relapse. Differences in emotional regulation skills influence how individuals cope with cravings, negative emotions, and environmental cues. An individual's belief in their ability to remain abstinent (self-efficacy) influences their treatment response. Individual differences in personality traits, such as impulsivity or sensation-seeking, may impact response to treatment. An individual's readiness to change, as described by the stages of change model, influences treatment engagement and progression. The presence of supportive social networks and a positive treatment environment can enhance treatment outcomes

(Malik et al., 2023). Understanding and addressing these psychological factors allows for the development of tailored and effective treatment interventions that address the specific needs of everyone. Incorporating psychological assessments and interventions into addiction treatment programs can contribute to improved outcomes and long-term recovery.

Co-occurring mental health conditions can also impact the effectiveness of addiction treatment. The presence of co-occurring mental health conditions, also known as dual diagnosis or comorbidity, introduces variability in treatment responses for drug addiction. Individuals with both substance use disorders and mental health issues may require integrated and specialized interventions to address the complexity of their conditions. Identifying and assessing co-occurring mental health conditions alongside substance use disorders can be challenging. Integrated treatment models that address both substance use and mental health issues concurrently are often more effective. Medication management may involve a careful balance to address both substance use and mental health symptoms without exacerbating either condition. Co-occurring mental health conditions may impact an individual's engagement in substance use treatment. Trauma-informed approaches may be crucial, as many individuals with co-occurring conditions have a history of trauma. Cognitive-behavioral therapy (CBT) adapted for dual disorders can address both substance use and mental health issues. Providing a continuum of care that addresses various treatment needs, including mental health and substance use, is essential. Peer support models can be beneficial, especially when individuals with lived experience of both addiction and mental health challenges provide support (Davidson et al., 2012). Addressing the complexities of co-occurring mental health conditions is crucial for tailoring effective and comprehensive treatment approaches for individuals with dual diagnoses. The variability in treatment responses emphasizes the need for personalized, integrated, and multidisciplinary interventions.

Socioeconomic and environmental influences individual variability in treatment response. The presence of co-occurring mental health conditions, also known as dual diagnosis or comorbidity, introduces variability in treatment responses for drug addiction. Individuals with both substances use disorders and mental health issues may require integrated and specialized interventions to address the complexity of their conditions. Identifying and assessing co-occurring mental health conditions alongside substance use disorders can be challenging. Integrated treatment models that address both substance use and mental health issues concurrently are often more effective. Medication management may involve a careful balance to address both substance use and mental health symptoms without exacerbating either condition. Co-occurring mental health conditions may impact an individual's engagement in substance use treatment. Trauma-informed approaches may be crucial, as many individuals with co-occurring conditions have a history of trauma. Cognitive-behavioral therapy (CBT) adapted for dual disorders can address both substance use and mental health issues. Providing a continuum of care that addresses various treatment needs, including mental health and substance use, is essential. Peer support models can be beneficial, especially when individuals with lived experience of both addiction and mental health challenges provide support (Davidson et al., 2012). Addressing the complexities of co-occurring mental health conditions is crucial for tailoring effective and comprehensive treatment approaches for individuals with dual diagnoses. The variability in treatment responses emphasizes the need for personalized, integrated, and multidisciplinary interventions.

Pharmacogenetics, i.e., genetic variations in drug-metabolizing enzymes can impact an individual's response to medications used in addiction treatment. Pharmacogenetics refers to the study of how an individual's genetic makeup influences their response to drugs. Understanding pharmacogenetic variability can be crucial in the treatment of drug addiction, as it can help tailor interventions to an individual's specific genetic profile. Variations in genes that encode drug-metabolizing enzymes, such as those in the cytochrome P450 family, can affect the rate at which drugs are metabolized in the body. Differences in drug metabolism can lead to variations in drug levels, potentially influencing treatment efficacy and the likelihood of side effects. Genetic variations in neurotransmitter receptors, such as those involved in the reward pathway (e.g., dopamine receptors), can impact an individual's susceptibility to drug addiction and response to treatment. Polymorphisms in opioid receptors, for example, may affect the effectiveness of medications used in opioid addiction treatment.

Understanding a patient's genetic profile can help clinicians develop personalized treatment plans. For example, certain genetic variations may make an individual more responsive to specific medications or more prone to adverse reactions. Pharmacogenetics can be particularly relevant in medication-assisted treatment for drug addiction. Drugs such as methadone, buprenorphine, and naltrexone are commonly used, and their effectiveness may vary based on genetic factors (Haile et al., 2007). Integrating genetic information into addiction treatment plans has the potential to enhance therapeutic outcomes and minimize adverse effects. However, it is crucial to approach this field with caution, taking into account ethical considerations and the need for ongoing research.

b. Co-occurring Mental Health Disorders: The co-occurrence of mental health disorders and substance abuse, often referred to as co-occurring disorders or dual diagnosis, is a common and complex phenomenon. The relationship between mental health disorders and drug abuse is bidirectional, with each condition influencing and exacerbating the other. It's important to recognize that co-occurring disorders are highly individualized, and the relationship between mental health and substance abuse can vary widely among individuals. Effective treatment requires a personalized and comprehensive approach that considers the unique needs and challenges of each person. Seeking professional help from mental health and addiction specialists is crucial in this regard, for a comprehensive and tailored treatment plan.

Self-medication in the context of drug abuse refers to the practice of using substances, such as drugs or alcohol, without professional guidance to alleviate physical or psychological symptoms. Individuals may engage in self-medication for various reasons, including the desire to manage stress, cope with emotional issues, alleviate pain, or address mental health symptoms. It's important to note that self-medication can lead to serious health consequences and may contribute to the development of substance use disorders. Many individuals who engage in self-medication often have underlying issues such as mental health disorders, trauma, or chronic pain. Instead of seeking professional help, they may turn to substances as a way to cope with these challenges. Self-medication may provide temporary relief from symptoms, but it doesn't address the root causes of the issues. As a result, individuals may find themselves trapped in a cycle of using substances to numb or escape from their problems (Holborn et al., 2023).

The use of drugs or alcohol without proper medical supervision increases the risk of developing a substance use disorder. Over time, the body can develop tolerance, leading to an increased need for the substance to achieve the same effects. Self-medication can have severe health consequences, including physical and mental health issues, increased risk of accidents, impaired cognitive function, and damage to vital organs. Self-medication can interfere with the effectiveness of prescribed medications or therapeutic interventions. Substances may interact negatively with prescribed drugs, making treatment less effective or causing harmful side effects. The use of illicit substances for self-medication can lead to legal consequences. Possession and use of illegal drugs can result in legal trouble and further complicate an individual's life (Ruiz, 2010). Individuals who engage in self-medication may experience social stigma and isolation, as their coping mechanism involves secrecy and avoidance of seeking help. It's crucial for individuals struggling with issues that lead to self-medication to seek professional help. Mental health professionals, doctors, and addiction specialists can provide appropriate assessments, diagnoses, and treatment plans to address underlying issues and help individuals develop healthier coping mechanisms.

Increased vulnerability to drug abuse is observed in individuals with mental health disorder. For example, conditions like depression or post-traumatic stress disorder may impair an individual's ability to cope with stressors, making them more likely to turn to substances for relief. Self-Medication: Individuals with mental health disorders may turn to drugs or alcohol as a way to self-medicate and alleviate their symptoms. Substances can provide temporary relief from anxiety, depression, or other mental health issues, leading to a higher risk of developing a substance use disorder. Many individuals experience both mental health disorders and substance use disorders simultaneously, a condition known as dual diagnosis or co-occurring disorders. The presence of one condition can exacerbate the other, making treatment more complex. There may be shared biological and genetic factors that contribute to both mental health disorders and substance abuse. Some individuals may have a genetic predisposition that increases their susceptibility to both conditions (Dhinsa et al., 2023).

Environmental factors, such as trauma, chronic stress, or a history of abuse, can contribute to the development of both mental health disorders and substance abuse. These stressors may act as trigg.rs for individuals to engage in drug use. Mental health disorders often involve imbalances in neurotransmitters and brain chemistry. Substance abuse can further disrupt these systems, creating a cycle of dependence and worsening mental health symptoms. The stigma surrounding mental health disorders may lead to social isolation, making individuals more vulnerable to substance abuse as a coping mechanism (Axinn et al., 2023). The use of substances can temporarily relieve feelings of isolation or marginalization. Individuals with mental health disorders may face challenges in accessing appropriate mental health care. If their mental health needs are not addressed, they may be more likely to turn to substances as a form of self-help. It's essential to approach mental health and substance abuse treatment holistically, addressing both aspects simultaneously. Integrated treatment programs that target both mental health and substance use disorders have been shown to be more effective in promoting long-term recovery.

Shared risk factors play a significant role in the development of both mental health disorders and substance abuse. These risk factors can contribute to a complex interplay between the two, often leading to a co-occurrence of mental health and substance use disorders. Genetic predispositions can influence an individual's susceptibility to both mental health disorders and substance abuse. Some individuals may have a family history of both conditions, suggesting a shared genetic vulnerability. Both mental health disorders and substance abuse involve changes in brain structure and function. Neurobiological factors, such as imbalances in neurotransmitters like dopamine and serotonin, can contribute to the development of both conditions. Adverse childhood experiences, including trauma, neglect, or abuse, are associated with an increased risk of developing both mental health disorders and substance abuse later in life. High levels of chronic stress, socioeconomic factors, and environmental stressors can contribute to the development of both mental health disorders and substance abuse. Difficult life circumstances may lead individuals to seek relief through substance use (van Draanen et al., 2022).

Individuals who have experienced trauma, whether in childhood or later in life, are at a higher risk of developing both mental health disorders (such as PTSD) and substance use disorders as a way to cope with the psychological impact of trauma. Social factors, such as isolation, lack of social support, or feelings of loneliness, can contribute to the development of mental health disorders and substance abuse. Substance use may be a way to cope with social difficulties. Traits like impulsivity and a tendency toward risk-taking are associated with an increased risk of both mental health disorders and substance abuse. Individuals with these traits may be more prone to engaging in risky behaviors, including substance use. Certain personality traits or psychological factors, such as low self-esteem, a negative self-image, or difficulties in emotion regulation, can contribute to the development of both mental health disorders and substance abuse (Alhammad et al., 2022). Addressing these shared risk factors is crucial in preventing and treating the co-occurrence of mental health and substance use disorders. Integrated treatment approaches that simultaneously target mental health and substance abuse issues can be more effective in promoting recovery and preventing relapse. Early intervention, support, and a comprehensive understanding of these shared risk factors are key components of successful prevention and treatment strategies.

Drug abuse and mental health disorders can often affect similar neurotransmitter systems in the brain. Neurotransmitters are chemical messengers that play a crucial role in communication between nerve cells (neurons) in the brain. The imbalances or dysregulation of certain neurotransmitter systems are associated with both substance use disorders and mental health disorders. Many drugs of abuse, including stimulants like cocaine and amphetamines, as well as some opioids, can increase dopamine levels in the brain. This contributes to the reinforcing effects of these substances, creating a reward pathway that reinforces drug-seeking behavior. Dysregulation of the dopamine system is implicated in several mental health disorders, including schizophrenia, bipolar disorder, and attention-deficit/hyperactivity disorder (Ciucă Anghel et al., 2023). Some drugs, such as MDMA (ecstasy) and hallucinogens, can affect serotonin levels. MDMA, for example, can cause a release of serotonin and inhibit its reuptake, leading to mood-altering effects. Serotonin imbalances are associated with mood disorders, such as depression and anxiety. Selective serotonin reuptake inhibitors (SSRIs) are a class of antidepressant medications that target the serotonin system (Poian & Chiavegatto, 2023).

Drugs like benzodiazepines and alcohol enhance the inhibitory effects of GABA, leading to sedation and relaxation. This can contribute to their abuse potential. GABA is an inhibitory neurotransmitter, and its dysfunction is linked to anxiety disorders and other mood disorders. Stimulant drugs like cocaine and methamphetamine can increase glutamate release, affecting brain function and contributing to addictive behaviors. Dysregulation of the glutamate system is implicated in conditions like schizophrenia and mood disorders. Opioids, both prescription and illicit, mimic the effects of endorphins, which are natural pain-relieving compounds produced by the body. This contributes to the addictive nature of opioid drugs. Endorphins are involved in the regulation of mood and stress response, and their dysregulation is linked to conditions like depression. The interplay between neurotransmitter systems in the brain is complex, and the effects of drug abuse and mental health disorders on these systems can vary depending on the specific substance or disorder (Engin, 2023; Ciucă Anghel et al., 2023). Understanding these neurobiological aspects is crucial for developing effective treatments and interventions for both substance use and mental health issues. It's worth noting that these explanations are simplified, and the actual neurobiology involved can be more intricate.

Individuals with co-occurring disorders often face greater challenges in treatment. Indeed, individuals with co-occurring disorders, also known as dual diagnosis or comorbidity, face unique and often more complex challenges in treatment compared to those with a single disorder. Co-occurring disorders refer to the presence of both a substance use disorder and a mental health disorder in an individual. Identifying and diagnosing co-occurring disorders can be challenging due to overlapping symptoms. The presence of one disorder can mask or mimic symptoms of the other, leading to difficulties in accurately assessing the individual's needs. Individuals with co-occurring disorders benefit from integrated treatment approaches that address both the substance use and mental health aspects simultaneously (Agterberg et al., 2020). However, many treatment settings historically have been separating, requiring collaboration between mental health and substance abuse treatment providers.

Co-occurring disorders are associated with a higher risk of relapse. If one aspect of the disorder is treated while the other is neglected, the untreated disorder may contribute to a relapse in the treated condition. Medication management becomes more complex in the presence of co-occurring disorders. The potential interactions between psychiatric medications and substances of abuse need careful consideration. Individuals with co-occurring disorders may face increased stigma and discrimination. There can be a lack of understanding about the interconnected nature of mental health and substance use disorders, leading to misconceptions and bias. Co-occurring disorders can lead to lower treatment engagement and adherence. The individual may struggle to engage fully in treatment due to the severity of symptoms, cognitive impairment, or the reinforcing effects of substances. Polypharmacy, or the use of multiple medications, may become a concern in the treatment of co-occurring disorders. Balancing the need for psychiatric medications with potential risks of substance interactions requires careful monitoring (Padwa et al., 2015). Establishing trust and a therapeutic alliance can be more challenging when individuals are dealing with both mental health and substance use issues. A comprehensive, non-judgmental approach is crucial to building a therapeutic relationship. Co-occurring disorders often arise in the context of challenging social and environmental factors, such as poverty, homelessness, or a lack of social support. Addressing these factors is integral to effective treatment. To address these challenges, an integrated and comprehensive treatment approach is recommended. This involves collaboration between mental health professionals, addiction specialists, and other relevant healthcare providers. Tailoring treatment plans to the unique needs of individuals with co-occurring disorders can significantly improve outcomes and enhance the individual's overall well-being.

Drug abuse can hinder the recovery process for individuals with mental health disorders. The relationship between substance abuse and mental health is complex, and each can exacerbate the challenges faced by individuals dealing with both issues. Substance abuse can interfere with the effectiveness of mental health treatments. The use of drugs or alcohol can undermine the therapeutic benefits of medications and counseling, making it more difficult for individuals to experience symptom relief. Drug abuse can exacerbate existing mental health symptoms or trigger the onset of new symptoms. This can lead to increased distress, impairment, and a more challenging recovery process. Individuals with mental health disorders who engage in substance abuse are at a higher risk of relapse. The use of substances can become a coping mechanism for managing stress, anxiety, or depressive symptoms, making it harder for individuals to maintain stability in their mental health. Co-occurring substance use disorders complicate treatment planning (Spencer et al., 2023). Mental health professionals need to address both the mental health and substance abuse aspects, often requiring an integrated treatment approach. Failure to address both issues simultaneously can hinder progress.

Substance abuse can impair cognitive function, making it more challenging for individuals to engage in therapeutic processes, learn new coping skills, and make informed decisions about their mental health treatment. Substance abuse is associated with an increased risk of suicidal ideation and self-harming behaviors, particularly in individuals with mental health disorders. This poses a significant risk to the individual's safety and complicates the treatment process. The consequences of substance abuse, including social isolation, strained relationships, and legal issues, can create additional stressors that negatively impact mental health. Dealing with the fallout from substance abuse can divert attention and resources away from the recovery process (Martinelli et al., 2023). Substance abuse can lead to financial difficulties, which may limit individuals' access to necessary mental health care and support services. Financial strain can become a barrier to recovery and hinder the ability to maintain mental health stability.

Addressing both mental health and substance use disorders concurrently is essential for an effective recovery process. Integrated treatment approaches that consider the interconnected nature of these conditions can provide individuals with the best chance of achieving and maintaining recovery. Seeking professional help from healthcare providers, addiction specialists, and mental health professionals is crucial for individuals facing these challenges. Co-occurring disorders are often associated with increased severity of symptoms . The interaction between substance abuse and mental health conditions can lead to a complex set of challenges, amplifying the impact on an individual's overall well-being. Substance abuse and mental health disorders can exacerbate each other. The symptoms of one disorder may intensify the symptoms of the other, creating a cycle of mutual reinforcement. The presence of co-occurring disorders can complicate the diagnosis and treatment of each condition. Identifying specific symptoms and their origins becomes more challenging, requiring a comprehensive assessment. Individuals with co-occurring disorders are at a higher risk of relapse compared to those with only one disorder. Substance use can be triggered by mental health symptoms, and vice versa, leading to a cycle of repeated relapses. Co-occurring disorders often result in impaired social, occupational, and daily functioning. The combined impact of both disorders can make it more difficult for individuals to maintain stability in various aspects of their lives (Andersson et al., 2023).

Individuals with co-occurring disorders may be less likely to engage in and adhere to treatment plans. The complexity of addressing both substance use and mental health issues simultaneously can be overwhelming, leading to reduced treatment effectiveness. The presence of co-occurring disorders may subject individuals to a dual stigma—stigmatization related to both mental health and substance use. This stigma can contribute to feelings of shame and reluctance to seek help. Co-occurring disorders can render individuals more vulnerable to the negative consequences of both substance abuse and mental health disorders. This increased vulnerability can impact various aspects of an individual's life, including relationships, employment, and overall quality of life. Managing medications for co-occurring disorders can be complex. Individuals may be prescribed multiple medications for mental health and substance use, leading to potential interactions and side effects (Keramatian et al., 2023). Addressing co-occurring disorders requires a comprehensive and integrated treatment approach. This approach involves collaboration between mental health professionals, addiction specialists, and other healthcare providers to develop tailored treatment plans that address the unique needs of individuals with both conditions. Integrated treatment has been shown to be more effective in promoting long-term recovery and improving overall functioning in individuals with co-occurring disorders.

Certain mental health disorders are more commonly associated with specific types of substance abuse. The relationship between mental health and substance use is complex, and various factors, including the specific symptoms of the mental health disorder and the effects of substances, contribute to these associations. Individuals with depression may be more prone to alcohol abuse. Alcohol is a depressant that can temporarily alleviate feelings of sadness or low mood. Excessive alcohol consumption can exacerbate depressive symptoms, interfere with treatment, and increase the risk of developing an alcohol use disorder. Benzodiazepines, such as Xanax or Valium, are commonly misused by individuals with anxiety disorders. These drugs have calming effects and are sometimes used as a form of self-medication. Benzodiazepine misuse can lead to dependence, addiction, and worsen anxiety symptoms. Abrupt cessation can also result in withdrawal symptoms (Fernández et al., 2023).

Individuals with Attention-Deficit/Hyperactivity Disorder (ADHD) may be at higher risk of stimulant abuse. Stimulant medications like Adderall or Ritalin, when misused, can produce feelings of focus and alertness. Misuse of stimulants can lead to dependence, cardiovascular issues, and exacerbation of ADHD symptoms. Individuals without ADHD who misuse stimulants may experience adverse effects. There is a higher prevalence of cannabis use among individuals with schizophrenia. Some may use cannabis to self-medicate or alleviate symptoms. Cannabis use can interfere with antipsychotic medications, increase the risk of psychosis, and worsen cognitive impairment in individuals with schizophrenia. Individuals with PTSD may be more susceptible to opioid abuse. Opioids can provide a temporary escape from distressing memories and emotional pain. Opioid abuse can lead to dependence, addiction, and pose significant health risks. It may also interfere with the processing of trauma in therapeutic settings (Halladay et al., 2023). Individuals with eating disorders, such as anorexia or bulimia, may misuse stimulants or diuretics to control weight. Misuse of these substances can lead to cardiovascular issues, electrolyte imbalances, and worsen the physical and psychological consequences of eating disorders. It's important to note that these associations are not universal, and individuals may have unique experiences. Additionally, substance abuse can contribute to the development of mental health disorders and vice versa, creating a complex interplay between the two. Effective treatment often involves addressing both the mental health and substance use aspects simultaneously in a comprehensive and integrated manner.

Co-occurring disorders are prevalent in substance abuse treatment settings. Co-occurring disorders refer to the presence of both a substance use disorder and a mental health disorder in an individual. The coexistence of these conditions is common, and individuals with co-occurring disorders often face unique challenges that require specialized treatment approaches. Research consistently shows a high prevalence of co-occurring disorders among individuals seeking treatment for substance abuse. Many individuals with substance use disorders also meet criteria for one or more mental health disorders. Substance use and mental health disorders can mutually reinforce each other. Substance use may be a way to cope with the symptoms of a mental health disorder, and the use of substances can contribute to the development or exacerbation of mental health symptoms. Individuals with mental health disorders may engage in substance abuse as a form of self-medication to alleviate symptoms such as anxiety, depression, or trauma-related distress. The presence of co-occurring disorders adds complexity to the treatment process. Addressing both substance use and mental health issues simultaneously requires a comprehensive and integrated approach to ensure effective outcomes (Dauber et al., 2018).

Individuals with co-occurring disorders are at a higher risk of relapse compared to those with a single disorder. Without simultaneous treatment for both conditions, untreated mental health symptoms can contribute to a return to substance use. Coordinating and managing medications for both substance use and mental health disorders can be challenging. The potential interactions between psychiatric medications and substances of abuse need careful consideration. Co-occurring disorders are often associated with increased severity of symptoms, leading to greater impairment in functioning. This can impact various aspects of an individual's life, including relationships, employment, and overall quality of life. Individuals with co-occurring disorders may face a dual stigma related to both substance use and mental health. Stigma can create barriers to seeking help and may impact the individual's willingness to engage in treatment (Rush & Koegl, 2008). Addressing co-occurring disorders requires a comprehensive assessment, individualized treatment planning, and collaboration between mental health professionals and addiction specialists. Integrated treatment models that simultaneously address both substance use and mental health issues have been shown to be more effective in promoting recovery and improving overall well-being.

c. Ethical Considerations in Pharmacotherapy: The pharmacotherapy of drug abuse involves the use of medications to assist individuals in overcoming substance use disorders. Individuals should be fully informed about the purpose, risks, benefits, and alternatives of pharmacotherapy. Informed consent is crucial, and individuals have the right to make autonomous decisions regarding their treatment. Providers must ensure that individuals understand the potential side effects, goals of the pharmacotherapy, and any potential risks associated with the medications. Respecting the autonomy of individuals seeking treatment is fundamental. This includes involving them in treatment decisions, considering their preferences, and respecting their right to refuse or discontinue pharmacotherapy. Providers should engage in shared decision-making, taking into account the individual's values and preferences while providing information to support informed choices. Protecting the confidentiality of individuals receiving pharmacotherapy is essential. Substance use disorders are often stigmatized, and breaches of confidentiality can have significant consequences. Providers must adhere to strict confidentiality standards, ensuring that information about a person's treatment is shared only with those authorized by the individual or required by law (Jonnalagadda et al., 2021).

Ensuring equitable access to pharmacotherapy is crucial to promoting justice. This involves addressing barriers to treatment, such as financial constraints or systemic inequalities. Providers should strive to make pharmacotherapy options accessible to individuals from diverse backgrounds, socioeconomic statuses, and communities. Pharmacotherapy decisions should involve a careful consideration of the risks and benefits. Providers must strive to maximize benefits while minimizing potential harm. Ongoing assessment and monitoring are critical to ensuring that the benefits of pharmacotherapy continue to outweigh potential risks, and adjustments to the treatment plan may be needed. Recognizing and respecting diverse cultural backgrounds is essential for ethical practice. Providers should be culturally competent, acknowledging the influence of culture on individual attitudes toward pharmacotherapy. Providers must be aware of cultural nuances, beliefs, and practices that may impact an individual's acceptance of pharmacotherapy (Duthie et al., 2023). Regular assessment of the effectiveness of pharmacotherapy is essential. If discontinuation of medication is considered, individuals should be informed about the process, potential withdrawal effects, and alternative options. Providers must monitor individuals closely, adjusting treatment plans based on ongoing assessments of progress and addressing withdrawal concerns if medication discontinuation is planned. Coercion in treatment decisions is ethically problematic. Individuals should not be pressured or forced into pharmacotherapy against their will. Providers must ensure that individuals feel empowered to make decisions about their treatment, and coercion or undue influence should be avoided (Sarkar & Balhara, 2023). In summary, ethical considerations in the pharmacotherapy of drug abuse involve respecting autonomy, ensuring informed consent, maintaining confidentiality, promoting equitable access, balancing risks and benefits, being culturally competent, conducting ongoing assessments, and avoiding coercion. Ethical practice in pharmacotherapy supports the well-being and rights of individuals seeking treatment for substance use disorders.

d. Adherence and Compliance: Adherence and compliance are crucial factors in the successful treatment of drug abuse. Adherence refers to the extent to which individuals follow the prescribed treatment plan, including taking medications as directed, attending therapy sessions, and engaging in recommended lifestyle changes. For individuals prescribed medications to manage substance use disorders, adherence is vital. Missing doses or discontinuing medications without consulting healthcare providers can impact treatment effectiveness. Barriers to medication adherence may include concerns about side effects, forgetfulness, stigma, financial constraints, or a lack of perceived benefits. Healthcare providers should address these concerns during treatment. Regular attendance at therapy or counseling sessions is a critical component of substance abuse treatment. Therapy provides individuals with coping skills, support, and strategies to address the underlying issues contributing to substance use. Factors such as transportation issues, work commitments, and mental health symptoms may affect an individual's ability to attend sessions regularly. Flexibility in scheduling and the consideration of virtual therapy options can help overcome these challenges (Lai et al., 2023).

Adherence extends beyond medications and therapy to include engagement in support groups, educational programs, and other supportive services. These elements contribute to a comprehensive and holistic approach to treatment. Some individuals may face barriers to participation, such as lack of awareness, social anxiety, or a perceived lack of time. Providers should actively encourage and facilitate engagement in these services. Lifestyle modifications, such as adopting healthier habits, avoiding triggers, and building a supportive social network, are integral to sustained recovery. Adherence to these changes enhances long-term success. Individuals may struggle with implementing lifestyle changes due to external pressures, lack of motivation, or the influence of the social environment. Setting realistic goals and providing ongoing support can address these challenges. Regular monitoring of progress and follow-up appointments with healthcare providers are essential to evaluate treatment effectiveness, adjust interventions as needed, and address emerging issues. Factors such as a lack of access to healthcare, fear of judgment, or a perceived lack of progress may affect an individual's willingness to engage in regular monitoring. Open communication and a non-judgmental approach can help overcome these challenges (Shalaeva et al., 2023). Providing individuals with information about their condition, treatment options, and the rationale behind recommendations empowers them to actively participate in their care. Limited health literacy, misunderstanding treatment goals, or skepticism about the effectiveness of interventions may hinder adherence. Clear and culturally sensitive communication can address these challenges. Having a plan for crisis management and relapse prevention is crucial. Individuals should be educated in recognizing early warning signs, accessing support during crises, and developing strategies to prevent relapse. Overcoming denial, recognizing relapse triggers, and actively implementing relapse prevention strategies can be challenging. Regularly revisiting and updating the relapse prevention plan supports ongoing adherence. Ensuring adherence and compliance with the treatment of drug abuse requires a collaborative and patient-centered approach. Healthcare providers, along with mental health professionals and support networks, play key roles in addressing barriers, promoting understanding, and fostering a therapeutic alliance that encourages individuals to actively engage in their recovery journey (Pinto et al., 2023).

Combination Therapies and Personalized Treatment: Combination therapies and personalized treatment plans are increasingly recognized as effective approaches in addressing drug abuse and substance use disorders. These approaches acknowledge the heterogeneity of individuals and the complex nature of substance abuse, recognizing that what works for one person may not work for another. A thorough assessment of an individual's medical, psychological, and social factors is essential to tailor treatment to their specific needs. This includes understanding the severity of the substance use disorder, co-occurring mental health conditions, and any other relevant factors. Healthcare providers conduct comprehensive assessments to identify unique challenges and strengths, which inform the development of a personalized treatment plan. Medications can play a crucial role in the treatment of substance use disorders. Depending on the substance involved and individual factors, medications may be prescribed to manage withdrawal symptoms, cravings, or co-occurring mental health conditions. Personalized treatment plans may involve the use of medications like methadone, buprenorphine, naltrexone, or acamprosate, depending on the specific substance and individual needs.

Various behavioral therapies can be effective in addressing the psychological aspects of substance use disorders. These interventions help individuals develop coping skills, identify triggers, and modify unhealthy behaviors. Cognitive-behavioral therapy (CBT), contingency management, motivational enhancement therapy, and dialectical behavior therapy (DBT) are among the behavioral interventions that may be incorporated into personalized treatment plans. Counseling and psychotherapy address underlying psychological issues, trauma, and co-occurring mental health disorders contributing to substance abuse. These interventions help individuals gain insight, develop healthier coping mechanisms, and improve overall well-being. Psychotherapeutic approaches, such as individual counseling, group therapy, or family therapy, are integrated based on the individual's needs and preferences. Supportive services, such as case management, vocational training, housing assistance, and legal support, can address the broader social determinants of substance use disorders. These services help create a stable and supportive environment for recovery. Personalized treatment plans may involve collaboration with social workers, case managers, and community organizations to address the individual's unique social and environmental challenges (Craft et al., 2023).

Peer support, such as 12-step programs or peer recovery support services, can provide individuals with a sense of community, shared experiences, and ongoing encouragement during their recovery journey. Including peer support in a personalized treatment plan can enhance social connectedness and reduce feelings of isolation. Holistic interventions, including mindfulness, yoga, and exercise, can contribute to overall well-being and stress reduction. These approaches address the interconnected nature of physical and mental health. Personalized treatment plans may incorporate holistic practices based on individual preferences and cultural considerations. Ongoing assessment and monitoring of an individual's progress are critical. Treatment plans should be flexible and subject to adjustment based on the individual's response to interventions and changing needs. Regular check-ins with healthcare providers and treatment teams help ensure that the treatment plan remains aligned with the individual's goals and evolving circumstances. Individuals with co-occurring mental health and substance use disorders require integrated treatment that addresses both conditions simultaneously. Personalized treatment plans for dual diagnosis may involve a combination of psychiatric medications, counseling, and specialized interventions designed to address the complexity of both disorders (Watts et al., 2023).

Cultural factors play a significant role in shaping individuals' beliefs, preferences, and approaches to treatment. Culturally competent care ensures that interventions are respectful, relevant, and inclusive. Implementation: Personalized treatment plans should consider cultural factors, taking into account the individual's background, values, and cultural preferences. Combination therapies and personalized treatment plans reflect a comprehensive and individualized approach to addressing drug abuse (Nguemeni Tiako et al., 2023). By tailoring interventions to the unique needs and circumstances of each person, these approaches increase the likelihood of successful outcomes in the journey toward recovery. Regular collaboration between healthcare providers, mental health professionals, and support networks is essential to adapt treatment plans as needed and provide ongoing encouragement and guidance.

Integration with Behavioral Interventions: The integration of drug addiction treatment with behavioral interventions is a comprehensive and effective approach that addresses both the physical aspects of addiction and the underlying behavioral and psychological factors that contribute to substance abuse. Behavioral interventions play a crucial role in helping individuals develop coping strategies, modify unhealthy behaviors, and build the skills necessary for sustained recovery. Cognitive-Behavioral Therapy (CBT) is a widely used behavioral intervention that helps individuals identify and change negative thought patterns and behaviors associated with substance abuse. It is effective in treating a range of substance use disorders. CBT can be integrated into drug addiction treatment programs as individual or group therapy sessions. It focuses on addressing distorted thinking, enhancing coping skills, and preventing relapse. Contingency management is a behavioral intervention that involves providing tangible rewards or incentives for positive behaviors, such as abstinence from drugs. It reinforces pro-recovery behaviors. This intervention can be integrated into treatment programs, offering rewards such as vouchers, prizes, or privileges for achieving and maintaining abstinence (Aklin et al., 2023).

Motivational Enhancement Therapy (MET) is a therapeutic approach that focuses on enhancing an individual's motivation to change by exploring and resolving ambivalence. It is often used to engage individuals in the early stages of treatment. MET can be integrated into drug addiction treatment by helping individuals explore their motivations for change, set goals, and strengthen their commitment to recovery. DBT is a comprehensive therapy that combines cognitive-behavioral techniques with mindfulness strategies. It is particularly useful for individuals with co-occurring substance use and mental health disorders. DBT can be integrated into treatment to address emotional dysregulation, impulsive behaviors, and difficulties in interpersonal relationships that contribute to substance abuse. Role in Integration: Involving families in treatment is crucial, as family dynamics can influence substance use. Family therapy addresses communication patterns, codependency issues, and provides support for the individual in recovery. Family therapy sessions can be incorporated into drug addiction treatment, involving family members in the recovery process and fostering a supportive environment (Magill et al., 2023).

Many individuals benefit from mutual support groups based on the 12-step model, such as Alcoholics Anonymous or Narcotics Anonymous. 12-step facilitation helps individuals engage with and derive support from these groups. Treatment programs can integrate 12-step facilitation by introducing individuals to these groups, discussing the principles, and helping them navigate the steps. Skills training focuses on teaching practical skills to enhance an individual's ability to cope with stress, manage emotions, and navigate social situations without resorting to substance use. Skill-building sessions can be integrated into drug addiction treatment to equip individuals with tools for handling challenging situations and preventing relapse. Relapse prevention strategies are essential to help individuals identify triggers, develop coping skills, and create a plan to maintain abstinence in the face of challenges. Relapse prevention can be integrated into drug addiction treatment through specific sessions or modules focused on recognizing and managing high-risk situations (Wolitzky-Taylor, 2023).

Many individuals with substance use disorders have a history of trauma. Trauma-informed care recognizes the impact of trauma on addiction and focuses on creating a safe and supportive treatment environment. Behavioral interventions within a trauma-informed framework address trauma-related issues, fostering healing and reducing the likelihood of substance use as a coping mechanism. Peer support, such as recovery coaching or peer mentorship, provides individuals with lived experience in recovery. Peer support reinforces positive behaviors, offers understanding, and promotes a sense of community. Peer support can be integrated into treatment programs by involving individuals in recovery as mentors, sponsors, or support group facilitators. The integration of drug addiction treatment with behavioral interventions requires a collaborative and individualized approach. Treatment programs should assess the unique needs of each individual and tailor behavioral interventions accordingly. A combination of these interventions, customized to address specific challenges and goals, enhances the overall effectiveness of drug addiction treatment and supports individuals in achieving lasting recovery. Regular collaboration between healthcare providers, mental health professionals, and support networks is essential to adapt treatment plans as needed and provide ongoing encouragement and guidance.

Future Directions and Emerging Trends: The field of drug addiction treatment is dynamic, and several future directions and emerging trends are shaping the way substance use disorders are addressed. These trends reflect advances in research, changes in societal attitudes, and innovations in healthcare. Tailoring treatment approaches based on an individual's unique genetic, biological, and psychosocial characteristics. Precision medicine aims to improve treatment outcomes by identifying the most effective interventions for specific individuals, reducing trial-and-error approaches. Expanding the use of telehealth and digital tools to provide remote access to treatment services, counseling, and support (Jordan et al., 2023) is a new approach, enhancing accessibility, especially in underserved areas, and offering flexibility in receiving treatment, particularly during times of public health crises.

Utilizing virtual reality (VR) technology for therapeutic interventions, exposure therapy, and skills training provides immersive and controlled environments for practicing coping skills, addressing cravings, and facilitating desensitization. Exploring and developing interventions that target specific neurobiological mechanisms involved in addiction. Advancements in understanding the neural circuitry of addiction may lead to novel pharmacotherapies and neuromodulation approaches. Developing new medications and refining existing ones to address various aspects of substance use disorders, including cravings, withdrawal symptoms, and relapse prevention facilitates continual research which aims to improve the efficacy, safety, and accessibility of medication-assisted treatments (MAT) for diverse substances (Marom et al., 2023). Promoting integration between mental health, primary care, and substance use disorder treatment to address co-occurring conditions comprehensively. Integrated care models improve coordination, enhance treatment engagement, and provide holistic support for individuals with complex needs.

Fostering environments are crucial that reduce stigma associated with substance use disorders and implementing trauma-informed care principles. It creates more supportive and empathetic treatment settings, recognizing the impact of trauma, and addressing the root causes of substance use. Empowering communities and leveraging peer support in the delivery of substance use disorder services recognizes the importance of community connections and the value of individuals with lived experience in supporting others through recovery. Addressing social and environmental factors that contribute to substance use, such as poverty, housing instability, and lack of access to education and employment address the broader societal issues that impact substance use can improve treatment outcomes and promote long-term recovery (Razaghi et al., 2023).

Expanding harm reduction strategies, including supervised consumption sites, needle exchange programs, and naloxone distribution should be strictly regulated. This would in turn reduce the negative consequences of substance use, preventing overdoses, and engaging individuals who may not be ready for traditional abstinence-focused treatment. Ensuring cultural competence in treatment settings and tailoring interventions to meet the diverse needs of individuals from various backgrounds is important (Kaviyani et al., 2023). It also helps to recognize respect cultural differences can enhance engagement, increase treatment retention, and improve outcomes.

Shifting policies toward decriminalization, diversion programs, and alternative approaches to incarceration for individuals with substance use disorders. Reducing the punitive aspects of the legal system can improve access to treatment, decrease stigma, and focus on public health approaches. These future directions and emerging trends highlight the evolving landscape of drug addiction treatment, emphasizing a shift toward more personalized, accessible, and comprehensive approaches. The integration of research findings, advancements in technology, and a greater understanding of the social determinants of substance use will likely continue to shape the field and improve outcomes for individuals seeking recovery from addiction. The pursuit of novel molecular pathways for drug addiction treatment represents a cutting-edge approach to address the complex neurobiological underpinnings of substance use disorders. Researchers are exploring innovative targets within the brain's intricate molecular landscape to identify key signaling pathways and neurochemical processes implicated in addiction. This endeavor involves investigating neurotransmitter systems, epigenetic modifications, neuroinflammatory responses, and neuroplasticity mechanisms. By delving into these novel molecular pathways, scientists aim to uncover potential therapeutic targets for drug development, paving the way for precision medicine in addiction treatment. This research not only holds promise for developing more effective pharmacotherapies but also contributes to a deeper understanding of the molecular basis of addiction, offering new insights into personalized and targeted interventions for individuals grappling with substance use disorders (Malik et al., 2023).

CHAPTER 11

CURRENT ADVANCEMENTS IN THE DIAGNOSTICS OF DRUG ADDICTION

"Anyone can give up; it is the easiest thing in the world to do. But to hold it together when everyone would expect you to fall apart, now that is true strength."
~ Chris Bradford

Immense challenges and resilience are required during the recovery process. Giving up or succumbing to the difficulties of overcoming addiction might seem like the path of least resistance, as it often involves coping with intense cravings, withdrawal symptoms, and potential relapses. This chapter explores that how evolving landscape of drug addiction diagnostics is marked by cutting-edge advancements that delve into the intricate nuances of neurobiology and behavioral science, offering more refined and targeted approaches to understanding and identifying substance use disorders. In the dynamic field of drug addiction diagnostics, current advancements showcase a convergence of technological innovations and neuroscientific insights, propelling the development of more accurate, personalized, and comprehensive tools for the assessment and diagnosis of individuals grappling with addictive behaviors.

Treating drug addiction poses several challenges, reflecting the complex nature of substance use disorders and the diverse factors influencing addiction. Stigmatization of individuals with substance use disorders can hinder their willingness to seek help and contribute to a lack of understanding among healthcare providers and the general public. Stigma may result in delayed or inadequate treatment, perpetuating the cycle of addiction. There is often a shortage of treatment facilities, particularly in certain geographic areas, leading to long waiting lists and limited access to evidence-based interventions. Delayed treatment can exacerbate the severity of addiction, increase the risk of overdose, and impede recovery efforts. Many individuals with substance use disorders also have co-occurring mental health conditions such as depression, anxiety, or trauma. Treating both addiction and co-occurring disorders concurrently is complex but crucial for successful outcomes. Failure to address underlying mental health issues may contribute to relapse

Biomarkers for Substance Use: Identifying biochemical markers in bodily fluids is a valuable approach for assessing drug addiction, providing insights into the physiological changes associated with substance use. Various substances and their metabolites can be detected in bodily fluids, such as blood, urine, and saliva, offering objective measures for diagnostic and monitoring purposes.

i. Urine biomarkers play a pivotal role in the diagnosis and monitoring of drug addiction, providing a non-invasive and widely utilized method for detecting the presence of substances and their metabolites. Various drugs, including opioids, cocaine, amphetamines, and cannabinoids, leave identifiable traces in urine, reflecting recent usage. Urine drug tests are commonly employed in clinical, forensic, and employment settings due to their convenience, reliability, and established protocols. Detection windows vary depending on the substance, with some tests capturing drug use within hours to days. Creatinine levels are often measured alongside drug screening to assess sample dilution. These urine biomarkers not only aid in confirming recent drug exposure but also contribute to treatment planning, intervention strategies, and the overall management of individuals with drug addiction. Despite their utility, it is important to consider the limitations of urine biomarkers, such as the potential for adulteration or the inability to provide a precise timeline of drug use. Integrating urine biomarker analysis with comprehensive clinical assessments enhances the understanding of an individual's substance use patterns, facilitating more informed and tailored approaches to addiction care. Urine biomarker analysis is widely employed in clinical and forensic settings due to its reliability and established protocols. This approach not only facilitates the detection of recent drug use but also supports treatment planning, monitoring, and interventions, contributing to comprehensive care for individuals grappling with drug addiction (Bharat et al., 2023). A few urine biomarkers associated with specific drugs are enlisted:

Morphine and Codeine: Metabolites of opioids like heroin are detectable in urine. Morphine is a major metabolite, and its presence indicates recent opioid use.

Oxycodone and Methadone: Prescription opioids, such as oxycodone and methadone, leave unique metabolites, like oxymorphone and EDDP (2-ethylidene-1,5-dimethyl-3,3-diphenylpyrrolidine).

Benzoylecgonine: Cocaine is rapidly metabolized in the body, and benzoylecgonine is its major urinary metabolite. Detection of benzoylecgonine indicates recent cocaine use.

Amphetamine and Methamphetamine: Urine tests can identify amphetamine and methamphetamine, commonly used stimulants. These drugs and their metabolites can be detected for a certain period after use.

THC-COOH: Tetrahydrocannabinol (THC), the psychoactive component in cannabis, is converted to its inactive metabolite THC-COOH. Detection of THC-COOH in urine signifies recent cannabis use.

Oxazepam, Nordiazepam, Temazepam: Different benzodiazepines have distinct metabolites, and urine tests can identify these metabolites to confirm recent use.

JWH-018, JWH-073: Some synthetic cannabinoids leave specific metabolites in urine, such as JWH-018 and JWH-073, which are commonly used markers for synthetic cannabinoid use.

Phencyclidine (PCP) and Its Metabolites: PCP and its metabolites, like 4-hydroxyphencyclidine (4-OH-PCP), can be detected in urine, indicating recent use of this dissociative hallucinogenic drug.

Secobarbital, Butalbital: Barbiturates, a class of sedative-hypnotic drugs, leave specific metabolites such as secobarbital and butalbital, detectable in urine.

EDDP (2-ethylidene-1,5-dimethyl-3,3-diphenylpyrrolidine): Methadone, used in opioid substitution therapy, is identified through the detection of its metabolite EDDP in urine.

Nortriptyline, Amitriptyline: Some tricyclic antidepressants leave identifiable metabolites in urine, such as nortriptyline and amitriptyline.

Ethyl Glucuronide (EtG), Ethyl Sulfate (EtS): Ethyl glucuronide and ethyl sulfate are alcohol metabolites that can be detected in urine for an extended period, providing insights into recent alcohol consumption.

Cotinine: Nicotine metabolizes into cotinine, which can be identified in urine. Cotinine levels reflect recent exposure to tobacco or nicotine-containing products.

It's essential to note that the detection windows for these biomarkers can vary, and factors such as hydration levels, metabolism, and individual variations can influence test results. Additionally, advances in analytical techniques continually improve the sensitivity and specificity of urine drug tests, enhancing their accuracy in identifying and monitoring substance use in individuals with drug addiction.

ii. Blood Biomarkers: Blood biomarkers in drug addiction play a pivotal role in providing objective and clinically relevant information about the impact of substance use on an individual's physiological health. These biomarkers offer a window into recent drug exposure, with tests capable of detecting specific substances and their metabolites, such as opioids, cocaine, cannabinoids, and more. Beyond confirming drug presence, blood biomarkers also illuminate potential consequences on organ systems. Liver function markers, including ALT, AST, and GGT, indicate possible hepatotoxicity linked to chronic substance abuse. Kidney function markers like BUN and creatinine help assess renal health. Cardiovascular biomarkers, such as troponin and CK, provide insights into potential cardiac strain associated with stimulant use. Inflammatory markers, hormones, electrolytes, and coagulation parameters offer a holistic view of the physiological repercussions of drug addiction. Monitoring these blood biomarkers not only aids in diagnosis but also guides tailored treatment plans, enabling healthcare professionals to address the specific health challenges individuals face in their journey towards recovery (Nazari et al., 2022). Few blood biomarkers are enlisted:

Drug and Metabolite Levels: Blood tests can detect the presence of drugs and their metabolites, offering information about recent substance use. This includes opioids, cocaine, amphetamines, cannabinoids, and other substances.

Alanine Aminotransferase (ALT) and Aspartate Aminotransferase (AST): Elevated levels may indicate liver damage, common in chronic substance abuse.

Gamma-Glutamyl Transferase (GGT): A marker of liver dysfunction associated with alcohol abuse.

Blood Urea Nitrogen (BUN) and Creatinine: Abnormal levels may suggest impaired kidney function, influenced by certain drugs and substances.

Troponin and Creatine Kinase (CK): Elevated levels may indicate cardiovascular strain or damage, particularly associated with stimulant drug use.

White Blood Cell Count (WBC), Red Blood Cell Count (RBC), Platelet Count: Changes can provide information about overall health and potential drug-related effects on the hematological system.

C-reactive Protein (CRP) and Interleukin-6 (IL-6): Elevated levels may indicate inflammation induced by chronic drug use.

Cortisol and Adrenaline: Dysregulation due to chronic substance use can impact the body's stress response system.

Thyroid Hormones: Substance abuse may affect thyroid function, leading to changes in hormone levels.

Sodium, Potassium, Calcium: Imbalances can occur due to dehydration or other physiological changes associated with drug use.

Arterial Blood Gas (ABG): Measures oxygen and carbon dioxide levels, providing information about respiratory function influenced by certain drugs.

Cholesterol, Triglycerides, High-Density Lipoprotein (HDL), Low-Density Lipoprotein (LDL): Substance abuse may impact lipid metabolism, leading to changes in the lipid profile.

Prothrombin Time (PT), Activated Partial Thromboplastin Time (APTT): Changes can occur with certain drug use and may affect blood clotting.

These blood biomarkers collectively contribute to a comprehensive understanding of the health implications of drug addiction. Regular monitoring of these markers enables healthcare professionals to assess organ function, identify potential complications, and tailor interventions to address the specific needs of individuals with substance use disorders. Advances in laboratory techniques continue to enhance the accuracy and sensitivity of blood biomarker assessments, further improving the precision of diagnostic and monitoring processes in the context of drug addiction.

iii. Saliva Biomarkers: Saliva biomarkers represent a non-invasive and convenient means of assessing drug addiction, offering real-time insights into recent substance use. With the ability to detect a variety of drugs and their metabolites, saliva biomarkers provide a comprehensive overview of an individual's drug exposure. Key substances, such as cannabinoids, cocaine, opioids, amphetamines, benzodiazepines, and alcohol, leave identifiable traces in saliva, enabling quick and efficient testing. The non-invasive nature of saliva collection makes it particularly advantageous for scenarios requiring immediate or frequent monitoring, such as roadside drug testing or workplace screenings. While saliva biomarkers offer simplicity and ease of collection, factors like detection windows and the potential for oral contamination should be considered. Overall, these biomarkers contribute significantly to the comprehensive diagnostic toolkit for drug addiction, aiding in timely interventions and personalized treatment strategies (Shreya et al., 2023). Key saliva biomarkers for drug addiction include:

THC-COOH (Cannabis): Tetrahydrocannabinol (THC), the psychoactive component in cannabis, is metabolized into THC-COOH, which can be detected in saliva. This biomarker is indicative of recent cannabis use.

Cocaine and Metabolites: Saliva tests can identify cocaine and its metabolites, such as benzoylecgonine, offering insights into recent cocaine use.

Opioids: Certain opioids and their metabolites, including morphine, can be detected in saliva. Saliva tests provide a non-invasive means of assessing opioid exposure.

Amphetamines and Methamphetamines: Amphetamines and methamphetamines, common stimulants, leave traces in saliva, allowing for the detection of recent use.

Benzodiazepines: Saliva tests can identify the presence of benzodiazepines and their metabolites, aiding in the assessment of sedative-hypnotic drug use.

Alcohol Biomarkers: Ethyl glucuronide (EtG) and ethyl sulfate (EtS) are alcohol metabolites detectable in saliva, providing information about recent alcohol consumption.

Nicotine and Cotinine: Nicotine and its metabolite cotinine can be measured in saliva, offering insights into tobacco or nicotine product use.

Illicit Drugs: Saliva biomarkers can detect various other illicit substances, including methadone, phencyclidine (PCP), and synthetic cannabinoids, providing a comprehensive assessment of drug exposure.

The advantages of saliva biomarkers include non-invasiveness, ease of collection, and reduced discomfort for the individual being tested. Saliva tests are particularly useful in settings where immediate or frequent monitoring is required, such as roadside drug testing or workplace screenings. While saliva biomarkers offer advantages in terms of simplicity and convenience, their detection windows may be shorter compared to urine or blood tests. Additionally, factors such as oral contamination or dilution can impact the accuracy of results. Despite these considerations, saliva biomarkers play a valuable role in the multifaceted approach to drug addiction detection and monitoring.

iv. Hair Biomarkers: Hair biomarkers serve as a valuable tool for assessing drug addiction, providing a unique retrospective perspective on an individual's substance use history. As hair grows, it incorporates substances and their metabolites, creating a chronological record of drug exposure over an extended period. Hair testing offers a longer detection window compared to other biological specimens like urine or blood. Depending on the length of hair sampled, it can provide insights into drug use patterns over several months to even years. Hair biomarkers can identify a wide range of substances, including illicit drugs such as cannabinoids, cocaine, opioids, amphetamines, and methamphetamines. Prescription medications and their metabolites can also be detected (Wade et al., 2023).

Drugs and their metabolites become trapped in the hair matrix during growth, providing a stable and durable record of substance exposure. This allows for the identification of chronic or repeated drug use. Hair testing allows for quantitative analysis, providing information not only on the presence or absence of substances but also on the concentration levels. This quantitative data can offer insights into the intensity and frequency of drug use. Collecting hair samples is a non-invasive procedure, and it does not require specialized handling or immediate testing. This makes it a practical and accessible method for assessing historical drug exposure. Hair biomarkers are commonly employed in forensic investigations and workplace drug testing, where a comprehensive understanding of an individual's drug use history is crucial for legal or employment-related decisions.

While hair testing provides a wealth of information, it is important to consider external contamination and variations in hair growth rates among individuals. Proper sample collection and preparation are essential to ensure accurate and reliable results. The use of hair biomarkers raises ethical and legal considerations, particularly regarding privacy and consent. Clear communication with individuals undergoing testing is essential to address these concerns. In summary, hair biomarkers offer a unique and informative perspective on an individual's drug exposure history, making them a valuable tool in the comprehensive assessment of drug addiction. While considerations such as detection windows and potential challenges exist, the non-invasiveness and long-term retrospective capabilities of hair testing contribute to its widespread use in various contexts, ranging from clinical settings to legal and employment-related scenarios.

v. Neurotransmitter Levels: Neurotransmitter levels serve as critical biomarkers for drug addiction, offering insights into the neurobiological changes associated with substance use. Neurotransmitters are chemical messengers that play a key role in communication between nerve cells in the brain. Chronic drug use can profoundly affect the balance and function of neurotransmitter systems, contributing to addictive behaviors. Dopamine is central to the brain's reward system, and its dysregulation is a hallmark of addiction. Many drugs, including cocaine, amphetamines, and opioids, increase dopamine levels, contributing to the reinforcing effects of substance use. Monitoring changes in dopamine levels or its metabolites can provide insights into the reward system's activity and the reinforcing effects of drugs.

Serotonin is involved in mood regulation, and its dysregulation is linked to conditions like depression and anxiety, often co-occurring with substance use disorders. Alterations in serotonin levels may indicate the impact of drug use on mood regulation and mental health. Glutamate is the primary excitatory neurotransmitter in the brain and is involved in learning and memory processes. Chronic drug use can affect glutamate transmission, contributing to drug-seeking behavior. Changes in glutamate levels may reflect neuroadaptive responses to chronic drug exposure and may influence cravings and relapse. GABA is the primary inhibitory neurotransmitter, and its dysregulation is implicated in withdrawal symptoms and heightened anxiety associated with drug dependence. Monitoring GABA levels can provide insights into the neurobiological adaptations that occur during drug withdrawal and the development of tolerance. Norepinephrine is involved in the body's stress response and arousal. Changes in norepinephrine levels are associated with the heightened stress response seen in addiction.

Dysregulation of norepinephrine may indicate the impact of chronic drug use on stress pathways and the development of stress-related cravings. Endorphins are endogenous opioids involved in pain modulation and pleasure. Chronic drug use can affect endorphin release, contributing to the development of opioid dependence. Assessing endorphin levels may provide insights into the neurochemical adaptations associated with opioid addiction (Abdullah et al., 2022; Wei et al., 2020; Volkow et al., 2019). Monitoring neurotransmitter levels as biomarkers in drug addiction helps researchers and clinicians understand the neurobiological mechanisms underlying substance use disorders. Advances in neuroimaging techniques and neurochemical assays allow for more precise measurement of neurotransmitter levels, enhancing our ability to characterize the neurobiology of addiction and develop targeted interventions to restore normal neurotransmitter function.

vi. Inflammatory Markers: Inflammatory markers serve as important biomarkers in the context of drug addiction, reflecting the intricate interplay between chronic substance use and the immune system. Prolonged drug abuse can induce systemic inflammation, impacting various organs and contributing to the progression of addiction-related disorders. Elevated C-Reactive Protein (CRP)levels are associated with systemic inflammation and are often observed in individuals with substance use disorders. Chronic drug use, especially opioids and stimulants, can contribute to increased CRP levels. Monitoring CRP provides insights into the overall inflammatory state and may indicate the systemic consequences of chronic substance abuse. IL-6 and IL-1β are pro-inflammatory cytokines involved in the immune response. Changes in their levels are linked to drug-induced neuroinflammation and the modulation of reward pathways. Elevated levels of interleukins may signify neuroinflammatory processes associated with chronic drug use and could contribute to mood disorders and addiction-related behaviors (Morcuende et al., 2021).

TNF-α is another pro-inflammatory cytokine associated with chronic drug use, particularly opioids and cocaine. It plays a role in the regulation of inflammation and immune responses. Measuring TNF-α levels helps assess the impact of drug-induced inflammation on physiological systems and its potential contribution to organ damage. Monocyte Chemoattractant Protein-1 (MCP-1) is a chemokine involved in the recruitment of immune cells. Elevated levels are observed in conditions associated with chronic drug use. Monitoring MCP-1 provides information on the recruitment of immune cells to sites of inflammation, which can be relevant in addiction-related organ damage. Proteins such as fibrinogen and serum amyloid A (SAA) are acute-phase reactants whose levels increase in response to inflammation. Elevated levels are observed in individuals with substance use disorders. Assessing acute-phase proteins contributes to understanding the systemic inflammatory response associated with chronic drug use (Wang et al., 2023).

Chronic drug use can lead to oxidative stress, contributing to inflammation and tissue damage. Markers such as malondialdehyde (MDA) and reactive oxygen species (ROS) are indicators of oxidative stress. Measuring oxidative stress markers helps evaluate the impact of drug-induced oxidative damage and inflammation on cellular health. The identification and monitoring of inflammatory markers provide a window into the broader health consequences of drug addiction. Beyond their role in inflammation, these markers are implicated in psychiatric comorbidities, cardiovascular complications, and neurodegenerative changes associated with chronic substance abuse. Understanding the inflammatory profile in individuals with drug addiction has implications for tailored interventions, including anti-inflammatory strategies, to mitigate the health risks associated with prolonged substance use.

vii. Hormones: Cortisol and adrenaline (epinephrine) play crucial roles as biomarkers in the context of drug addiction, serving as indicators of the complex interplay between chronic substance use and the stress response system. These stress hormones are integral components of the body's neuroendocrine system and are responsive to various psychoactive substances. Cortisol, often referred to as the "stress hormone," is released in response to stressors, including those induced by drug withdrawal and chronic substance use. Dysregulation of the hypothalamic-pituitary-adrenal (HPA) axis, which governs cortisol release, is observed in individuals with substance use disorders. Monitoring cortisol levels provides insights into the stress response system's activation, reflecting the psychological and physiological stress associated with drug addiction. Elevated cortisol levels may signify chronic stress, withdrawal symptoms, and disruptions in circadian rhythms commonly observed in addiction (Fitzpatrick-Schmidt et al., 2023).

Adrenaline is a key mediator of the body's "fight or flight" response, mobilizing energy resources in response to stress. Chronic drug use, especially stimulants like cocaine and amphetamines, can enhance adrenaline release, contributing to heightened arousal and increased heart rate. Elevated adrenaline levels may indicate the activation of the sympathetic nervous system, reflecting the physiological arousal and hyperstimulation associated with stimulant drug use. Monitoring adrenaline provides insights into the acute effects of drugs on the cardiovascular and central nervous systems. Synergistic Effects: Cortisol and adrenaline often work in tandem to orchestrate the body's stress response. Chronic drug use can dysregulate this interplay, leading to persistent activation of stress pathways. Examining the balance between cortisol and adrenaline levels helps unravel the intricate dynamics of the stress response in individuals with substance use disorders. Imbalances may contribute to the perpetuation of addictive behaviors and complicate the management of withdrawal symptoms.

Elevated cortisol and adrenaline levels are associated with chronic stress, which, in turn, increases the risk of relapse in individuals recovering from addiction. Monitoring stress hormone levels during addiction treatment can aid in identifying individuals at a higher risk of relapse, informing the development of targeted interventions to manage stress and improve long-term outcomes. In summary, cortisol and adrenaline serve as dynamic biomarkers reflecting the intricate connections between chronic substance use, stress responses, and the neuroendocrine system in drug addiction. Monitoring these stress hormones contributes to a deeper understanding of the physiological and psychological challenges individuals face during addiction and recovery, guiding personalized treatment strategies that address both the neurobiological and behavioral aspects of substance use disorders.

viii. Metabolic Markers: Metabolic markers play a significant role as biomarkers in the context of drug addiction, reflecting the impact of substance use on various metabolic processes in the body. Chronic drug abuse can lead to alterations in metabolism, affecting energy balance, nutrient utilization, and overall physiological health. Changes in Body Mass Index (BMI) i.e., body weight and composition are common in individuals with substance use disorders. Both weight loss and gain can occur, depending on the type of drug used. Monitoring BMI provides insights into nutritional status, metabolic health, and potential complications related to weight fluctuations, such as malnutrition or obesity. Some drugs, particularly stimulants like cocaine and methamphetamines, can affect glucose metabolism and insulin sensitivity. Opioids may influence glucose homeostasis as well. Assessing glucose and insulin levels helps identify metabolic disturbances and insulin resistance associated with certain substances, contributing to the understanding of the metabolic consequences of drug addiction (Ghantarchyan et al., 2023). Chronic drug use, including certain opioids and stimulants, can influence lipid metabolism, leading to changes in cholesterol and triglyceride levels. Monitoring lipid profiles provides information about cardiovascular risk factors and potential metabolic complications associated with substance abuse. Role in Addiction: Many drugs, particularly those metabolized by the liver, can impact liver function. Chronic alcohol and certain drugs contribute to liver enzyme elevations. Elevated liver enzymes, such as alanine aminotransferase (ALT), aspartate aminotransferase (AST), and gamma-glutamyl transferase (GGT), indicate potential liver damage and play a role in assessing the hepatic consequences of substance use. Substance abuse can affect thyroid function, influencing the levels of thyroid hormones such as thyroxine (T4) and triiodothyronine (T3). Assessing thyroid hormone levels helps identify potential disruptions in metabolism and energy regulation associated with drug addiction (Zhuo et al., 2019). Monitoring these metabolic markers provides a comprehensive view of the physiological impact of drug addiction on the body. It aids in identifying potential complications, guiding interventions to address metabolic disturbances, and improving overall healthcare for individuals with substance use disorders.

ix. Genetic and Epigenetic Markers: Genetic and epigenetic markers play crucial roles in understanding the susceptibility, development, and progression of drug addiction. These markers provide insights into the interplay between genetic factors and environmental influences, shedding light on the underlying biological mechanisms of substance use disorders. Genetic variations in enzymes responsible for drug metabolism, such as cytochrome P450 enzymes, can influence an individual's response to specific substances. Variants in these genes may impact the rate of drug metabolism and contribute to variability in drug effects. Genetic variations in receptors targeted by drugs, such as dopamine receptors in the case of stimulants, can influence an individual's susceptibility to the reinforcing effects of substances. Specific genes, such as those involved in neurotransmitter regulation (e.g., DRD2, OPRM1), have been identified as risk factors for addiction. Variations in these genes may contribute to individual differences in vulnerability to substance use disorders (Picci et al., 2022).

Epigenetic modifications, such as DNA methylation, can regulate gene expression. Changes in DNA methylation patterns at specific gene loci associated with addiction-related pathways may influence susceptibility to substance abuse. Epigenetic modifications of histone proteins can alter chromatin structure and gene expression. Histone acetylation or methylation in regions related to reward pathways and stress responses may be implicated in addiction. MicroRNAs (miRNAs) are small non-coding RNAs that regulate gene expression post-transcriptionally. Altered expression of miRNAs in response to drug exposure can impact the expression of genes involved in addiction-related processes. The interplay between genetic factors and environmental influences is crucial in addiction susceptibility. Certain genetic variants may confer increased vulnerability to substance use disorders, particularly in the presence of specific environmental stressors or exposures. Genes involved in the stress response, such as those regulated by the hypothalamic-pituitary-adrenal (HPA) axis, may show altered expression in individuals exposed to chronic stress or trauma, contributing to addiction risk (Gim et al., 2023).

BDNF (Brain-Derived Neurotrophic Factor) is involved in neuroplasticity and synaptic function. Genetic variations in BDNF may impact neural circuits related to reward and motivation, influencing susceptibility to addiction. FosB and ΔFosB genes are associated with long-term changes in neuronal activity and have been implicated in the development of addiction-related behaviors. Understanding the role of genetic and epigenetic markers in drug addiction is critical for personalized approaches to prevention and treatment. These markers not only contribute to the identification of individuals at higher risk but also offer insights into potential targets for therapeutic interventions. Advances in genomic and epigenomic research continue to enhance our understanding of the complex interplay between genetics, epigenetics, and environmental factors in the etiology of drug addiction (de Lucca et al., 2023). Identifying and interpreting these biochemical markers in bodily fluids requires a multidisciplinary approach involving clinicians, laboratory specialists, and addiction experts. Integrating this information with clinical assessments contributes to a comprehensive understanding of an individual's substance use history, aiding in diagnosis, treatment planning, and ongoing monitoring in the context of addiction care.

Integration of biomarker data for comprehensive diagnostics in drug abuse holds immense promise for advancing comprehensive diagnostics in the field of drug abuse. By combining information from various biomarkers, researchers and clinicians gain a more holistic understanding of the complex interplay between biological, psychological, and environmental factors contributing to substance use disorders. Comprehensive diagnostic approaches leverage multiple types of biomarkers, including genetic, epigenetic, neurochemical, and metabolic markers, to provide a nuanced and personalized assessment of an individual's vulnerability to addiction, the progression of the disorder, and potential treatment outcomes (Grove et al., 2023). The integration of genetic and epigenetic markers allows for a more precise characterization of an individual's predisposition to drug abuse. Genetic variations influencing drug metabolism, receptor sensitivity, and overall susceptibility to addiction can be combined with epigenetic modifications that reflect environmental influences on gene expression. This multifaceted approach enables the identification of specific genetic and epigenetic signatures associated with increased risk, potentially facilitating early intervention and targeted prevention strategies. Moreover, the integration of neurochemical markers, such as neurotransmitter levels and stress hormones, provides insights into the neurobiological changes occurring in response to chronic substance use. Monitoring changes in these markers aids in understanding the impact of drugs on the central nervous system and helps guide interventions tailored to address neurochemical imbalances (Murnane et al., 2023).

Incorporating metabolic markers further enhances the comprehensiveness of diagnostics by offering information on the physiological consequences of drug abuse. Metabolic markers can reveal alterations in glucose homeostasis, lipid metabolism, and liver function, providing a broader perspective on the systemic effects of substance use. This integration allows for the identification of potential co-occurring health conditions and guides the development of interventions that address both addiction and associated metabolic complications (Bodaghi et al., 2023). By amalgamating diverse biomarker data, comprehensive diagnostics not only improve the accuracy of addiction assessments but also pave the way for precision medicine approaches, where treatment plans can be tailored based on an individual's unique biological profile. As research in biomarker science continues to advance, the integration of diverse data sources will play a pivotal role in refining diagnostic tools and advancing personalized treatment strategies for individuals affected by drug abuse.

Neuroimaging Techniques: Neuroimaging techniques play a pivotal role in comprehensive diagnostics for drug abuse, offering valuable insights into the structural and functional alterations within the brain associated with substance use disorders. These advanced imaging technologies provide a non-invasive means to examine the impact of drugs on neural circuits, aiding in the identification, characterization, and treatment of addiction.

Functional Magnetic Resonance Imaging (fMRI) plays a crucial role in comprehensive diagnostics for drug abuse, offering a powerful tool to investigate the neural correlates of addiction. fMRI enables researchers and clinicians to observe and analyze changes in blood flow and oxygenation levels in the brain, providing insights into functional brain activity associated with drug use. fMRI is instrumental in mapping brain regions involved in reward processing, such as the nucleus accumbens and ventral tegmental area. These areas are central to the brain's reward circuit, implicated in the reinforcing effects of drugs. Aberrant activation patterns in these regions can serve as biomarkers, indicating dysregulation of reward pathways and potential susceptibility to addictive behaviors. fMRI is employed to study responses to drug-related cues and cues associated with drug reward. This helps in understanding the neural mechanisms underlying craving and the risk of relapse. Altered activation in regions like the prefrontal cortex, amygdala, and hippocampus during cue exposure can be indicative of heightened craving and vulnerability to relapse (Pollard et al., 2023).

fMRI is utilized to investigate the neural processes underlying decision-making and impulse control, which are often impaired in individuals with substance use disorders. Dysfunctional activation in prefrontal regions, such as the dorsolateral prefrontal cortex, can indicate compromised executive functions, contributing to impulsive behaviors and poor decision-making associated with drug addiction. Emotional dysregulation is a common feature in addiction. fMRI helps study emotional processing circuits, including the amygdala and prefrontal regions. Abnormal responses in these regions may signify emotional dysregulation, contributing to the development and maintenance of addictive behaviors. Resting-state fMRI explores intrinsic connectivity networks (Wang et al., 2023), revealing patterns of functional connectivity between brain regions even in the absence of explicit tasks. Altered resting-state connectivity, such as disruptions in the default mode network, can provide information about the brain's functional organization and may be associated with addiction-related behaviors.

fMRI can be integrated into neurofeedback interventions, allowing individuals to regulate their own brain activity. This approach holds promise for addiction treatment by targeting specific neural circuits. Neurofeedback based on fMRI data enables individuals to learn self-regulation strategies (Vargas et al., 2023), potentially aiding in the modification of maladaptive brain patterns associated with drug abuse. fMRI contributes significantly to the comprehensive diagnostics of drug abuse by providing a window into the neural underpinnings of addiction-related behaviors. The information obtained from fMRI studies enhances our understanding of the complex neurobiology of substance use disorders, facilitating the development of targeted interventions and personalized treatment strategies for individuals struggling with drug addiction.

Structural Magnetic Resonance Imaging (sMRI) is a valuable tool for comprehensive diagnostics in drug abuse, offering insights into the structural integrity and anatomical changes within the brain associated with substance use disorders. By visualizing and quantifying alterations in brain structures, sMRI provides crucial information for understanding the impact of drug abuse on neural morphology. sMRI allows for the visualization of gray matter structures, such as the hippocampus, amygdala, and prefrontal cortex, which are implicated in addiction-related processes. Reductions in gray matter volume in specific regions may indicate neurodegenerative changes associated with chronic substance use, providing insights into cognitive and emotional dysregulation. sMRI, particularly diffusion tensor imaging (DTI), enables the examination of white matter tracts, assessing their integrity and connectivity. Disruptions in white matter integrity, commonly observed in fiber bundles like the corpus callosum, may signify impaired communication between brain regions involved in addiction-related behaviors and cognitive functions (Vargas et al., 2023).

sMRI is instrumental in mapping regions of brain atrophy, which may result from neurotoxic effects of certain substances, especially alcohol and methamphetamines. The extent and location of atrophy can serve as biomarkers of structural damage, informing the severity and progression of neural consequences associated with substance abuse. Enlargement of cerebral ventricles, often detected through sMRI, is indicative of overall brain volume loss. Ventricular enlargement can be a biomarker of generalized brain atrophy and may correlate with cognitive deficits observed in individuals with substance use disorders. The hippocampus is crucial for memory and learning processes, and sMRI enables the detection of structural changes in this region. Biomarker Implications: Hippocampal atrophy or alterations in volume may be associated with memory deficits and cognitive impairments observed in individuals with substance use disorders, particularly in chronic alcohol abuse (Wadsley et al.,2023).

sMRI can measure cortical thickness, providing information about changes in the outer layer of the brain associated with cognitive functions. Reduced cortical thickness, especially in prefrontal regions, may be indicative of impaired executive functions and decision-making, common features in addiction. sMRI helps localize structural abnormalities, lesions, or focal damage resulting from drug-induced neurotoxicity. The precise localization of structural abnormalities aids in understanding the specific brain regions affected by substance use, contributing to targeted interventions and treatment planning. sMRI is an essential component of comprehensive diagnostics in drug abuse, providing critical structural information that complements functional and molecular assessments. The structural insights obtained through sMRI contribute to a more comprehensive understanding of the neural consequences of substance use disorders, guiding interventions, and facilitating personalized treatment strategies for individuals affected by drug abuse.

Positron Emission Tomography (PET) is a powerful imaging technique that plays a vital role in comprehensive diagnostics for drug abuse. PET allows for the visualization and quantification of molecular and cellular processes within the brain, providing valuable insights into neurochemical and metabolic changes associated with substance use disorders. Dopamine receptor imaging in the brain could be performed by PET, particularly the D2 receptors in the striatum. Changes in dopamine receptor availability are associated with reward processing and are crucial in understanding the neurobiological basis of addiction. Altered dopamine receptor binding is observed in various substance use disorders, including those involving stimulants and opioids. PET allows for the imaging of serotonin receptors, providing insights into the serotonergic system. Dysregulation of serotonin receptors is implicated in mood disorders and can be relevant in the context of substance abuse, particularly substances like MDMA (ecstasy) that affect serotonin transmission (Nerella et al., 2023).

PET with 18F-fluorodeoxyglucose (FDG) can measure glucose metabolism in the brain, providing information about regional cerebral metabolic rates. Altered glucose metabolism patterns are indicative of changes in neuronal activity and are observed in individuals with substance use disorders. This can help identify brain regions affected by chronic drug use. PET can image opioid receptors, offering insights into the endogenous opioid system. Changes in opioid receptor availability may be associated with opioid use disorders and can be relevant for understanding the neurobiology of opioid addiction. PET imaging with radioligands targeting microglial activation can assess neuroinflammation. Chronic drug use can lead to neuroinflammation, and PET can identify regions of increased microglial activation (Rong et al., 2023). This information is crucial for understanding the consequences of prolonged substance abuse on brain health.

PET can be utilized to image tau and amyloid aggregates, which are associated with neurodegenerative processes. In certain cases, individuals with substance use disorders may exhibit accelerated neurodegeneration. PET imaging of tau and amyloid provides insights into potential comorbidities and long-term consequences of drug abuse. PET can image neurotransmitter transporters, such as the dopamine transporter (DAT) and serotonin transporter (SERT). Changes in transporter availability are indicative of alterations in neurotransmitter reuptake mechanisms, which can be associated with specific drugs of abuse. PET imaging, with its ability to probe molecular and functional changes in the brain, enhances the understanding of the neurobiology of addiction. By providing quantitative data on neurotransmitter systems, metabolic activity, and neuroinflammatory processes, PET contributes to a comprehensive assessment of the neural consequences of drug abuse. This information is crucial for tailoring interventions, monitoring treatment responses, and advancing our understanding of the complex relationship between substance use and brain function.

Single-Photon Emission Computed Tomography (SPECT) is a valuable imaging technique that contributes to comprehensive diagnostics in drug abuse. SPECT provides insights into cerebral perfusion, allowing for the assessment of blood flow and functional activity in the brain. SPECT is particularly useful for imaging cerebral perfusion, providing information about regional blood flow in the brain. Altered perfusion patterns can indicate changes in neural activity, helping to identify regions affected by chronic drug use and offering insights into the functional consequences of substance abuse. SPECT can help identify focal brain lesions or abnormalities resulting from drug-induced neurotoxicity.

The detection of structural abnormalities aids in understanding the specific brain regions affected by substance use, contributing to targeted interventions and treatment planning. SPECT allows for the exploration of regional brain function by assessing blood flow in specific brain areas associated with addiction. Changes in perfusion in regions such as the prefrontal cortex, striatum, and limbic system may provide insights into the neurobiological underpinnings of addiction-related behaviors (Hussain et al., 2022). SPECT is well-suited for assessing prefrontal cortex function, which is crucial for decision-making, impulse control, and emotional regulation. Dysfunctional perfusion in the prefrontal cortex may contribute to impaired executive functions observed in individuals with substance use disorders, impacting their ability to make informed decisions. SPECT can identify regional changes in blood flow associated with acute or chronic drug use. Variations in blood flow patterns may provide information about the acute effects of drugs on the central nervous system and contribute to the understanding of substance-specific neuronal responses. SPECT can be used to assess thalamic function, a region involved in relaying sensory and motor signals and implicated in addiction. Altered thalamic perfusion may be associated with sensory and motor disturbances observed in individuals with substance use disorders, influencing their experiences and responses to drugs. SPECT can be employed to monitor changes in cerebral perfusion in response to addiction treatment. Tracking improvements or alterations in regional blood flow during treatment provides valuable feedback on the effectiveness of interventions and aids in refining therapeutic strategies (Murnane et al., 2023).

SPECT, with its ability to assess regional cerebral perfusion, complements other neuroimaging techniques in offering a comprehensive view of the neurobiological consequences of drug abuse. By providing functional insights into brain activity and blood flow patterns, SPECT contributes to the understanding of addiction-related changes, guiding diagnostics, and facilitating targeted interventions for individuals affected by substance use disorders.

Diffusion Tensor Imaging (DTI) is a specialized magnetic resonance imaging (MRI) technique that plays a significant role in comprehensive diagnostics for drug abuse. DTI allows for the visualization and quantification of white matter tracts in the brain by measuring the diffusion of water molecules. This imaging modality provides insights into the structural connectivity and integrity of neural pathways, offering valuable information about the impact of drug abuse on the brain's white matter. DTI is particularly well-suited for assessing white matter integrity by examining the microstructural properties of fiber bundles. Disruptions in white matter integrity, such as alterations in fractional anisotropy (FA) and mean diffusivity (MD), may indicate structural changes associated with chronic drug use, affecting communication between brain regions.

DTI enables the identification of abnormalities in specific fiber tracts, including those connecting regions implicated in addiction. Changes in the integrity of major fiber tracts, such as the corpus callosum, fornix, and cingulum bundle, can be indicative of alterations in connectivity related to substance use. DTI contributes to mapping the structural connectivity of the brain by visualizing the pathways of white matter tracts. Altered connectivity patterns may be associated with disruptions in neural circuits implicated in reward processing, decision-making, and impulse control, providing insights into addiction-related behaviors. DTI allows for the assessment of longitudinal changes in white matter microstructure over the course of substance use and abstinence. Biomarker Implications: Monitoring longitudinal changes provides information about the progression of structural alterations associated with drug abuse and potential recovery trajectories (Gaudreault et al., 2023).

DTI is instrumental in investigating the connectivity between cortical and subcortical structures, revealing the impact of substance use on critical neural pathways. Changes in connectivity between the prefrontal cortex and subcortical regions, such as the striatum, may contribute to executive dysfunction and impaired impulse control in individuals with substance use disorders. DTI provides quantitative measures of axonal integrity, offering insights into the condition of neural pathways. Disruptions in axonal integrity, reflected in metrics like axial diffusivity and radial diffusivity, may indicate degenerative processes associated with chronic drug use. DTI findings can be correlated with behavioral measures, such as cognitive performance and impulsivity. Associations between white matter alterations and behavioral outcomes provide a bridge between structural changes and functional consequences, enhancing our understanding of the neural basis of addiction. DTI, as part of comprehensive neuroimaging assessments, contributes crucial information about the structural consequences of drug abuse on the brain's white matter architecture. The detailed insights provided by DTI enhance the understanding of neural connectivity disruptions and guide the development of targeted interventions and personalized treatment strategies for individuals affected by substance use disorders (Hampton et al., 2023).

Advances in neuroimaging have significantly enhanced our understanding of addiction mechanisms by providing unprecedented insights into the neural processes underlying substance use disorders. These technological developments have allowed researchers and clinicians to investigate the complex interplay of neurotransmitters, neural circuits, and structural changes associated with addiction. High-resolution structural imaging techniques, such as ultra-high-field magnetic resonance imaging (MRI), offer detailed views of brain anatomy, enabling the identification of subtle structural alterations associated with addiction. These advancements help researchers pinpoint specific brain regions affected by chronic drug use and provide a more accurate assessment of neuroanatomical changes, contributing to a comprehensive understanding of addiction-related neural adaptations (Murnane et al., 2023).

Functional connectivity mapping using resting-state fMRI has become more sophisticated, allowing researchers to examine how different brain regions communicate and coordinate during rest (Dong et al., 2023). This advancement has provided insights into the disruptions in functional connectivity networks associated with addiction, revealing alterations in the default mode network, salience network, and other circuits implicated in reward processing and decision-making. PET imaging with radioligands targeting specific neurotransmitter systems, such as dopamine, serotonin, and opioid receptors, has become more precise and sensitive (Murnane et al., 2023). Improved neurotransmitter-specific imaging has facilitated a deeper understanding of how drugs of abuse directly affect receptor availability, synaptic transmission, and reward circuitry, shedding light on the neurochemical basis of addiction.

Advancement: Advanced diffusion imaging techniques, including diffusion spectrum imaging (DSI) and high-angular-resolution diffusion imaging (HARDI), offer more detailed information about white matter tracts (Obara et al., 2023). These techniques allow for a finer assessment of white matter integrity, offering insights into the structural connectivity disruptions associated with drug abuse and their implications for neural communication. Integration of multiple neuroimaging modalities, such as combining structural MRI, functional MRI, PET, and DTI data, enables a comprehensive examination of the neurobiological changes in addiction (Vermeulen et al., 2022). Multimodal imaging approaches provide a holistic view of how different aspects of brain structure and function interact in individuals with substance use disorders, offering a more nuanced understanding of addiction mechanisms. Machine learning algorithms and computational models are increasingly applied to neuroimaging data to identify patterns, predict treatment outcomes, and classify individuals based on their addiction vulnerability. These approaches enhance the extraction of meaningful information from complex neuroimaging datasets, paving the way for personalized diagnostics, treatment planning, and outcome prediction in addiction research. Real-time fMRI and neurofeedback technologies allow individuals to observe and modulate their brain activity, providing a novel tool for addiction treatment (Bloom et al., 2023). Real-time neurofeedback has applications in addiction therapy by enabling individuals to learn self-regulation strategies, potentially aiding in the modification of maladaptive brain patterns associated with substance use. These advances collectively contribute to a more nuanced understanding of addiction mechanisms, moving beyond the traditional focus on specific brain regions to consider complex network dynamics and individual variability. As technology continues to evolve, neuroimaging will likely play a central role in uncovering the intricate neurobiology of addiction, guiding the development of targeted interventions and personalized treatment strategies.

Behavioral Assessments and Psychometric Tools: Behavioral assessments and psychometric tools are essential components of comprehensive diagnostics in drug abuse, providing valuable information about an individual's behavior, psychological functioning, and the impact of substance use on various domains. These assessments aid in understanding the severity of substance use disorders, co-occurring mental health issues, and treatment needs. Addiction Severity Index (ASI) assesses the severity of problems in various life domains, including drug and alcohol use, medical, employment, and legal issues (Lindner et al., 2024). It provides a comprehensive profile of an individual's substance use and associated problems, guiding treatment planning and resource allocation.

Drug Abuse Screening Test (DAST-10) is a self-report tool that assesses the extent of drug use and identifies individuals at risk for substance use disorders (V et al., 2023). It is a quick and effective screening tool used in various settings to identify individuals who may require further assessment and intervention. Alcohol Use Disorders Identification Test (AUDIT) is a screening tool specifically designed to identify individuals with hazardous or harmful alcohol use (Duffy et al., 2023). It assesses alcohol consumption patterns, dependence symptoms, and negative consequences, aiding in the identification of alcohol-related issues. Severity of Dependence Scale (SDS) evaluates the severity of dependence on specific substances (Rotermann, 2023). It provides a quantitative measure of substance dependence, assisting in treatment planning and monitoring changes in dependence severity over time.

Beck Depression Inventory (BDI) and Beck Anxiety Inventory (BAI) are self-report measures assessing the severity of depression and anxiety symptoms, respectively (do Nascimento et al., 2023). These tools help identify co-occurring mental health issues common in individuals with substance use disorders, informing integrated treatment approaches. Substance Use Risk Profile Scale (SURPS) assesses personality traits associated with substance use risk, including sensation-seeking, impulsivity, anxiety sensitivity, and hopelessness (Mahu et al., 2023). It provides insights into individual vulnerabilities that may contribute to substance use and can guide targeted prevention and intervention strategies. Timeline Follow-Back (TLFB) is a retrospective calendar-based method used to gather detailed information about an individual's substance use over a specific period (McCann et al., 2024). It aids in assessing patterns of substance use, identifying triggers, and evaluating changes in use over time, supporting treatment planning and monitoring.

CAGE Questionnaire is a brief screening tool for identifying alcohol-related issues (Edwards et al., 2023). It consists of four questions related to cutting down on drinking, annoyance by criticism, guilt about drinking, and eye-openers. A positive score suggests the need for further assessment. Kessler Psychological Distress Scale (K10) assesses psychological distress and is widely used to screen for mental health issues (Landry et al., 2023). It helps identify individuals with elevated levels of distress, facilitating early intervention for co-occurring mental health and substance use disorders. Michigan Alcohol Screening Test (MAST) is a self-report tool designed to assess alcohol-related problems (Woodward et al., 2023). It evaluates the consequences of alcohol use, providing a comprehensive overview of an individual's relationship with alcohol and guiding intervention strategies.

These behavioral assessments and psychometric tools, when used in combination with clinical interviews and other diagnostic measures, contribute to a comprehensive understanding of an individual's substance use and associated challenges. They assist clinicians in tailoring treatment plans, monitoring progress, and addressing co-occurring issues to improve overall outcomes in the context of drug abuse.

Emerging Technologies: Emerging technologies are revolutionizing comprehensive diagnostics in drug abuse, offering innovative tools to enhance understanding, assessment, and treatment of substance use disorders. Technologies such as mobile health (mHealth) applications, wearable devices, and digital phenotyping leverage real-time data collection to monitor and analyze individuals' behaviors, moods, and physiological responses related to substance use. Virtual reality (VR) and neuroimaging techniques provide novel insights into the neurobiological underpinnings of addiction, allowing for more precise diagnostics. Additionally, advances in machine learning and artificial intelligence enable the integration of diverse data sources for predictive analytics and personalized treatment approaches. These technologies not only enhance the accuracy of diagnostic assessments but also pave the way for more targeted and effective interventions in the evolving landscape of drug abuse.

Smartphone applications and digital phenotyping leverage sensors and behavioral data to monitor and analyze patterns related to substance use, mood, and daily activities. Neurofeedback and brain-computer interfaces are technologies that provide real-time feedback on brain activity, allowing individuals to self-regulate neural patterns associated with substance use. Virtual Reality (VR) and Augmented Reality (AR) platforms are used for immersive experiences and simulations, aiding in exposure therapy, relapse prevention, and behavioral interventions. Wearable technologies and biosensors monitor physiological parameters and detect biomarkers associated with substance use (Yuan et al., 2023). These emerging technologies represent a dynamic field with ongoing developments. As the research and applications in these areas progress, new references and studies will continue to contribute to the understanding and implementation of comprehensive diagnostics in drug abuse.

Challenges and Considerations: Comprehensive diagnostics in drug abuse face several challenges and considerations that span biological, psychological, social, and technological dimensions. Stigma associated with substance use remains a significant hurdle, influencing the accuracy of self-reported data. The diversity of substances and the prevalence of polydrug use introduce complexity, making it challenging to develop universal diagnostic criteria. Individual differences, cultural variations, and disparities in access to diagnostics and treatment also pose considerable challenges. The dynamic nature of drug trends, ethical concerns regarding privacy, and the integration of biological and behavioral data further contribute to the complexity of comprehensive diagnostics in drug abuse. Navigating these challenges necessitates a multidisciplinary approach that considers the evolving nature of substance use and acknowledges the diverse factors influencing addiction (Mardani et al., 2023).

Stigma associated with substance use can hinder accurate self-reporting and disclosure of drug use, leading to underreporting and biased diagnostic assessments. Many individuals engage in polydrug use, complicating diagnostic efforts by introducing multiple substances with varying effects and interactions. Substance use disorders manifest differently across individuals, and the heterogeneity of symptoms can make it challenging to develop universal diagnostic criteria. Cultural variations in drug use patterns and expressions of distress may not be adequately captured by standardized diagnostic tools, emphasizing the need for cultural sensitivity. Disparities in access to comprehensive diagnostics and treatment services can limit the effectiveness of interventions, particularly in underserved populations (Swimmer & Sandelich, 2024). Rapid changes in drug markets and the emergence of novel substances pose challenges for diagnostic tools that may not capture evolving patterns of substance use.

The dynamic nature of drug trends, including the rise of designer drugs and novel psychoactive substances, can outpace the development of diagnostic tools. Ethical concerns related to privacy, confidentiality, and potential legal implications need careful consideration in the design and implementation of comprehensive diagnostics. Integrating biological and behavioral data poses challenges in terms of standardization, interpretation, and ensuring the ethical use of sensitive information. The use of emerging technologies for diagnostics introduces concerns related to data security, privacy, and the responsible use of technology (Mintz Hemed et al., 2023). Comprehensive diagnostics in drug abuse face several challenges and considerations that span biological, psychological, social, and technological domains. These challenges can impact the accuracy and effectiveness of assessments and necessitate careful consideration in the development and implementation of diagnostic strategies. Addressing these challenges and considerations requires a multidisciplinary and holistic approach to drug abuse diagnostics, taking into account the diverse factors influencing substance use and its associated disorders. It also highlights the importance of ongoing research, collaboration, and adaptability in the field of addiction diagnostics.

Future Directions: Future directions in comprehensive diagnostics for drug abuse hold exciting possibilities for advancing our understanding and refining assessment methodologies. The integration of precision medicine, incorporating genetic, epigenetic, and neurobiological markers, promises more individualized approaches. The use of advanced technologies, such as virtual reality for immersive simulations and ecological momentary assessment through mobile health applications, offers real-time insights into individuals' behaviors and environmental factors. Multimodal assessment approaches that combine biological, psychological, and behavioral data may provide a more holistic understanding. Additionally, the application of big data analytics and the exploration of cognitive and emotional assessments showcase promising avenues for refining diagnostics. These future-oriented endeavors reflect a dynamic landscape where innovation and multidisciplinary collaboration aim to enhance the accuracy and effectiveness of drug abuse diagnostics.

Tailoring diagnostic approaches based on individual characteristics, including genetic, epigenetic, and neurobiological markers, to enhance precision medicine in addiction treatment. Advancing the integration of neuroimaging techniques with other advanced technologies, such as machine learning and real-time neurofeedback, for more accurate and dynamic diagnostics. Utilizing mobile technologies and ecological momentary assessment to collect real-time data on individuals' behaviors, moods, and environmental factors for more ecologically valid diagnostics. Developing and implementing multimodal assessment approaches that combine biological, psychological, and behavioral data to provide a comprehensive understanding of substance use disorders. Leveraging big data analytics and integrating data from diverse sources (genetic, clinical, behavioral) to identify patterns, risk factors, and treatment responses on a large scale. Expanding the use of virtual reality as a diagnostic tool and therapeutic intervention to simulate real-world scenarios and assess and treat substance use disorders. Further refining cognitive and emotional assessments to better understand decision-making processes, impulsivity, and emotional regulation in the context of substance use. Conducting longitudinal studies to investigate developmental trajectories of substance use disorders, identifying critical periods for intervention and personalized treatment strategies. Incorporating global perspectives and adapting diagnostic tools to different cultural contexts to enhance the validity and reliability of assessments worldwide.

Focusing on the development of diagnostics that facilitate early identification of risk factors and the implementation of preventive and early intervention strategies. The field of comprehensive diagnostics in drug abuse is continuously evolving, and several future directions show promise for advancing our understanding and assessment of substance use disorders. These future directions represent a dynamic and evolving landscape in the field of drug abuse diagnostics, with ongoing research and innovations expected to shape the next generation of assessment tools and interventions.

CHAPTER 12

CURRENT ADVANCEMENTS IN THE PHARMACOTHERAPY OF DRUG ADDICTION

"Sometimes, you can only find Heaven by slowly backing away from Hell."
~ Carrie Fisher

Finding peace and positive change may require a deliberate and measured distancing from the detrimental behaviors, substances, and environments that contribute to the individual's struggles. Even when someone is mired in the difficulties of addiction, a pathway to a better life exists through a patient and step-by-step retreat from the negative elements that contribute to their challenges. The ever-evolving landscape of drug addiction treatment is marked by groundbreaking advancements in pharmacotherapy, ushering in a new era of precision and effectiveness in addressing the complexities of substance use disorders. At the forefront of combating drug addiction, current advancements in pharmacotherapy present a paradigm shift, leveraging cutting-edge research and innovative medications to provide more targeted and personalized interventions for individuals navigating the challenges of substance abuse.

Current advancements in the pharmacotherapy of drug addiction reflect a multifaceted approach aimed at addressing various substance use disorders. Notable progress has been made in the treatment of opioid use disorder (OUD) with medications such as buprenorphine/naloxone and extended-release naltrexone, offering effective options for managing withdrawal symptoms and preventing relapse. In alcohol use disorder (AUD), medications like acamprosate and naltrexone continue to play pivotal roles in supporting abstinence and reducing cravings. Research is exploring novel medications, including GABAB receptor agonists and orexin receptor antagonists, suggesting promising avenues for tackling addiction to substances like alcohol and cocaine. Personalized medicine approaches, incorporating pharmacogenetics, contribute to tailoring treatments based on individual genetic factors. These advancements underscore the ongoing commitment to improving the efficacy and accessibility of pharmacotherapy in addressing the complex challenges of drug addiction.

Need for novel therapeutic approaches: The need for novel therapeutic options in the pharmacotherapy of drug addiction is underscored by several factors. First and foremost, the chronic nature of addiction involves complex neurobiological changes, making it challenging to achieve sustained recovery with existing treatments. Moreover, current medications may not be equally effective across different substances of abuse, highlighting the necessity for substance-specific interventions. Additionally, the high prevalence of relapse, even with available treatments, emphasizes the need for medications that target diverse aspects of addiction, including cravings, withdrawal symptoms, and underlying neurobiological mechanisms. Novel therapeutic options are crucial for addressing the limitations of existing medications, enhancing treatment outcomes, and providing tailored solutions for individuals with co-occurring disorders or unique clinical profiles. Furthermore, considering the diverse nature of substance use disorders, including emerging trends and designer drugs, there is a growing imperative to develop medications that can adapt to evolving patterns of drug abuse. Overall, the development of novel pharmacotherapies is essential for advancing the field, improving treatment efficacy, and addressing the nuanced challenges associated with drug addiction.

Challenges in current pharmacotherapy for drug addiction: The current pharmacotherapy for drug addiction faces several challenges that impact its efficacy and implementation. These challenges contribute to the complexity of treating substance use disorders and highlight areas for improvement in addiction treatment. The neurobiological complexity of drug addiction presents a formidable challenge in the current landscape of pharmacotherapy. Addiction is characterized by intricate changes in neural circuits, neurotransmitter systems, and molecular pathways that vary not only across different substances of abuse but also among individuals. The heterogeneity of these neurobiological changes poses a significant obstacle to the development of universal medications that can effectively target the diverse manifestations of addiction. The dynamic nature of neuroplasticity further complicates this challenge, as the brain undergoes continuous structural and functional alterations in response to chronic drug exposure. These dynamic changes, occurring at various levels of the nervous system, necessitate a comprehensive understanding to inform the development of pharmacotherapies capable of adapting to the evolving neurobiological landscape of addiction.

Individual variability in the neurobiological response to drugs, influenced by genetic factors and environmental cues, adds another layer of complexity. The interplay between reward and aversion pathways, the comorbidity of addiction with mental health disorders, and the interconnected nature of neural circuits regulating motivation and decision-making further contribute to the intricate neurobiological tapestry of addiction. Overcoming the challenge of neurobiological complexity requires a multidisciplinary approach, leveraging advancements in neuroscientific research, molecular biology, and systems neuroscience. Additionally, the development of personalized medicine strategies that tailor pharmacotherapies to individual neurobiological profiles holds promise for addressing the diverse and dynamic nature of addiction-related neuroadaptations.

i. Substance-specific variability: Substance-specific variability poses a significant challenge in the current landscape of pharmacotherapy for drug addiction. Different substances of abuse induce distinct neurobiological adaptations and behavioral responses, necessitating tailored interventions for effective treatment. For example, medications that prove effective for opioid use disorder may not exhibit the same efficacy in treating alcohol or stimulant addiction. This variability arises from the diverse pharmacological actions of different drugs, affecting various neurotransmitter systems, receptors, and neural circuits. The complexity of substance-specific effects extends beyond neurobiology to behavioral and psychological aspects. The reinforcing properties, withdrawal symptoms, and patterns of use differ markedly between substances, demanding a nuanced understanding of each addiction phenotype. Current pharmacotherapies often struggle to address this diversity, leading to a lack of universal medications that can effectively target the intricate mechanisms underlying addiction to various substances. Additionally, the prevalence of polydrug use further complicates the treatment landscape. Individuals may simultaneously misuse multiple substances, amplifying the challenge of developing pharmacotherapies capable of addressing the complexities associated with different drugs. Overcoming substance-specific variability requires a comprehensive approach that considers the unique characteristics of each substance of abuse. Tailoring pharmacotherapies to the specific neurobiological and behavioral features of individual addictions represents a crucial step in addressing the diverse challenges posed by substance-specific variability in the current pharmacotherapy of drug addiction.

The lack of universal medications for different substances of abuse is a significant challenge in the field of pharmacotherapy for drug addiction. Each substance, whether it be opioids, alcohol, stimulants, or others, elicits distinct neurobiological and behavioral responses. The pharmacological mechanisms of action, the neural pathways involved, and the subjective experiences of addiction vary widely across different classes of substances. Consequently, a one-size-fits-all approach to medication development is inadequate, and there is a pressing need for tailored interventions that consider the specific characteristics of each substance. One key reason for this lack of universality is the diverse neurochemical impact of different drugs. For instance, medications effective in mitigating opioid cravings and withdrawal symptoms may not necessarily address the underlying mechanisms of alcohol dependence.

The variations in neurotransmitter systems affected by different substances require targeted pharmacotherapies to address the specific challenges associated with each type of addiction. Additionally, the heterogeneity of addiction presentations among individuals further complicates the development of universal medications. Factors such as genetic predispositions, co-occurring mental health disorders, and environmental influences contribute to the individualized nature of addiction, making it challenging to identify a single pharmacological approach that can effectively address all cases. Overcoming the lack of universal medications involves advancing research into the distinct neurobiological underpinnings of each substance of abuse. Tailoring pharmacotherapies to specific substances, while also considering individual differences, holds promise for improving treatment outcomes and addressing the diverse challenges posed by the varied nature of drug addiction. Substance-specific variations in treatment responses represent a critical challenge in the field of drug addiction pharmacotherapy, emphasizing the need for tailored interventions. Different substances of abuse, such as opioids, alcohol, stimulants, and cannabinoids, exert unique pharmacological effects on the brain, resulting in diverse patterns of addiction and response to treatment. The variations in neurobiological mechanisms, withdrawal symptoms, and reinforcing properties of each substance underscore the importance of developing targeted pharmacotherapies to address the specific challenges associated with different types of addiction. For example, medications that effectively manage cravings and withdrawal symptoms in opioid use disorder may not necessarily be suitable for addressing the distinct features of alcohol dependence.

The complexities arising from substance-specific responses extend beyond neurobiology to behavioral and psychological dimensions. Factors such as the reinforcing effects, cognitive impairments, and comorbid mental health conditions differ across substances, necessitating interventions that account for this diversity. Tailored interventions become crucial not only for addressing the specific effects of substances but also for optimizing treatment outcomes based on individual variability. Genetic factors, co-occurring mental health disorders, and environmental influences contribute to the unique presentation of addiction in each individual. Therefore, a personalized medicine approach that considers both substance-specific characteristics and individual differences is essential for developing effective and targeted pharmacotherapies. Overcoming substance-specific variations in treatment responses requires a nuanced understanding of the neurobiological and behavioral intricacies associated with each substance of abuse. Research efforts focused on identifying substance-specific treatment targets and advancing personalized medicine strategies hold promise for improving the precision and effectiveness of interventions in the complex landscape of drug addiction.

ii. Craving and withdrawal management: The management of craving and withdrawal symptoms poses a significant challenge in the current landscape of pharmacotherapy for drug addiction. Cravings, intense desires to use substances, and withdrawal symptoms, the physiological and psychological reactions when substance use is reduced or discontinued, are primary drivers of relapse and can undermine treatment success. Addressing these challenges requires medications that effectively modulate the neurobiological mechanisms underpinning cravings and withdrawal, yet developing such pharmacotherapies remains complex for several reasons. Craving and withdrawal involve diverse neurobiological responses depending on the substance of abuse. Variability in how different drugs impact neurotransmitter systems and neural circuits complicates the development of universally effective medications.

Withdrawal symptoms can vary across substances and exhibit different temporal patterns. The need for medications capable of addressing both acute withdrawal and protracted symptoms presents a multifaceted challenge. Craving is influenced by both the positive reinforcement of substance use and the negative reinforcement associated with avoiding withdrawal. Medications must address the dual nature of craving to comprehensively manage the motivational aspects of addiction. Craving and withdrawal responses exhibit considerable individual variability influenced by genetic, psychological, and environmental factors. Tailoring pharmacotherapies to individual profiles is challenging but crucial for optimizing treatment outcomes. Individuals often engage in polydrug use, complicating the development of medications effective across multiple substances. Co-occurring mental health disorders further add complexity, requiring integrated approaches to address both addiction and psychiatric symptoms.

Adherence to daily medication regimens can be challenging for individuals with addiction, affecting the consistent management of cravings and withdrawal symptoms. The development of long-acting formulations and innovative delivery methods aims to enhance treatment adherence. Addressing the challenge of craving and withdrawal management in pharmacotherapy involves a comprehensive understanding of the neurobiology of addiction and the development of medications that target specific aspects of this complex process. Advancements in personalized medicine, incorporating genetic and individualized treatment approaches, offer potential solutions to optimize treatment efficacy and improve outcomes for individuals struggling with drug addiction. One of the notable challenges in the current landscape of pharmacotherapy for drug addiction is the limited efficacy in managing both acute and protracted withdrawal symptoms. Withdrawal symptoms, which emerge when substance use is reduced or discontinued, can vary in intensity and duration depending on the type of drug and individual factors. Effective pharmacotherapies need to address both the immediate, acute symptoms and the more prolonged, protracted symptoms that can persist for weeks or even months. However, several factors contribute to the challenge of providing comprehensive relief. Different substances of abuse elicit distinct withdrawal symptoms, each requiring tailored interventions. Medications that effectively manage withdrawal from one substance may not be equally efficacious for others, necessitating a substance-specific approach.

Withdrawal symptoms evolve over time, with acute symptoms giving way to protracted symptoms in some cases. Developing medications capable of addressing the dynamic nature of withdrawal throughout its various phases presents a complex treatment challenge. Individuals exhibit considerable variability in their withdrawal experiences, influenced by genetic, psychological, and environmental factors. Tailoring pharmacotherapies to accommodate individual differences is crucial for optimizing treatment outcomes and addressing the diversity of withdrawal presentations. While acute withdrawal mechanisms are relatively well understood, the neurobiological basis of protracted withdrawal is less clear. Research gaps in understanding protracted withdrawal hinder the development of targeted medications for this phase. Co-occurring mental health disorders can complicate the management of withdrawal symptoms. Integrated approaches that address both addiction and psychiatric symptoms are essential for comprehensive treatment.

Achieving a balance between alleviating withdrawal symptoms and minimizing the risk of relapse is challenging. Medications should provide relief without reintroducing substances of abuse or hindering the recovery process. Addressing the limited efficacy in managing both acute and protracted withdrawal symptoms requires ongoing research into the neurobiological mechanisms involved and the development of pharmacotherapies that can adapt to the evolving nature of withdrawal throughout the recovery process. Advances in personalized medicine and substance-specific treatment strategies offer promising avenues for enhancing the effectiveness of withdrawal management in drug addiction pharmacotherapy.

Developing medications that robustly reduce cravings across various substances of abuse is a formidable challenge in the field of pharmacotherapy for drug addiction. Cravings, intense desires to use substances, play a pivotal role in driving relapse and can significantly impede the recovery process. However, addressing cravings universally across different classes of drugs presents several complex challenges. Different substances of abuse activate distinct neurobiological pathways and neurotransmitter systems. Developing medications that effectively modulate cravings requires a nuanced understanding of the diverse neurobiological underpinnings associated with each substance.

Craving intensity varies not only between substances but also among individuals using the same substance. Identifying universal pharmacological targets to address this variability and the multitude of triggers associated with cravings is challenging. Craving is influenced by both the positive reinforcement of substance use and the negative reinforcement associated with avoiding withdrawal. Medications must address the dual nature of craving, considering both the rewarding and aversive aspects of the addiction experience. Individuals often engage in polydrug use, complicating the development of medications effective across multiple substances. Co-occurring mental health disorders may exacerbate cravings, requiring integrated treatment approaches. Genetic, psychological, and environmental factors contribute to individual variability in treatment response. Tailoring medications to accommodate this variability is essential for optimizing treatment outcomes. Cravings are often triggered by specific environmental cues, stressors, or social situations. Developing medications that can address both the biological and environmental triggers of cravings is a multifaceted challenge. Cravings can be dynamic, fluctuating in intensity and frequency over the course of recovery. Medications need to adapt to the changing nature of cravings throughout the recovery process. Achieving a balance between effectively reducing cravings and managing potential side effects or risks associated with medications is crucial. Medications should not compromise overall well-being or introduce new risks. Addressing these challenges requires a comprehensive understanding of the neurobiology of craving, innovative research methodologies, and the development of targeted pharmacotherapies that can address the complexities associated with cravings across a spectrum of substances of abuse. Advances in personalized medicine and substance-specific treatment strategies hold promise for improving the precision and effectiveness of interventions targeting cravings in drug addiction.

iii. High rates of relapse: High rates of relapse represent a significant challenge in the current landscape of pharmacotherapy for drug addiction. Relapse, defined as the recurrence of drug use after a period of abstinence, is a common and often complex aspect of addiction recovery. Addressing this challenge requires a nuanced understanding of the factors contributing to relapse and the development of pharmacotherapies that can effectively mitigate the risk. Several factors contribute to the high rates of relapse in addiction pharmacotherapy. Addiction induces enduring neurobiological changes that persist even after cessation of substance use. Medications may not fully reverse or address these changes, leaving individuals vulnerable to relapse. Environmental cues associated with past drug use can trigger cravings and prompt relapse. Pharmacotherapies may not adequately address the diverse contextual and situational triggers that contribute to relapse.

Individuals with addiction often have co-occurring mental health disorders, which can complicate treatment and increase the risk of relapse. Integrated treatment strategies targeting both addiction and mental health are essential for reducing relapse rates. Response to pharmacotherapy varies among individuals, influenced by genetic, psychological, and environmental factors. Tailoring interventions to individual profiles is crucial for optimizing treatment outcomes and preventing relapse. The duration and completeness of pharmacotherapy treatment may impact its effectiveness in preventing relapse. Inadequate treatment duration or premature discontinuation of medications can contribute to relapse. Social and peer influences can significantly impact relapse, especially in individuals with a history of substance use within social circles. Addressing these external influences requires comprehensive treatment approaches. Stigma surrounding addiction and insufficient social support can hinder recovery efforts and contribute to relapse. Integrating psychosocial support alongside pharmacotherapy is crucial for addressing these challenges. Individuals engaging in polydrug use face additional challenges in treatment. Developing medications that effectively address cravings and withdrawal symptoms across multiple substances is complex. To address the challenge of high relapse rates, ongoing research efforts focus on refining existing pharmacotherapies, developing novel medications, and exploring integrated treatment approaches that encompass both pharmacotherapy and psychosocial interventions. Enhancing treatment adherence, tailoring interventions to individual needs, and addressing the multifaceted nature of addiction contribute to more effective strategies for reducing relapse in the context of drug addiction pharmacotherapy.

The persistent high rates of relapse, despite the availability of pharmacotherapies, underscore the complexity of addiction and the challenges in achieving sustained recovery. Several factors contribute to this ongoing issue. Addiction is a multifaceted and chronic disorder, involving complex interactions between biological, psychological, and social factors. Pharmacotherapies may address specific aspects of addiction but may not comprehensively target all contributing factors. Individuals exhibit substantial variability in their response to pharmacotherapies due to genetic, environmental, and personal factors. Tailoring treatments to the unique needs and characteristics of each individual is challenging but crucial for improving outcomes.

Environmental cues and triggers associated with past substance use can evoke cravings and contribute to relapse. Pharmacotherapies may not effectively mitigate the impact of environmental factors on relapse risk. Chronic substance use induces enduring changes in the brain's neurobiology, contributing to the persistence of addictive behaviors. Pharmacotherapies may not fully reverse or address these underlying neurobiological changes. The presence of co-occurring mental health disorders complicates the treatment landscape and increases the risk of relapse. Integrated approaches that address both addiction and mental health are essential for reducing relapse rates. Medication adherence can be challenging for individuals with addiction, impacting the effectiveness of pharmacotherapies. Strategies to improve adherence, such as long-acting formulations or support systems, are crucial for sustained treatment benefits. Pharmacotherapies are often more effective when combined with comprehensive behavioral interventions. The absence or limited availability of such interventions may contribute to higher relapse rates. Stigma surrounding addiction can impact treatment-seeking behavior and support systems, influencing relapse rates.

Addressing societal attitudes and enhancing social support are vital components of a comprehensive approach. Addiction is a highly individualized condition, and a one-size-fits-all approach may not be sufficient. Holistic and individualized treatment plans that address the specific needs of each person are crucial for reducing relapse rates. Addressing the persistent high rates of relapse requires ongoing research, a deeper understanding of addiction's complexity, and the development of more targeted and personalized treatment strategies. Integrating pharmacotherapies with comprehensive behavioral interventions, social support systems, and addressing underlying neurobiological changes are essential components of a holistic approach to reduce relapse in individuals with substance use disorders.

The need for more effective medications to prevent relapse and sustain long-term recovery is a central challenge in the field of addiction treatment. Despite the availability of some pharmacotherapies, relapse rates remain high, emphasizing the urgency for innovative and targeted interventions. Several key factors highlight the demand for improved medications. Existing pharmacotherapies, while helpful for some individuals, may not provide sufficient efficacy across all substances of abuse and for every individual. The variable response to current medications underscores the need for more tailored and potent interventions. Addiction induces profound neurobiological changes that persist during abstinence, contributing to the vulnerability to relapse. Developing medications that more comprehensively address these underlying neurobiological changes is crucial for sustaining recovery. Cravings and withdrawal symptoms, which often drive relapse, have both rewarding and aversive components. Medications need to effectively manage both aspects to reduce the likelihood of relapse. Environmental cues and triggers play a significant role in relapse, and medications should be designed to better mitigate the impact of these triggers. Improved medications should address the complexity of external factors contributing to relapse. Individuals frequently engage in polydrug use, necessitating medications that can address cravings and withdrawal symptoms across various substances. Co-occurring mental health disorders must also be considered in the development of more effective medications. The development of extended-release and long-acting formulations can improve treatment adherence by reducing the burden of daily dosing. Such formulations can contribute to sustained medication effects, helping prevent relapse over more extended periods.

Advancements in personalized medicine can facilitate the identification of individuals who are more likely to respond to specific medications. Tailoring interventions based on an individual's genetic, neurobiological, and behavioral profile enhances treatment effectiveness. Medications should be integrated with evidence-based behavioral therapies to provide a comprehensive approach to relapse prevention. Combining pharmacotherapy with behavioral interventions can address both the biological and psychological aspects of addiction. Stigma associated with addiction can deter individuals from seeking and adhering to treatment. Medications that are more acceptable and have fewer social barriers can improve treatment engagement and contribute to sustained recovery. Increased investment in research and development is essential for exploring novel targets and mechanisms for medications. Continued efforts to discover and refine pharmacotherapies will enhance the arsenal of effective treatments. Addressing the need for more effective medications to prevent relapse and sustain long-term recovery requires a comprehensive, multidisciplinary approach that integrates advancements in neuroscience, pharmacology, and personalized medicine. Ongoing research, innovation, and collaboration across these domains are essential to meet the challenges posed by addiction and enhance the effectiveness of pharmacotherapies in promoting sustained recovery.

iv. Co-occurring disorders: The presence of co-occurring disorders, where individuals experience both substance use disorders and mental health disorders simultaneously, poses a significant challenge in the current landscape of pharmacotherapy for drug addiction. Several factors contribute to the complexity of addressing co-occurring disorders with medications. Co-occurring disorders involve the interplay of substance use disorders and various mental health conditions such as depression, anxiety, bipolar disorder, or schizophrenia. The diverse range of comorbidities requires a nuanced and multifaceted approach in developing pharmacotherapies. Substance use and mental health disorders often exert a bidirectional influence on each other, complicating the understanding and treatment of both conditions. Medications must consider the interconnected nature of these disorders and provide comprehensive treatment that addresses both aspects simultaneously. Individuals with co-occurring disorders may exhibit variable responses to medications due to the heterogeneity of symptoms and underlying neurobiological factors. Tailoring pharmacotherapies to the specific needs and characteristics of each individual becomes crucial for optimizing treatment outcomes. Individuals with co-occurring disorders may be prescribed medications for both the substance use disorder and the mental health condition. The potential interactions between these medications need to be carefully considered to avoid adverse effects or reduced efficacy. Historically, mental health and addiction treatment have been separate entities, leading to fragmented care. Developing medications that can integrate the treatment of both disorders seamlessly is essential for improving overall outcomes.

Many individuals with co-occurring disorders have a history of trauma, which can complicate treatment and contribute to substance use as a coping mechanism. Pharmacotherapies should consider the underlying trauma and incorporate trauma-informed care principles. Stigma surrounding mental health and addiction can create barriers to seeking and receiving appropriate treatment. Medications that are more widely accepted and destigmatized can improve treatment engagement for individuals with co- occurring disorders. The presence of multiple conditions may lead to polypharmacy, where individuals are prescribed multiple medications. Managing polypharmacy and ensuring adherence to complex medication regimens can be challenging. Integrated treatment approaches that combine pharmacotherapy with evidence-based psychotherapies and psychosocial interventions are crucial. An integrated approach addresses both the substance use and mental health aspects comprehensively. Individuals with co-occurring disorders often require long-term, comprehensive care that extends beyond acute treatment phases. Developing medications that support a continuum of care, including relapse prevention and maintenance of mental health stability, is essential. Addressing the challenge of co-occurring disorders in pharmacotherapy requires a holistic and integrated approach that considers the complexity of both conditions. The development of medications should align with a broader treatment framework that recognizes the interconnected nature of substance use and mental health disorders, emphasizing individualized, evidence-based care to optimize outcomes for individuals facing these complex challenges.

The limited availability of medications suitable for individuals with co-occurring mental health disorders can present significant challenges in managing their conditions effectively. Co-occurring disorders, also known as comorbid or dual disorders, refer to the presence of both a mental health disorder and a substance use disorder or two or more mental health disorders in an individual. Here are some challenges and considerations associated with the limited availability of medications for individuals with co-occurring mental health disorders. Individuals with co-occurring disorders often have complex treatment needs that require a comprehensive and integrated approach. Medication can be a crucial component of this treatment, addressing both mental health and substance use symptoms.

Limited medication options may increase the risk of adverse interactions between drugs used to treat mental health disorders and substances of abuse. This can compromise treatment effectiveness and safety. People with co-occurring disorders may have unique responses to medications due to the interplay of different conditions. Finding the right combination and dosage of medications for each individual can be challenging. Stigma associated with mental health and substance use disorders can contribute to a lack of resources and attention in terms of medication development and accessibility. This may result in fewer treatment options for individuals with co-occurring disorders. Limited research and development in the area of co-occurring disorders may contribute to a lack of innovative medications tailored to address the specific needs of this population. The treatment of co-occurring disorders may involve multiple medications, leading to concerns about polypharmacy—taking several medications simultaneously.

This can increase the risk of side effects and medication non-adherence. Regulatory hurdles and challenges in obtaining approval for medications that target co-occurring disorders may slow down the availability of new and effective treatments. Addressing the issue of limited availability of medications for individuals with co-occurring mental health disorders requires a multi-faceted approach. This includes increased research and development efforts, improved access to integrated treatment programs, reduced stigma, and a holistic understanding of the complexities involved in treating co-occurring disorders. Additionally, healthcare providers should engage in ongoing education to stay informed about the latest evidence-based practices and treatment options.

Integrating treatments for individuals with both addiction and co-existing psychiatric conditions, also known as co-occurring disorders or dual diagnosis, can be challenging due to several factors. Here are some key challenges associated with integrating treatments for addiction and psychiatric conditions. Mental health and addiction treatment services are often provided by separate systems, leading to fragmentation of care. Lack of coordination between these services can result in disjointed and less effective treatment. Stigma surrounding mental health and addiction issues can hinder collaboration between mental health and addiction treatment providers. This can create barriers to integrated care and lead to a lack of understanding and empathy for individuals with co-occurring disorders.

Identifying and accurately diagnosing both the addiction and psychiatric conditions can be challenging. Symptoms may overlap, making it difficult to determine the primary and secondary issues. This can impact the choice of appropriate interventions. Individuals with co-occurring disorders may require multiple medications to address both mental health and addiction issues. Managing polypharmacy (multiple medications) presents challenges in terms of potential drug interactions, side effects, and adherence. Many healthcare professionals may lack training and expertise in both addiction and mental health treatment. Integrated care requires a multidisciplinary approach with providers who have a comprehensive understanding of both domains. Communication between mental health and addiction treatment providers, as well as between different healthcare systems, can be challenging. Information sharing is crucial for providing coordinated and effective care, but barriers such as privacy concerns and lack of standardized communication protocols can impede this. Integrated treatment models that address both addiction and psychiatric conditions are not universally implemented. The absence of standardized approaches can result in variations in care quality and effectiveness. Limited access to comprehensive services that address both addiction and mental health issues can impede the delivery of integrated care. This includes a lack of facilities that offer dual diagnosis treatment programs. Reimbursement policies and funding mechanisms may not adequately support integrated care models. This can hinder the implementation and sustainability of programs that aim to address both addiction and mental health simultaneously.

Individuals with co-occurring disorders may be at higher risk of relapse, and treatment resistance may be more common. Comprehensive and tailored interventions are needed to address these challenges effectively. Addressing these challenges requires a systemic and collaborative effort involving policymakers, healthcare providers, educators, and advocacy groups. Developing integrated treatment models, increasing training opportunities, reducing stigma, and improving communication and coordination among various healthcare sectors are crucial steps toward providing effective care for individuals with co-occurring disorders.

v. Treatment adherence: Treatment adherence poses a significant challenge in the current pharmacotherapy for drug addiction. Adherence refers to the extent to which individuals follow the prescribed treatment plan, including taking medications as directed and participating in other recommended therapeutic interventions. Here are several factors contributing to the challenge of treatment adherence in pharmacotherapy for drug addiction. Stigma associated with addiction may lead individuals to deny or downplay the severity of their condition. This attitude can hinder acceptance of pharmacotherapy as a legitimate and effective treatment, impacting adherence. Some pharmacotherapies for drug addiction involve complex medication regimens. This complexity, including dosing schedules and potential side effects, can be a barrier to adherence, especially for individuals with co-occurring mental health disorders. Medications used in addiction treatment may have side effects that individuals find unpleasant or intolerable. This can lead to non-adherence, as individuals may be reluctant to continue taking medications that cause discomfort. Addiction often affects an individual's motivation and ability to engage in treatment. Low motivation can result in non-adherence, as individuals may not see the immediate benefits of taking medications or attending therapy sessions. Social and environmental factors, such as a lack of support from family or friends, unstable living conditions, or exposure to environments that trigger cravings, can negatively impact adherence to pharmacotherapy. Limited access to medications, whether due to financial constraints, geographic barriers, or healthcare system limitations, can compromise treatment adherence. This is particularly relevant for medications like methadone or buprenorphine used in opioid addiction treatment.

Inadequate patient education about the benefits of pharmacotherapy, potential side effects, and the importance of adherence can contribute to non-adherence. Lack of understanding may lead individuals to discontinue medication without consulting their healthcare providers. Individuals with co-occurring mental health disorders may face additional challenges in adhering to pharmacotherapy. Mental health symptoms can interfere with the ability to consistently follow treatment plans. Discontinuity in treatment, such as gaps in therapy sessions or disruptions in the supply of medications, can lead to non-adherence. Consistent and uninterrupted access to treatment is essential for achieving positive outcomes. Pre-existing negative attitudes toward medications, whether due to past experiences or cultural beliefs, can influence adherence. Some individuals may resist relying on medications for their addiction treatment.

Addressing treatment adherence in pharmacotherapy for drug addiction requires a comprehensive and individualized approach. Strategies may include improving patient education, reducing stigma, simplifying medication regimens when possible, providing adequate support systems, addressing social determinants of health, and implementing interventions to enhance motivation and engagement in treatment. Additionally, ongoing communication between healthcare providers and individuals in treatment is crucial to monitor and address adherence challenges as they arise. Poor adherence to medication regimens, especially with daily dosing, is a common and significant challenge across various medical conditions, including mental health disorders, chronic illnesses, and addiction treatment. Several factors contribute to this issue. Forgetting to take medications is a common reason for poor adherence. Individuals may lead busy lives, and incorporating daily medication into a routine can be challenging. Medication regimens that involve multiple pills, varying dosages, or specific instructions may be difficult for individuals to follow consistently. Unpleasant side effects can discourage individuals from adhering to their prescribed medication regimens. If the perceived negative effects outweigh the perceived benefits, adherence may suffer. Some medications may not produce immediate noticeable effects. If individuals do not perceive improvements quickly, they may question the need for continued adherence.

Stigma associated with certain conditions or medications can impact adherence. Individuals may avoid taking medications due to concerns about judgment from others or internalized stigma. Conditions that affect cognitive function, such as mental health disorders or aging-related cognitive decline, can impact an individual's ability to remember and manage their medication regimen. Limited access to medications or financial constraints can lead to inconsistent adherence. Issues with insurance coverage or the high cost of medications may result in skipped doses. Conditions such as depression can affect motivation and energy levels, making it difficult for individuals to prioritize their medication adherence. Medications that require specific conditions for administration, such as fasting or avoiding certain foods, may be challenging for individuals to incorporate into their daily routines.

Lack of support from family, friends, or healthcare providers can contribute to poor adherence. A supportive environment can positively influence a person's commitment to their medication regimen. Simplify medication regimens whenever possible to reduce the burden on individuals are essential. Clear and comprehensive education about the importance of medication adherence, potential side effects, and expected benefits should be provided. The use of reminder systems, such as alarms, pill organizers, or smartphone apps, must be encouraged to help individuals remember to take their medications. Regular follow-up appointments must be conducted to monitor progress, address concerns, and make necessary adjustments to the treatment plan. Behavioral interventions, such as cognitive-behavioral therapy or motivational interviewing must be conducted, to address psychological barriers to adherence. Family members and support systems must be involved in the treatment process to create a supportive environment for adherence. Active monitoring and management of side effects, and consideration of alternative medications if side effects are a significant barrier must be taken into account.

Collaboration with individuals to address any barriers to medication access, including insurance coverage and affordability concerns, would be very helpful in this regard. By adopting a patient-centered and individualized approach, healthcare providers can work with individuals to overcome the specific challenges contributing to poor adherence and promote better medication management. Non-adherence to prescribed treatment regimens presents a formidable challenge with far-reaching implications for treatment outcomes and the risk of relapse. In medical contexts, particularly mental health disorders, non-adherence disrupts the delicate balance that medication seeks to establish. Failure to consistently take prescribed psychiatric medications can lead to a worsening of symptoms, impeding progress toward stability. The nuanced interplay between these medications and an individual's mental health underscores the importance of adherence in achieving therapeutic goals. The consequences extend beyond symptom exacerbation to compromise the overall effectiveness of the treatment plan.

In substance use disorder treatment, non-adherence can be a critical factor contributing to an increased risk of relapse. Medications such as methadone or buprenorphine, integral components of opioid agonist therapy, help individuals manage withdrawal symptoms and cravings. However, irregular use or discontinuation of these medications can destabilize the progress made in overcoming substance dependence, heightening susceptibility to a return to drug use. The link between medication adherence and relapse underscores the need for comprehensive, individualized strategies that address the unique challenges individuals face in maintaining continuity with their prescribed treatments. Beyond the individual level, the impact of non-adherence reverberates through healthcare systems and public health. Increased healthcare utilization, often stemming from exacerbated symptoms or relapses, places a burden on medical resources and contributes to elevated costs. In infectious disease contexts, non-adherence to medication regimens may pose public health risks, fostering the spread of diseases and complicating efforts to control their transmission. Recognizing the multifaceted consequences of non-adherence is crucial for healthcare providers, policymakers, and individuals alike as they work collaboratively to develop interventions that support sustained adherence, improve treatment outcomes, and mitigate the risk of relapse.

vi. Stigma and accessibility: Stigma and accessibility represent formidable challenges in the current landscape of pharmacotherapy for drug addiction. The pervasive societal stigma attached to substance use disorders can deter individuals from seeking treatment and adhering to pharmacotherapeutic interventions. The stigma surrounding addiction often leads to feelings of shame and judgment, making individuals hesitant to disclose their struggles and engage with healthcare providers. This stigma can extend to pharmacotherapy itself, hindering acceptance of medications designed to assist in recovery. Consequently, the reluctance to embrace pharmacotherapy as a legitimate and effective component of addiction treatment can impede accessibility, exacerbating the challenge of addressing substance use disorders on a broader scale.

Accessibility is a critical concern in the implementation of pharmacotherapy for drug addiction. Disparities in access to healthcare services, including medication-assisted treatment (MAT), can be influenced by socioeconomic factors, geographic location, and systemic barriers. Limited availability of addiction specialists and treatment centers in certain regions may result in insufficient access to pharmacotherapeutic interventions. Additionally, disparities in insurance coverage and affordability of medications can further hinder accessibility. These barriers not only restrict the reach of pharmacotherapy but also perpetuate health inequalities, as marginalized populations may face additional challenges in obtaining the necessary support for their recovery through medication-based interventions. Efforts to address the challenge of stigma and accessibility in pharmacotherapy for drug addiction must be multifaceted. Public health campaigns aimed at destigmatizing addiction and promoting awareness about the efficacy of pharmacotherapeutic options can help shift societal perceptions. Additionally, improving the training of healthcare providers to deliver non-judgmental and culturally competent care is essential. Policy initiatives that expand access to addiction treatment services, including pharmacotherapy, and address systemic barriers such as insurance coverage gaps can contribute to a more equitable and accessible landscape for individuals seeking help for substance use disorders. By dismantling stigma and enhancing accessibility, the potential of pharmacotherapy to play a transformative role in addiction treatment can be fully realized, benefiting both individuals and communities at large

Stigmatization of medication-assisted treatments (MAT) for substance use disorders poses a significant obstacle to their acceptance and utilization. MAT, which often involves medications like methadone, buprenorphine, or naltrexone, is an evidence-based approach that effectively helps individuals manage cravings and withdrawal symptoms, supporting them in achieving and maintaining recovery. However, societal stigma surrounding addiction can extend to MAT, contributing to negative perceptions and biases. Individuals undergoing MAT may encounter judgment and misconceptions that label them as merely substituting one addiction for another, perpetuating the misconception that medication-based interventions are not legitimate forms of treatment.

This stigmatization not only impacts the individuals seeking MAT but also influences healthcare providers and policymakers, shaping their attitudes and approaches to addiction treatment. Clinicians may hesitate to recommend MAT due to concerns about patient judgment or societal disapproval, limiting access to these proven therapeutic options. Public health campaigns and educational initiatives are essential to challenge these stigmatizing beliefs, emphasizing the medical and evidence-based nature of MAT. Destigmatizing MAT requires a shift in public perception to recognize it as a valuable tool in the continuum of care for substance use disorders, rather than as a compromise or concession. Addressing stigmatization involves promoting understanding of the complex nature of addiction and the diverse range of effective treatments available. Combating stigma should also involve fostering empathy and compassion, recognizing that individuals seeking MAT are taking a proactive step towards recovery. By dismantling stigmatizing attitudes, society can contribute to a more supportive environment for individuals seeking MAT, encouraging greater acceptance of these evidence-based treatments and ultimately improving overall outcomes in the treatment of substance use disorders. Limited accessibility to pharmacotherapies for substance use disorders is exacerbated by pervasive stigma and systemic barriers, creating substantial challenges for individuals seeking evidence-based treatment. Stigma surrounding addiction often permeates healthcare systems, discouraging both individuals and healthcare providers from embracing pharmacotherapies as viable options. This societal bias can result in a lack of education about the effectiveness of medications like methadone, buprenorphine, or naltrexone, hindering their integration into mainstream addiction treatment protocols.

The reluctance to fully endorse these pharmacotherapies stems from deeply rooted misconceptions and biases, perpetuating the idea that medication-based interventions are not legitimate forms of treatment. Systemic barriers further contribute to limited accessibility, disproportionately affecting marginalized and underserved populations. Geographical disparities, where certain regions lack sufficient addiction treatment infrastructure, can impede access to pharmacotherapies. Additionally, disparities in insurance coverage and affordability create financial barriers, preventing many individuals from accessing essential medications. Systemic issues such as insufficient training for healthcare providers and a lack of integration between mental health and addiction services also hinder the widespread adoption of pharmacotherapies. Addressing limited accessibility requires dismantling societal stigma through targeted education and awareness campaigns and implementing policy changes that enhance the integration and affordability of pharmacotherapies within comprehensive addiction treatment frameworks.

Efforts to increase accessibility must involve a coordinated approach that addresses both societal attitudes and systemic deficiencies. By fostering a more informed and empathetic understanding of addiction treatment, and by implementing policies that prioritize equitable access, it is possible to break down these barriers and ensure that pharmacotherapies become more widely available to individuals in need. Ultimately, overcoming limited accessibility involves transforming societal perceptions and reforming healthcare systems to better align with evidence-based practices in addiction treatment.

vii. Risk of diversion and misuse: The risk of diversion and misuse poses a significant challenge in the current landscape of pharmacotherapy for drug addiction. Pharmacotherapeutic interventions, such as medications used in opioid agonist therapy (e.g., methadone, buprenorphine) or those targeting other substances, are crucial components of addiction treatment. However, the potential for diversion—when prescribed medications are redirected for non-medical use by individuals for whom they were not intended—and misuse can complicate the effective implementation of these interventions.

One prominent concern is the diversion of medications into illicit markets, where they may be sold or traded. This not only compromises the integrity of the treatment process but also contributes to the perpetuation of substance misuse within communities. The diversion of medications used in addiction treatment can have legal, social, and public health implications, raising challenges for regulatory bodies and law enforcement agencies. The risk of misuse is another facet of this challenge, involving the intentional use of prescribed medications in a manner inconsistent with medical advice. Patients may misuse medications to achieve a euphoric effect or to self-manage withdrawal symptoms. Misuse can undermine the therapeutic goals of pharmacotherapy and may lead to health complications or contribute to relapse.

To address the risk of diversion and misuse, healthcare providers must implement comprehensive strategies. This includes thorough patient assessments to identify individuals at higher risk, regular monitoring of medication adherence, and the incorporation of counseling and support services into treatment plans. Moreover, adopting tamper-resistant formulations, implementing secure dispensing practices, and promoting public education on the importance of proper medication use are essential components of mitigating the risks associated with diversion and misuse. Balancing the need for widespread access to effective pharmacotherapies with the imperative to prevent diversion and misuse requires a nuanced and collaborative approach. Striking this balance involves ongoing research, policy development, and education to ensure that pharmacotherapy remains a cornerstone of evidence-based addiction treatment while minimizing the potential risks associated with diversion and misuse. The potential for the diversion of medications, particularly those used in the treatment of substance use disorders, poses a complex challenge in healthcare and public health. Medications such as methadone and buprenorphine, employed in opioid agonist therapy, play a crucial role in stabilizing individuals and reducing cravings, contributing to recovery from opioid addiction. However, the inherent risk lies in the diversion of these medications into illicit markets, where they may be sold or traded for non medical use. The diversion not only undermines the efficacy of pharmacotherapy but also contributes to the perpetuation of substance misuse within communities.

One concern is that diverted medications may be used by individuals for whom they were not prescribed, potentially leading to unintended health consequences. This poses risks both for those who divert the medications and for those who may unknowingly consume them. Furthermore, the illegal distribution of medications can strain regulatory and law enforcement efforts to ensure the safe and controlled use of these substances. Addressing the potential for diversion requires a multi-faceted approach that balances the need for widespread access to effective treatments with the imperative to minimize the risks associated with illicit distribution. Efforts to mitigate the diversion of medications include the implementation of secure prescribing and dispensing practices, routine monitoring of patients in treatment, and the use of tamper-resistant formulations. Public health campaigns and educational initiatives can also play a role in raising awareness about the consequences of diverting medications and the importance of responsible use. Striking the right balance between ensuring access to essential medications for those in need and preventing diversion is crucial for optimizing the benefits of pharmacotherapy while safeguarding against potential misuse and illicit distribution.

Balancing accessibility to pharmacotherapies for substance use disorders with measures to prevent misuse and diversion is a delicate task that demands a comprehensive and nuanced approach. On one hand, ensuring widespread access to evidence-based treatments such as medications for opioid agonist therapy is crucial for addressing the complex challenges of addiction. These medications, like methadone and buprenorphine, play a pivotal role in stabilizing individuals, reducing cravings, and supporting recovery. On the other hand, the potential for misuse and diversion necessitates the implementation of rigorous safeguards to maintain the integrity of these treatments. Strategies for achieving this balance include adopting secure prescribing practices, employing tamper- resistant formulations, and implementing robust monitoring systems. Regular assessments of patients, along with the integration of counseling and support services, contribute to a more comprehensive approach that addresses both the medical and psychosocial aspects of addiction treatment. Furthermore, healthcare providers must engage in ongoing education and training to stay informed about best practices for prescribing and monitoring pharmacotherapies. Public awareness campaigns are also essential to foster a nuanced understanding of the benefits of these medications and the importance of responsible use. By emphasizing the medical nature of pharmacotherapy and its role in supporting recovery, such campaigns can help destigmatize treatment, reduce misconceptions, and encourage a supportive environment. Ultimately, striking the right balance between accessibility and measures to prevent misuse and diversion requires collaboration among healthcare professionals, policymakers, regulatory bodies, and the community to ensure that evidence-based treatments are accessible to those in need while minimizing the risks associated with diversion and misuse.

viii. Limited long-acting formulations: The limited availability of long-acting formulations poses a notable challenge in the current landscape of pharmacotherapy for drug addiction. In the context of substance use disorders, long-acting formulations provide sustained release of medication over an extended period, offering potential advantages such as improved adherence, reduced frequency of dosing, and a more stable pharmacological effect. However, the development and accessibility of long- acting formulations for addiction treatment have been relatively constrained compared to other therapeutic areas. One significant consequence of the limited availability of long-acting formulations is the potential impact on treatment adherence. Short-acting medications may necessitate more frequent dosing, increasing the likelihood of missed doses and compromising the consistency of treatment. Long- acting formulations, on the other hand, can contribute to improved adherence by minimizing the need for multiple daily administrations. This is particularly relevant in the context of opioid agonist therapy, where medications like methadone or buprenorphine could benefit from extended-release options to enhance treatment outcomes. The scarcity of long-acting formulations also restricts the range of options available to healthcare providers and individuals seeking treatment. A more diverse array of long-acting medications tailored to different substances of abuse would offer greater flexibility in addressing the unique needs of individuals with various addiction profiles. This limitation highlights the importance of ongoing research and development efforts to expand the repertoire of long-acting formulations for addiction pharmacotherapy. Addressing the challenge of limited long-acting formulations involves collaborative efforts among pharmaceutical companies, researchers, and healthcare providers. Increased investment in research to develop and refine long-acting formulations for various substances of abuse is critical. Additionally, regulatory frameworks and reimbursement structures should encourage the development and utilization of these formulations to optimize treatment outcomes and enhance the overall effectiveness of pharmacotherapy in the realm of addiction treatment.

The scarcity of long-acting or extended-release formulations for certain medications used in the treatment of drug addiction represents a significant challenge in the field of addiction pharmacotherapy. Many medications employed in substance use disorder treatment, such as those for opioid agonist therapy (e.g., methadone, buprenorphine), lack extended-release options. This scarcity limits the therapeutic choices available to healthcare providers and individuals seeking treatment, potentially impacting treatment adherence and overall effectiveness. One primary consequence of the limited availability of long-acting formulations is the potential for challenges in treatment adherence. Medications with shorter durations of action may require multiple daily administrations, introducing complexity and increasing the likelihood of missed doses. Long-acting formulations offer the advantage of sustained release, reducing the frequency of dosing and providing a more consistent pharmacological effect. This can be particularly crucial in addiction treatment, where maintaining steady medication levels is important for preventing relapse and promoting stabilization. The scarcity of long-acting formulations also affects the tailoring of treatment plans to individual needs. The one-size-fits-all approach may not adequately address the diverse profiles of individuals with substance use disorders. Having more options in terms of extended-release formulations would allow healthcare providers to better match medications to the specific needs and preferences of patients, enhancing the patient-centered nature of addiction treatment. Efforts to address the scarcity of long- acting formulations require increased research and development initiatives, along with incentives for pharmaceutical companies to invest in these formulations. Additionally, regulatory frameworks should encourage the timely approval and availability of extended-release options for medications used in addiction treatment. This would contribute to a more comprehensive and flexible pharmacotherapeutic approach, ultimately improving treatment outcomes and providing individuals with more tailored and accessible options for their recovery journey.

The development of sustained-release options to enhance treatment adherence for drug abuse faces several challenges that impact the effectiveness of pharmacotherapy interventions. One significant challenge is the complex pharmacokinetics of drugs of abuse. Many substances, such as opioids or stimulants, have rapid onset and short duration of action, making it challenging to design sustained- release formulations that maintain therapeutic levels in the body over an extended period. Another challenge lies in the diverse nature of drug abuse and individual variability in response to treatment. The optimal sustained-release formulation may vary between different substances of abuse and among individuals with varying addiction profiles. Designing formulations that accommodate this diversity poses a considerable challenge for researchers and pharmaceutical developers. The stigma surrounding drug abuse further complicates the development and acceptance of sustained-release options. Stigma may influence perceptions of medication-assisted treatment in general, and the introduction of novel formulations may face skepticism or resistance from both healthcare providers and individuals seeking treatment. Regulatory hurdles also contribute to the challenges in developing sustained-release options. The approval process for new formulations is rigorous, requiring extensive clinical trials and evidence of safety and efficacy. This process can be time-consuming and resource-intensive, delaying the availability of innovative treatment options. Moreover, financial considerations and market dynamics may affect the motivation of pharmaceutical companies to invest in sustained-release formulations for drug abuse treatment. The prevalence of generic versions of some medications may limit the financial incentives for companies to engage in the development of extended-release alternatives. To address these challenges, there is a need for increased research investment, collaboration between researchers and pharmaceutical companies, and regulatory frameworks that facilitate the development and approval of sustained-release options for drug abuse treatment. Public awareness campaigns and education initiatives can also play a role in destigmatizing medication-assisted treatment, fostering a more supportive environment for the introduction and acceptance of novel formulations. Ultimately, overcoming these challenges is essential to expanding the arsenal of effective treatments for individuals struggling with drug abuse and improving overall treatment adherence.

ix. Individual variability in treatment response: Individual variability in treatment response represents a significant challenge in the current landscape of pharmacotherapy for drug addiction. The diverse nature of substance use disorders, coupled with variations in genetic, biological, and psychosocial factors among individuals, contributes to a wide range of responses to pharmacological interventions. This heterogeneity poses challenges in tailoring treatment approaches to meet the unique needs of each patient, optimizing effectiveness, and minimizing the risk of adverse outcomes. One aspect of individual variability is the pharmacogenetic differences that influence how individuals metabolize and respond to medications. Genetic variations in drug-metabolizing enzymes and receptor systems can impact the efficacy and tolerability of pharmacotherapies. Identifying and understanding these genetic factors can aid in personalized treatment plans, but integrating genetic testing into routine clinical practice remains a challenge. Psychosocial factors, such as co-occurring mental health disorders, environmental stressors, and social support, also contribute to individual variability in treatment response. Patients with dual diagnoses or complex psychosocial challenges may experience different responses to pharmacotherapy compared to those without such complications. Tailoring treatment plans to address these factors is essential but requires a comprehensive understanding of each individual's unique circumstances. The dynamic nature of addiction itself adds another layer of complexity. The stage of addiction, the severity of dependence, and an individual's motivation for change can influence treatment response. Matching the appropriate medication and dosage to a person's specific addiction profile is an ongoing challenge, especially given the fluidity of substance use disorders. To address these challenges, a personalized and comprehensive approach to addiction treatment is crucial. This includes thorough assessments that consider genetic factors, mental health status, and psychosocial determinants. Regular monitoring and adjustments to treatment plans based on individual response and evolving circumstances are essential for optimizing outcomes. Moreover, ongoing research into the genetic and neurobiological underpinnings of addiction can contribute to the development of more targeted and effective pharmacotherapies that account for individual variability in treatment response.

Genetic and individual differences exert a profound impact on treatment responses, presenting a complex challenge in the current landscape of pharmacotherapy for drug addiction. Genetic variations among individuals can significantly influence how they metabolize and respond to medications used in addiction treatment. The field of pharmacogenomics seeks to understand how an individual's genetic makeup affects their response to drugs, including potential variations in drug efficacy, side effects, and overall treatment outcomes. However, integrating this knowledge into routine clinical practice and tailoring treatment plans accordingly remains a significant challenge. Individual differences extend beyond genetics to encompass diverse factors such as age, sex, co-occurring medical conditions, and psychosocial determinants. These factors contribute to the heterogeneity of treatment responses observed in individuals with substance use disorders. For example, individuals with co-occurring mental health disorders may experience different responses to pharmacotherapy compared to those without such comorbidities. Additionally, factors like stress, social support, and environmental influences play a pivotal role in shaping treatment outcomes, highlighting the need for personalized and holistic approaches to addiction treatment. Individuals at different stages of addiction, with varying levels of dependence and motivation for change, may respond differently to pharmacotherapy. Tailoring treatment plans to address these dynamic factors requires ongoing assessments and adjustments to ensure that interventions are aligned with the evolving needs of each individual. Addressing the challenge of genetic and individual differences in treatment responses requires an integrated and personalized approach to addiction care. Clinicians need to consider a range of factors, from genetic markers to psychosocial determinants, to develop treatment plans tailored to the unique characteristics of each patient. Advancements in pharmacogenomic research, along with ongoing efforts to understand the interplay of genetic and environmental influences, hold promise for refining and optimizing pharmacotherapy for drug addiction based on individual differences in treatment responses.

The need for personalized and adaptive treatment strategies stands out as a critical challenge in the current landscape of pharmacotherapy for drug addiction. Substance use disorders are highly heterogeneous, influenced by a myriad of genetic, environmental, and psychosocial factors. The one- size-fits-all approach often falls short in addressing the unique needs and characteristics of individuals struggling with addiction. Tailoring treatment to the specific profile of each patient is essential for optimizing outcomes, but implementing personalized and adaptive strategies faces several challenges. One major obstacle is the complexity of individual differences. Genetic variations, co-occurring mental health conditions, and diverse life circumstances contribute to the variability in how individuals respond to medications. Identifying and understanding these factors require comprehensive assessments, including genetic testing and detailed psychosocial evaluations. Integrating this wealth of information into treatment plans is a formidable task, particularly in routine clinical settings.

The dynamic nature of addiction further complicates the need for adaptability in treatment. Individuals may experience fluctuations in motivation, external stressors, and changes in their addiction severity over time. An effective treatment strategy must be flexible enough to adjust to these evolving circumstances, requiring ongoing monitoring and adjustments by healthcare providers. The current healthcare system's limitations, including time constraints during clinical visits and a lack of integrated data systems, hinder the seamless integration of personalized and adaptive treatment strategies. Additionally, there is a need for increased awareness and education among healthcare professionals about the benefits of personalized medicine in addiction treatment. Overcoming these challenges requires a concerted effort across multiple fronts. Increased research into the genetic and neurobiological underpinnings of addiction can contribute to the development of targeted pharmacotherapies. Integrating electronic health records and utilizing technology for real-time monitoring can enhance the adaptive nature of treatment plans. Comprehensive training programs for healthcare providers can ensure a more informed and skilled workforce capable of delivering personalized care. Addressing the need for personalized and adaptive treatment strategies is integral to advancing addiction pharmacotherapy. By acknowledging and navigating the complexities of individual differences, healthcare providers can offer more effective and tailored interventions, ultimately improving the prospects for recovery in individuals grappling with drug addiction.

Evolving Drug Trends: The dynamic nature of evolving drug trends presents a formidable challenge in the current landscape of pharmacotherapy for drug addiction. The patterns of substance use are constantly changing, with the emergence of new drugs and shifts in the prevalence of existing ones. This fluidity introduces complexities in the development and implementation of pharmacotherapeutic interventions that can effectively address the diverse array of substances individuals may be using. One challenge lies in keeping pharmacotherapy aligned with the specific pharmacological properties and mechanisms of action of novel and emerging drugs of abuse. The traditional focus of pharmacotherapy has often been on well-established substances, such as opioids or alcohol. However, the rise of synthetic drugs, novel psychoactive substances, and changing trends in polydrug use necessitate a swift and adaptable response to develop medications that can effectively target these newer substances. The rapid emergence of substances with varying potencies and modes of action makes it challenging for researchers and pharmaceutical companies to keep pace with the evolving landscape of drug trends. This lag in development can result in a lack of evidence-based pharmacotherapies for certain substances, leaving healthcare providers with limited options for treating individuals who are using these drugs. Furthermore, the prevalence of polydrug use, where individuals use multiple substances concurrently, adds complexity to the treatment landscape. Developing pharmacotherapies that can address the intricacies of polydrug use and the potential interactions between different substances presents an additional layer of challenge. To navigate the challenge of evolving drug trends, there is a need for increased research funding and a more nimble regulatory framework that can facilitate the timely development and approval of medications targeting emerging substances. Additionally, a comprehensive approach that combines pharmacotherapy with behavioral interventions and social support is crucial to address the multifaceted nature of substance use disorders. Ultimately, staying ahead of evolving drug trends in the context of pharmacotherapy requires a collaborative effort involving researchers, healthcare providers, policymakers, and pharmaceutical companies. By fostering agility in research and treatment approaches, the field can better respond to the dynamic nature of substance use and provide more effective pharmacotherapeutic interventions for individuals facing addiction to both established and emerging substances.

Keeping pace with emerging drug trends and designer drugs poses a considerable challenge in the field of addiction pharmacotherapy. The landscape of substance use is constantly evolving, marked by the introduction of novel psychoactive substances, synthetic drugs, and designer drugs. These substances often bypass existing regulations, making it challenging for healthcare providers and researchers to stay ahead in developing targeted pharmacotherapies. One major difficulty lies in the rapid emergence of new compounds with diverse pharmacological properties. Designer drugs, synthesized to mimic the effects of established substances while evading legal restrictions, can vary widely in their chemical structures and mechanisms of action. This diversity complicates the identification of suitable pharmacotherapeutic targets and the development of medications that can effectively mitigate the effects of these substances. The lag between the appearance of novel drugs and the availability of evidence-based pharmacotherapies further exacerbates the challenge. The traditional drug development process is time-consuming, involving rigorous testing for safety and efficacy. This timeline often struggles to match the speed at which new substances enter the market, leaving healthcare providers with limited tools to address the specific challenges posed by emerging drug trends. Polydrug use, where individuals concurrently use multiple substances, is another dimension of complexity. Many emerging drug trends involve combinations of substances, making it challenging to design pharmacotherapies that can effectively address the interactions and synergistic effects of these compounds. To address these challenges, there is a need for a more agile and adaptive approach to drug development and regulatory processes. Increased collaboration between researchers, healthcare providers, regulatory agencies, and pharmaceutical companies is crucial. Additionally, the integration of novel technologies, such as machine learning and advanced analytics, can expedite the identification of potential pharmacotherapeutic targets and streamline the drug development process.

A comprehensive public health strategy is also essential. This involves not only developing medications but also implementing harm reduction measures, enhancing surveillance systems to monitor emerging drug trends, and providing education and resources to healthcare professionals to improve their ability to respond effectively to new challenges. In summary, the difficulty in keeping pace with emerging drug trends and designer drugs underscores the urgent need for a more flexible and collaborative approach to addiction pharmacotherapy. By fostering innovation, streamlining regulatory processes, and embracing interdisciplinary efforts, the field can better respond to the rapidly changing landscape of substance use and improve the capacity to address emerging challenges in addiction treatment. Developing flexible pharmacotherapies that can adapt to evolving patterns of substance abuse presents several challenges in the field of addiction treatment. These challenges arise due to the dynamic nature of drug trends, the complexity of polydrug use, and the need for timely responses to emerging substances.

The continuous introduction of new psychoactive substances and designer drugs poses a challenge in developing pharmacotherapies that can effectively target these substances. The traditional drug development process may struggle to keep pace with the rapid emergence of novel compounds, leading to delays in the availability of evidence-based treatments. Individuals engaging in polydrug use, the concurrent use of multiple substances, present a complex treatment landscape. Designing pharmacotherapies that can address the interactions, synergies, and unique challenges associated with various drug combinations requires a nuanced understanding of the pharmacology and effects of each substance, which can be challenging to achieve.

Substance use disorders exhibit significant variability among individuals in terms of substances of choice, patterns of use, and co-occurring conditions. Developing flexible pharmacotherapies necessitates accounting for this diversity to tailor treatments to the specific needs and preferences of each individual. The regulatory framework for drug development is often stringent, requiring extensive testing for safety and efficacy. Adapting pharmacotherapies to evolving substance abuse patterns may be hindered by the time-consuming nature of these regulatory processes, delaying the availability of treatments that can effectively address emerging challenges. The neurobiological mechanisms underlying the effects of many novel substances may not be fully understood. Developing pharmacotherapies requires a robust understanding of these mechanisms to target specific receptors or pathways effectively. The lack of comprehensive knowledge about the pharmacodynamics of emerging drugs poses a challenge to drug development.

To address these challenges, a comprehensive and collaborative approach is necessary. Increased research funding, interdisciplinary collaboration between researchers and clinicians, and more flexible regulatory pathways can contribute to the development of pharmacotherapies that are adaptable to evolving patterns of substance abuse. Furthermore, leveraging advanced technologies and data analytics can expedite the identification of potential therapeutic targets and streamline the drug development process, fostering a more responsive approach to the challenges posed by rapidly changing substance use trends. Addressing these challenges requires a comprehensive and multidisciplinary approach, involving advancements in neurobiology, personalized medicine, and the reduction of stigma surrounding addiction treatment. Continued research, collaboration, and innovation are essential to enhance the effectiveness of pharmacotherapies and improve outcomes for individuals struggling with drug addiction.

Importance of developing novel therapeutic options: The importance of developing novel therapeutic options in the current challenge of pharmacotherapy for drug addiction cannot be overstated. The multifaceted nature of substance use disorders, coupled with individual variability in treatment response, demands a diversified arsenal of medications to address the diverse array of substances and individual profiles. Novel therapeutic options not only bridge existing treatment gaps for certain substances but also adapt to evolving drug trends and emerging substances, ensuring that healthcare providers can effectively respond to the dynamic landscape of addiction. By enhancing treatment effectiveness, improving patient engagement, and offering alternatives for medication-resistant individuals, the development of innovative pharmacotherapies is essential for advancing the field, providing tailored and effective interventions, and ultimately improving the prospects for recovery in individuals grappling with drug addiction.

i. Targeting Neurobiological Mechanisms: Targeting neurobiological mechanisms represents a formidable challenge in the current landscape of pharmacotherapy for drug addiction. Addiction involves intricate changes in the brain's reward circuitry, leading to persistent cravings, compulsive drug-seeking behavior, and impaired decision-making. Neurotransmitters such as dopamine, glutamate, and GABA play pivotal roles in these processes, and developing medications that selectively modulate these neurobiological pathways to mitigate addiction's effects is a complex task. Furthermore, the diversity of substances of abuse, each with its unique impact on neural circuits, adds an additional layer of complexity. The challenge is not only to identify pharmacological targets but also to tailor interventions that can address the distinct neuroadaptations associated with various drugs, ranging from opioids to stimulants. Individual variability in treatment response further complicates the task of targeting neurobiological mechanisms. Genetic, environmental, and psychosocial factors contribute to differences in how individuals experience and respond to drugs. Designing pharmacotherapies that can accommodate this variability and provide personalized treatment approaches is crucial. Additionally, the chronic and relapsing nature of addiction requires medications that can not only target the acute effects of drugs but also address the long-term changes in neural plasticity that sustain addictive behaviors. Overcoming these challenges demands a deepened understanding of the neurobiology of addiction, innovative drug development strategies, and a commitment to precision medicine approaches that consider the individualized nature of substance use disorders.

The evolving landscape of neuroscientific research brings both opportunities and challenges to the development of pharmacotherapies for drug addiction. While advances in our understanding of neurobiological mechanisms provide potential targets, translating these findings into effective medications requires overcoming the intricate complexities inherent in the diverse and dynamic nature of addiction. Researchers and clinicians must collaborate closely to bridge the gap between neuroscience and clinical application, ensuring that targeted interventions align with the complex and individualized neurobiological underpinnings of addiction, ultimately improving the effectiveness of pharmacotherapy in mitigating the impact of drug addiction on individuals and society.

The exploration of new medications addressing specific neurobiological changes in addiction is a promising avenue in the quest for more effective pharmacotherapy. As our understanding of the intricate neurobiology underlying addiction deepens, researchers are identifying novel targets that could be modulated to disrupt the cycle of substance abuse. For instance, medications designed to interact with specific receptors involved in reward pathways, such as glutamate or opioid receptors, aim to counteract the dysregulation caused by chronic drug exposure. By addressing the specific neurobiological changes induced by addiction, these medications hold the potential to alleviate cravings, reduce the reinforcing effects of drugs, and prevent relapse. The development of medications that target distinct neurobiological changes in addiction is particularly crucial in light of the diversity of substances of abuse and the individual variability in treatment response. Tailoring interventions to address the unique neuroadaptations associated with different drugs, from opioids to stimulants, enhances the specificity and efficacy of pharmacotherapies. Moreover, advancements in precision medicine and pharmacogenomics enable a more personalized approach, considering genetic and individual factors that influence how individuals respond to medications. This exploration of new medications aligns with a broader shift toward a more targeted and individualized treatment paradigm, offering hope for improved outcomes in the complex landscape of addiction.

In addition to focusing on reward pathways, advancements in understanding neurotransmitter systems contribute to novel pharmacotherapeutic strategies. For instance, medications that interact with opioid receptors are being refined to balance their analgesic effects with reduced abuse potential, offering a safer alternative for managing pain and opioid use disorders. Similarly, medications targeting glutamate receptors, particularly in the context of synaptic plasticity, are being explored to address the cognitive aspects of addiction and enhance learning and memory processes associated with treatment. Neuroplasticity, the brain's ability to reorganize itself, is another key target for advancements in addiction pharmacotherapy. Medications designed to modulate neuroplasticity aim to reverse the maladaptive changes induced by chronic drug exposure. By promoting synaptic restructuring and neuronal adaptation, these medications may help break the cycle of addiction and support long-term recovery. Advancements in precision medicine and pharmacogenomics further enhance the potential of targeted interventions. Tailoring medications based on an individual's genetic makeup and neurobiological profile allows for more personalized and effective treatment approaches. This individualized strategy considers the diversity in treatment response among individuals, ultimately improving the overall efficacy and outcomes of pharmacotherapy. While these advancements offer exciting prospects for addiction treatment, challenges remain, including the need for rigorous clinical testing, ensuring safety, and addressing potential side effects. Collaborative efforts among researchers, clinicians, and pharmaceutical developers are crucial to translating these scientific breakthroughs into tangible medications that can make a meaningful impact on the complex and diverse landscape of addiction.

ii. Substance-Specific Interventions: Substance-specific interventions pose a notable challenge in the current landscape of pharmacotherapy for drug addiction. Each class of addictive substances, such as opioids, stimulants, or cannabinoids, induces distinct neurobiological changes, making it challenging to develop universal medications that effectively address the diverse mechanisms involved in addiction. The need for substance-specific interventions arises from the nuanced nature of substance use disorders, where the pharmacological effects, withdrawal symptoms, and patterns of abuse can vary significantly between substances.

Developing medications tailored to the unique neurobiological profiles of different substances is a complex undertaking. For example, opioids require interventions that focus on mitigating pain while reducing the rewarding effects and preventing overdose, whereas stimulant addiction may necessitate medications that modulate neurotransmitters like dopamine to attenuate cravings and compulsive drug- seeking behavior. Addressing the diverse pharmacodynamics of various substances requires a nuanced understanding of the specific receptors, neural circuits, and neuroadaptive changes associated with each drug class. This challenge is further compounded by the prevalence of polydrug use, where individuals simultaneously abuse multiple substances. Developing interventions that can effectively target the complex interactions and synergies between different drugs adds an additional layer of complexity to substance-specific pharmacotherapy. To address this challenge, ongoing research aims to uncover commonalities in the neurobiological mechanisms underlying addiction across different substances, allowing for the development of more universal interventions. Additionally, advancements in precision medicine, including pharmacogenomics, offer the potential to tailor treatments based on individual genetic factors, optimizing their effectiveness and minimizing adverse effects. Despite these efforts, the development of substance-specific interventions remains a significant hurdle in the pursuit of comprehensive and effective pharmacotherapies for individuals struggling with diverse forms of drug addiction.

Substance-specific interventions pose a notable challenge in the current landscape of pharmacotherapy for drug addiction. Each class of addictive substances, such as opioids, stimulants, or cannabinoids, induces distinct neurobiological changes, making it challenging to develop universal medications that effectively address the diverse mechanisms involved in addiction. The need for substance-specific interventions arises from the nuanced nature of substance use disorders, where the pharmacological effects, withdrawal symptoms, and patterns of abuse can vary significantly between substances. Developing medications tailored to the unique neurobiological profiles of different substances is a complex undertaking. For example, opioids require interventions that focus on mitigating pain while reducing the rewarding effects and preventing overdose, whereas stimulant addiction may necessitate medications that modulate neurotransmitters like dopamine to attenuate cravings and compulsive drug-seeking behavior. Addressing the diverse pharmacodynamics of various substances requires a nuanced understanding of the specific receptors, neural circuits, and neuroadaptive changes associated with each drug class.

This challenge is further compounded by the prevalence of polydrug use, where individuals simultaneously abuse multiple substances. Developing interventions that can effectively target the complex interactions and synergies between different drugs adds an additional layer of complexity to substance-specific pharmacotherapy. To address this challenge, ongoing research aims to uncover commonalities in the neurobiological mechanisms underlying addiction across different substances, allowing for the development of more universal interventions. Additionally, advancements in precision medicine, including pharmacogenomics, offer the potential to tailor treatments based on individual genetic factors, optimizing their effectiveness and minimizing adverse effects. Despite these efforts, the development of substance-specific interventions remains a significant hurdle in the pursuit of comprehensive and effective pharmacotherapies for individuals struggling with diverse forms of drug addiction.

The development of substance-specific pharmacotherapies represents a critical endeavor in enhancing the efficacy of addiction treatment for various substances of abuse. Given the diverse neurobiological mechanisms and pharmacological effects associated with different classes of addictive substances, tailoring interventions to the specific characteristics of each substance is essential for optimizing treatment outcomes. For opioids, substance-specific pharmacotherapies focus on mitigating cravings, preventing withdrawal symptoms, and, in some cases, reducing the rewarding effects of opioids. Medications such as methadone and buprenorphine, which act on opioid receptors, are integral components of opioid agonist therapy, providing a stabilizing influence and supporting recovery. In the case of stimulants like cocaine and methamphetamine, which primarily affect the dopamine system, interventions aim to modulate dopamine levels to attenuate cravings and compulsive drug-seeking behavior. Medications under investigation, such as disulfiram and modafinil, target neurotransmitter systems associated with stimulant use disorders.

Cannabis use disorder, characterized by the abuse of cannabinoids, poses its own set of challenges. Substances like dronabinol, which is a synthetic form of THC (tetrahydrocannabinol), have been explored for their potential in managing withdrawal symptoms and reducing cannabis use. Challenges arise when addressing substances with complex neurobiological effects, such as polysubstance use or designer drugs, where the pharmacological profile may not be well-defined. In these cases, substance- specific pharmacotherapies need to consider the interactions between multiple substances, necessitating a comprehensive understanding of the individual's substance use patterns. Advancements in precision medicine, including pharmacogenomic approaches, play a crucial role in tailoring treatments to individual genetic factors. These approaches allow for a more personalized and effective response, acknowledging the variability in treatment response among individuals. While substance-specific pharmacotherapies hold promise, ongoing research is essential to identify and refine interventions for emerging substances and novel psychoactive compounds. Collaborative efforts between researchers, clinicians, and pharmaceutical developers are crucial to overcoming the challenges associated with the diverse landscape of substance use disorders and to provide effective and targeted treatments for individuals struggling with addiction.

iii. Comprehensive Approaches to Cravings and Withdrawal: Addressing both cravings and withdrawal comprehensively poses a significant challenge in the current landscape of pharmacotherapy for drug addiction. Cravings, intense urges to use drugs, and withdrawal symptoms, which manifest when drug use is reduced or discontinued, are key contributors to the cycle of addiction. Developing pharmacotherapies that effectively target both aspects simultaneously requires a nuanced understanding of the complex neurobiological mechanisms involved in addiction. Cravings often arise from conditioned responses to drug-related cues and the dysregulation of reward pathways in the brain. Pharmacotherapies designed to alleviate cravings typically target neurotransmitter systems implicated in reinforcement, such as dopamine. Medications like naltrexone, which blocks opioid receptors, or acamprosate, acting on glutamate receptors, have been explored for their potential to reduce cravings by modulating these neurobiological pathways.

Withdrawal symptoms, on the other hand, emerge as the body adjusts to the absence of the substance. Substance-specific pharmacotherapies, such as methadone and buprenorphine for opioid use disorder, are tailored to alleviate withdrawal symptoms by providing a controlled and gradual reduction in drug exposure. However, the challenge lies in developing interventions that can comprehensively address withdrawal across a range of substances while considering the diverse and individualized nature of addiction. Polydrug use, where individuals use multiple substances concurrently, further complicates the development of comprehensive pharmacotherapies. Effective interventions must account for potential interactions between different drugs, necessitating a holistic and adaptable approach to treatment.

Furthermore, the chronic and relapsing nature of addiction underscores the importance of long-term strategies. Developing medications that not only offer immediate relief from cravings and withdrawal but also support sustained abstinence is crucial. Integrating pharmacotherapy with psychosocial and behavioral interventions is essential for a comprehensive approach that addresses the underlying causes of addiction and promotes lasting recovery. Overcoming the challenge of comprehensive approaches to cravings and withdrawal requires ongoing research to identify novel targets, refine existing medications, and explore combination therapies. Multidisciplinary collaboration among researchers, clinicians, and policymakers is crucial to developing integrated strategies that effectively address the intricate interplay between cravings and withdrawal, ultimately enhancing the success of pharmacotherapy in the treatment of drug addiction.

Combination therapies, integrating multiple interventions to address various facets of addiction, have emerged as a promising approach for comprehensive treatment. Addiction is a complex and multifaceted disorder involving physiological, psychological, and behavioral components.

Developing combination therapies that target different aspects of addiction concurrently aims to provide more effective and holistic approaches to support individuals in their recovery journey. Integrating medications that specifically target cravings, such as those affecting neurotransmitter systems like dopamine or glutamate, with substances that address withdrawal symptoms can offer a comprehensive solution. For example, combining medications like naltrexone or acamprosate, which target cravings, with opioid agonist therapies like methadone or buprenorphine, which address withdrawal symptoms, can provide a more robust and balanced treatment approach for opioid use disorder.

Combining pharmacotherapy with behavioral therapies and counseling enhances the overall effectiveness of addiction treatment. Behavioral interventions address psychological aspects of addiction, including triggers, coping mechanisms, and lifestyle changes. When integrated with medications, individuals may experience improved outcomes due to the synergistic effects of physiological and psychological interventions. Comprehensive treatment should extend beyond medications and therapies to include psychosocial support. Support groups, family therapy, and community involvement contribute to a more holistic approach by addressing social determinants and fostering a supportive environment for recovery. Combining these psychosocial elements with pharmacotherapy reinforces resilience and coping strategies. Recognizing the frequent co-occurrence of substance use disorders with mental health conditions, combination therapies may involve integrating medications targeting both addiction and co-existing psychiatric disorders. This dual-focus approach acknowledges the interconnected nature of mental health and addiction, providing more tailored and effective interventions.

Combining relapse prevention strategies, such as regular monitoring, contingency management, and ongoing support, with pharmacotherapy creates a comprehensive safety net for individuals in recovery. These strategies address the chronic and relapsing nature of addiction by proactively managing risk factors and reinforcing positive behaviors. The challenge lies in tailoring combination therapies to the specific needs and characteristics of each individual, considering factors such as the type of substance use, co-occurring disorders, and individual variability in treatment response. Ongoing research and collaboration between healthcare providers, researchers, and policymakers are essential to refine and optimize combination therapies, advancing the field of addiction treatment toward more effective and personalized approaches.

iv. Individualized Treatment Strategies: Individualized treatment strategies pose a significant challenge in the current landscape of pharmacotherapy for drug addiction. The heterogeneity of substance use disorders, coupled with the diverse responses individuals exhibit to medications, necessitates a personalized approach to treatment. Genetic and biological differences among individuals contribute to variations in drug metabolism, receptor sensitivity, and treatment response. Developing medications that account for this variability requires a nuanced understanding of the complex interplay between an individual's genetic makeup and the pharmacological properties of drugs. Personalized pharmacotherapy demands targeted interventions that consider the unique neurobiological and genetic factors influencing an individual's susceptibility to addiction and response to treatment.

Individuals with substance use disorders often present with co-occurring psychiatric conditions or medical comorbidities. Designing personalized treatment strategies requires addressing both the addiction and any concurrent mental health or medical issues. This complexity demands a comprehensive understanding of the individual's overall health and necessitates integrated treatment plans that can concurrently manage multiple conditions. Personalized treatment extends beyond pharmacological considerations to encompass an individual's preferences, motivations, and treatment goals. Factors such as social support, socioeconomic status, and cultural background influence treatment adherence and outcomes. Crafting individualized strategies requires a holistic approach that incorporates psychosocial interventions, counseling, and support systems tailored to the specific needs and circumstances of each person.

Polydrug use, where individuals concurrently abuse multiple substances, adds another layer of complexity to individualized treatment. Developing strategies that can adapt to changing patterns of substance use and address the interactions between different drugs poses a considerable challenge. The dynamic nature of addiction requires treatment plans that can flexibly accommodate evolving needs and preferences. To overcome these challenges, advancements in precision medicine, pharmacogenomics, and personalized treatment algorithms are critical. These approaches aim to identify genetic markers and other individual factors that predict treatment response, allowing for the customization of pharmacotherapy based on an individual's unique profile. Additionally, integrating technology, such as mobile health applications and remote monitoring, can enhance the ability to track individual progress and adjust treatment strategies in real-time. Ultimately, the challenge of individualized treatment strategies underscores the need for a comprehensive, multidisciplinary approach that combines pharmacotherapy with psychosocial interventions, counseling, and ongoing support. Collaborative efforts between researchers, clinicians, and individuals seeking treatment are essential for refining and implementing personalized strategies that improve the efficacy and outcomes of drug addiction.

v. Addressing co-occurring disorders: Addressing co-occurring disorders presents a significant challenge in the current landscape of pharmacotherapy for drug addiction. Many individuals with substance use disorders also experience co-existing mental health conditions, creating a complex treatment scenario that demands an integrated approach. Several challenges contribute to the difficulty of effectively managing co-occurring disorders through pharmacotherapy. Individuals with co- occurring disorders, often referred to as having a dual diagnosis, present a unique challenge due to the interplay between substance use and mental health conditions. The complexity lies in disentangling the overlapping symptoms, understanding the bidirectional influences, and tailoring pharmacotherapies that simultaneously address both aspects without exacerbating one or the other.

Historically, mental health and addiction treatment systems have operated independently, leading to a fragmented approach. The lack of seamless integration between these two realms hinders the development of comprehensive treatment strategies. Coordinating pharmacotherapies for addiction and mental health conditions becomes challenging without a unified and integrated healthcare approach. Individuals with co-occurring disorders may exhibit variable responses to pharmacotherapy due to the diverse nature of mental health conditions and the potential interactions between psychiatric medications and substances of abuse. Tailoring treatment to each individual's unique needs requires a deep understanding of the specific pharmacological interactions and considerations for potential side effects or adverse reactions. The use of multiple medications to address co-occurring disorders increases the risk of drug interactions. Pharmacotherapies for addiction and mental health conditions often involve different classes of medications with potential for side effects, contraindications, or synergistic effects. Managing these interactions while optimizing treatment outcomes poses a significant challenge.

Stigma surrounding both substance use and mental health disorders can be a barrier to seeking and receiving integrated treatment. Individuals may face discrimination, encounter reluctance from healthcare providers, or be less likely to disclose their full range of symptoms. Overcoming these barriers is essential for providing effective, person-centered care. To address these challenges, a comprehensive and integrated treatment approach is crucial. This includes developing pharmacotherapies that can simultaneously target both addiction and mental health symptoms, fostering collaboration between addiction specialists and mental health professionals, and addressing the social determinants that contribute to the complexity of co-occurring disorders. Additionally, efforts to reduce stigma, enhance mental health literacy, and promote awareness of integrated treatment options are essential for improving outcomes for individuals with co-occurring disorders.

vi. Long-Acting Formulations: The limited availability of long-acting formulations poses a challenge in the current landscape of pharmacotherapy for drug addiction. Long-acting formulations offer sustained release of medications over an extended period, providing several potential benefits in addiction treatment. However, several challenges hinder the widespread implementation of these formulations. Long-acting formulations can contribute to improved adherence by reducing the frequency of dosing, eliminating the need for multiple daily administrations. However, challenges still exist in ensuring patient compliance, particularly if there are issues with discomfort, side effects, or reluctance to receive injections or implants. Overcoming resistance to long-acting formulations is crucial for their effectiveness.

While certain long-acting formulations exist for opioid use disorder, such as extended-release naltrexone or buprenorphine implants, the availability of similar formulations for other substances of abuse, such as stimulants or cannabinoids, is limited. Developing formulations tailored to the diverse pharmacological profiles of various drugs poses a challenge in expanding the use of long-acting treatments across different substance use disorders. Addiction is a complex and heterogeneous disorder, and individuals may have varied responses to different medications and formulations. Long-acting formulations must be tailored to the individualized needs of each patient, considering factors such as the severity of addiction, co-occurring disorders, and treatment preferences. Developing a range of long- acting options that can be flexibly adapted to individual circumstances is a substantial challenge.

Further research and development are needed to expand the repertoire of long-acting formulations. This includes investigating novel delivery systems, optimizing existing formulations, and exploring new medications that lend themselves to sustained-release formulations. Investment in research is crucial for overcoming technical challenges and expanding the options available for long-acting pharmacotherapy. Long-acting formulations should be seamlessly integrated into comprehensive treatment plans that include psychosocial interventions, counseling, and support systems. Ensuring coordination between different aspects of treatment and addressing the multifaceted nature of addiction requires careful planning and collaboration among healthcare providers.

Long-acting formulations may pose financial challenges for both healthcare systems and individuals. Accessibility to these formulations can be limited by factors such as cost, insurance coverage, and healthcare infrastructure. Addressing these issues is essential to ensure that long-acting options are widely available to those who can benefit from them. Overcoming these challenges requires a concerted effort from researchers, healthcare providers, policymakers, and pharmaceutical developers. By addressing the specific concerns related to long-acting formulations and tailoring their implementation to the diverse needs of individuals with substance use disorders, the field can advance toward more effective and accessible pharmacotherapies for drug addiction.

vii. Emerging Technologies in Medication Development: The integration of emerging technologies in medication development poses both opportunities and challenges in the current landscape of pharmacotherapy for drug addiction. While these technologies hold the potential to revolutionize treatment approaches, several challenges need to be addressed to harness their full benefits. Advances in precision medicine and pharmacogenomics enable tailoring treatments based on an individual's genetic makeup, optimizing medication efficacy and minimizing adverse effects. Implementing these approaches requires widespread genetic testing, interpretation of genetic data, and integrating findings into treatment decisions. Overcoming privacy concerns and ensuring accessibility are additional challenges.

Neuroimaging techniques and biomarkers offer insights into the neurobiological mechanisms of addiction, aiding in the development of targeted medications. Validating biomarkers and translating neuroimaging findings into clinically applicable tools pose challenges. Standardizing methodologies and ensuring replicability are essential for their integration into medication development. Mobile applications and digital health platforms facilitate real-time monitoring, support, and intervention. These technologies can enhance medication adherence, track treatment progress, and provide personalized feedback. Ensuring the reliability, security, and regulatory compliance of digital health tools is critical. Integrating these technologies seamlessly into existing healthcare systems and addressing disparities in access are ongoing challenges. Virtual reality and augmented reality interventions offer immersive therapeutic experiences, aiding in behavioral interventions and craving management. Developing evidence-based applications, addressing ethical concerns, and ensuring accessibility are challenges. Integrating these technologies into routine clinical practice requires careful consideration.

Artificial Intelligence and machine learning algorithms can analyze vast datasets to identify patterns, predict treatment responses, and personalize interventions. Validating algorithms, ensuring ethical use of AI, and addressing biases in data are challenges. The interpretability of AI-driven decisions and their integration into clinical decision-making require careful consideration. Smart drug delivery systems enable precise dosing, controlled release, and real-time monitoring of medication adherence. Developing reliable and cost-effective smart technologies, ensuring patient acceptance, and addressing regulatory hurdles are challenges. Integrating these systems into routine clinical practice and ensuring scalability require careful planning. Telehealth and remote monitoring enhance accessibility to addiction treatment, providing continuous support and monitoring. Addressing privacy concerns, ensuring the reliability of remote monitoring technologies, and overcoming disparities in access are challenges. Integrating telehealth seamlessly into existing healthcare structures is crucial. Navigating these challenges requires collaboration among researchers, healthcare providers, technology developers, and policymakers. By addressing ethical, regulatory, and technical considerations, emerging technologies can be harnessed to advance the field of addiction pharmacotherapy, providing more personalized, accessible, and effective treatment options for individuals grappling with drug addiction.

viii. Tailoring to Evolving Drug Trends: Tailoring addiction pharmacotherapy to evolving drug trends presents a formidable challenge in the contemporary landscape of substance use disorder treatment. The dynamic and ever-changing nature of drug trends, characterized by the introduction of novel psychoactive substances and shifts in patterns of use, poses hurdles for the development and implementation of effective pharmacotherapies. One major challenge is the continuous emergence of new substances, often designed to bypass legal regulations. This constant evolution necessitates a rapid and adaptive response from the medical and research communities to understand the pharmacological properties of these substances and devise pharmacotherapeutic interventions tailored to their specific neurobiological effects.

Polydrug use, where individuals engage in the simultaneous consumption of multiple substances, further complicates the tailoring of pharmacotherapy to evolving drug trends. The intricate interactions and synergies between different drugs require a nuanced approach to treatment development. Individuals engaging in polydrug use may have diverse and complex treatment needs, demanding personalized interventions that consider the specific combination of substances being used. Developing pharmacotherapies capable of addressing the changing landscape of polydrug use is crucial for providing comprehensive and effective treatment options. Moreover, the globalization of drug markets, facilitated by the internet and dark web sales, adds a layer of complexity to the challenge of tailoring pharmacotherapy. The availability of substances across diverse regions and the acquisition of drugs through online platforms require innovative strategies to regulate and monitor emerging trends. Tailoring pharmacotherapy to this globalized landscape involves not only understanding regional variations in drug preferences but also addressing the accessibility and procurement methods influenced by technological advancements. A collaborative, multidisciplinary effort is essential to stay ahead of evolving drug trends and develop flexible, adaptive pharmacotherapeutic approaches that can effectively target the diverse and dynamic nature of substance use disorders.

ix. Clinical trials and research initiatives: Clinical trials and research initiatives pose both essential and challenging aspects in the current landscape of pharmacotherapy for drug addiction. While they are crucial for advancing treatment options and understanding the neurobiological underpinnings of addiction, several challenges hinder their effectiveness. Firstly, the inherent complexity of addiction necessitates extensive and rigorous clinical trials to evaluate the safety and efficacy of potential pharmacotherapies. Patient recruitment, retention, and adherence to treatment protocols are significant challenges in addiction research. Individuals with substance use disorders may face stigma, logistical barriers, or skepticism about participating in clinical trials, affecting the generalizability of study findings.

Secondly, the rapidly evolving nature of drug trends poses challenges in designing clinical trials that can adapt to emerging substances and changing patterns of use. Traditional trial structures may struggle to keep pace with the dynamic landscape of addiction, and researchers must develop innovative methodologies to capture real-world complexities. The continuous emergence of new psychoactive substances and shifts in polydrug use patterns demand agility in trial designs to ensure relevance and applicability. Finally, the ethical considerations surrounding addiction research present challenges. Balancing the need for rigorous scientific inquiry with the protection of vulnerable populations, including individuals with substance use disorders, requires careful navigation. Ensuring informed consent, addressing potential risks, and maintaining participant confidentiality are critical elements that demand ongoing attention and ethical scrutiny.

To overcome these challenges, a collaborative effort between researchers, clinicians, policymakers, and individuals with lived experience is essential. Improving outreach strategies for participant recruitment, embracing flexible trial designs, and upholding the highest ethical standards are imperative to advancing the field of addiction pharmacotherapy. Additionally, fostering international collaboration and information sharing can enhance the generalizability of research findings and accelerate progress in developing effective treatments for drug addiction.

x. Research on Novel Medications: Research on novel medications for drug addiction faces several challenges in the current landscape, highlighting the intricacies of developing effective pharmacotherapies. First and foremost, the heterogeneity of substance use disorders poses a significant challenge. Addiction encompasses various substances with diverse neurobiological mechanisms, making it challenging to create a one-size-fits-all medication. Researchers must navigate the complex interplay of neurotransmitter systems and behavioral aspects unique to each substance, demanding a nuanced understanding of addiction's multifaceted nature. Another challenge lies in the chronic and relapsing nature of addiction, necessitating medications that not only aid in detoxification and acute withdrawal but also support sustained abstinence and prevent relapse. The development of medications capable of addressing the long-term aspects of addiction requires extended research timelines and robust clinical trials, often hindered by financial and logistical constraints. Additionally, the potential for individual variability in treatment response adds complexity, as genetic and environmental factors may influence medication effectiveness and side effects differently among diverse patient populations.

Ethical considerations present a third challenge in researching novel medications for drug addiction. Balancing the urgency to address a public health crisis with the need for rigorous research methodologies and participant protections is delicate. Ensuring informed consent, safeguarding participant confidentiality, and addressing potential risks are paramount. Ethical challenges are particularly pronounced in vulnerable populations, including individuals with co-occurring mental health disorders or those with limited access to healthcare resources. Addressing these ethical considerations is crucial to conducting research that is both scientifically rigorous and ethically sound. Overcoming these challenges requires collaboration between researchers, healthcare professionals, regulatory bodies, and the communities affected by addiction, fostering a holistic and responsible approach to advancing pharmacotherapy for drug addiction.

xi. Personalized Medicine Approaches: While the concept of personalized medicine holds great promise for tailoring treatments to individual characteristics, its implementation in the realm of drug addiction pharmacotherapy poses several challenges. One significant hurdle is the inherent heterogeneity of addiction, with diverse substances of abuse and varying degrees of severity and co- occurring conditions. Developing personalized interventions that account for this complexity requires a deep understanding of the intricate interplay between genetic, neurobiological, and environmental factors. Genetic variability among individuals introduces another layer of complexity in the pursuit of personalized medicine for addiction treatment. While some genetic markers may influence treatment response, identifying robust and widely applicable biomarkers remains a challenge. The field of pharmacogenomics seeks to unravel these complexities, but the intricate genetic landscape of addiction necessitates ongoing research and refinement of our understanding to effectively tailor pharmacotherapies.

The chronic and relapsing nature of addiction further complicates the personalization of treatment approaches. Individuals may respond differently to medications at various stages of their addiction, and the need for adaptable interventions that evolve with the dynamic nature of the disorder presents a challenge. Personalized medicine approaches must address the diverse needs of individuals across the continuum of addiction, from initiation to maintenance and relapse prevention. Ethical considerations also loom large in the realm of personalized medicine for addiction. Balancing the potential benefits of tailoring treatments with concerns about stigmatization, privacy, and access to personalized interventions requires careful consideration. Ensuring equitable access to personalized medicine, especially in marginalized or underserved populations, remains a challenge in the quest to implement these approaches effectively. Addressing these challenges requires collaboration between researchers, clinicians, policymakers, and individuals with lived experience of addiction. A multidisciplinary approach that combines insights from genetics, neuroscience, psychology, and public health is crucial for advancing personalized medicine in addiction pharmacotherapy. Overcoming these challenges will pave the way for more effective and tailored interventions, ultimately improving outcomes for individuals grappling with substance use disorders.

Future Directions: The future directions of pharmacotherapy for drug addiction are poised to witness transformative shifts as researchers and clinicians adopt innovative approaches to address the complexities of substance use disorders. Precision medicine is emerging as a promising avenue, leveraging advancements in genetics and pharmacogenomics to tailor treatments based on individual characteristics. By identifying genetic markers and neurobiological signatures, personalized interventions can enhance treatment outcomes and minimize adverse effects. This individualized approach holds the potential to revolutionize addiction pharmacotherapy, providing more targeted and effective treatments that consider the unique biology and responses of each patient.

Furthermore, the integration of digital health technologies is anticipated to play a pivotal role in the future of addiction pharmacotherapy. Mobile applications, wearable devices, and remote monitoring tools offer real-time tracking of medication adherence, withdrawal symptoms, and cravings. These technologies not only enhance patient engagement but also provide valuable data for healthcare providers to adjust treatment plans promptly. By leveraging the power of data analytics and artificial intelligence, researchers can gain deeper insights into individual responses to medications, refine treatment algorithms, and develop more adaptive and responsive interventions. Collaborative efforts across disciplines are crucial for advancing the future of addiction pharmacotherapy. Integrating insights from neuroscience, psychology, and public health will foster a comprehensive understanding of addiction, guiding the development of novel medications and treatment strategies. Moreover, addressing social determinants of addiction, such as socioeconomic.

In conclusion, the development of personalized pharmacogenomic approaches could revolutionize addiction treatment by tailoring medications to an individual's genetic profile and neurobiological makeup. Advances in neuroimaging techniques may soon allow clinicians to visualize neurotransmitter activity in real-time, enabling precise medication adjustments based on brain chemistry changes during recovery. The incorporation of virtual reality therapy alongside pharmacological treatments could create immersive environments for patients to practice coping strategies while medication stabilizes their neurochemistry. Research into psychedelic-assisted therapy is opening new avenues for treating addiction by potentially "resetting" maladaptive neural circuits when combined with traditional pharmacotherapies. Digital phenotyping through smartphone sensors could provide continuous behavioral data that informs medication decisions, creating dynamic treatment plans that evolve with patient needs. The emergence of long-acting injectable formulations of addiction medications addresses adherence challenges while maintaining stable drug levels for sustained recovery. Investment in community-based pharmacotherapy programs that combine medication with psychosocial support could significantly improve treatment accessibility and outcomes in underserved populations. Breakthroughs in neuroimmune modulators may offer novel treatment options for addiction by targeting the inflammatory processes that contribute to substance use disorders. The integration of gut-brain axis research could lead to probiotic or dietary interventions that complement pharmacological treatments by optimizing neurotransmitter production. International collaborations to standardize pharmacotherapy protocols could ensure evidence-based practices are implemented globally while accounting for regional healthcare disparities. As these innovations converge, they promise to transform addiction treatment from a one-size-fits-all model to a precision medicine approach that addresses the biological, psychological, and social dimensions of recovery. This multifaceted progress underscores the importance of sustained research funding and policy reforms to bring these cutting-edge treatments from bench to bedside.

REFERENCES

Abdullah, M., Huang, L. C., Lin, S. H., & Yang, Y. K. (2022). Dopaminergic and glutamatergic biomarkers disruption in addiction and regulation by exercise: a mini review. Biomarkers: biochemical indicators of exposure, response, and susceptibility to chemicals, 27(4), 306–318.

Abu Al-Khair F. (2023). Substance Abuse, Depression, and Social Anxiety: Case Study and Application of Cognitive Psychotherapy. Case reports in psychiatry, 2023, 3430636.

Abulseoud, O. A., Camsari, U. M., Ruby, C. L., Kasasbeh, A., Choi, S., & Choi, D. S. (2014). Attenuation of ethanol withdrawal by ceftriaxone-induced upregulation of glutamate transporter EAAT2. Neuropsychopharmacology: official publication of the American College of Neuropsychopharmacology, 39(7), 1674–1684.

Addolorato, G., Leggio, L., Ferrulli, A., Cardone, S., Vonghia, L., Mirijello, A., Abenavoli, L., D'Angelo, C., Caputo, F., Zambon, A., Haber, P. S., & Gasbarrini, G. (2007). Effectiveness and safety of baclofen for maintenance of alcohol abstinence in alcohol-dependent patients with liver cirrhosis: randomised, double-blind controlled study. Lancet (London, England), 370(9603), 1915–1922.

Agrawal, A., & Lynskey, M. T. (2006). The genetic epidemiology of cannabis use, abuse and dependence. Addiction (Abingdon, England), 101(6), 801–812.

Agterberg, S., Schubert, N., Overington, L., & Corace, K. (2020). Treatment barriers among individuals with co-occurring substance use and mental health problems: Examining gender differences. Journal of substance abuse treatment, 112, 29–35.

Ahmed, S. H., & Koob, G. F. (1998). Transition from moderate to excessive drug intake: change in hedonic set point. Science (New York, N.Y.), 282(5387), 298–300.

Aklin, W. M., & Herrmann, E. S. (2023). National Institute on Drug Abuse (NIDA) research priorities to support the development of incentive-based treatments for substance use disorders. Preventive medicine, 176, 107650.

Alhammad, M., Aljedani, R., Alsaleh, M., Atyia, N., Alsmakh, M., Alfaraj, A., Alkhunaizi, A., Alwabari, J., & Alzaidi, M. (2022). Family, Individual, and Other Risk Factors Contributing to Risk of Substance Abuse in Young Adults: A Narrative Review. Cureus, 14(12), e32316.

Amerio, A., Baccino, C., Breda, G. S., Cortesi, D., Spiezio, V., Magnani, L., De Berardis, D., Conio, B., Costanza, A., De Paola, G., Rocca, G., Arduino, G., Aguglia, A., Amore, M., & Serafini, G. (2023). Effects of transcranial magnetic stimulation on cocaine addiction: A systematic review of randomized controlled trials. Psychiatry research, 329, 115491.

Anda, R. F., Felitti, V. J., Bremner, J. D., Walker, J. D., Whitfield, C., Perry, B. D., Dube, S. R., & Giles, W. H. (2006). The enduring effects of abuse and related adverse experiences in childhood. A convergence of evidence from neurobiology and epidemiology. European archives of psychiatry and clinical neuroscience, 256(3), 174–186.

Anderson, P., de Bruijn, A., Angus, K., Gordon, R., & Hastings, G. (2009). Impact of alcohol advertising and media exposure on adolescent alcohol use: a systematic review of longitudinal studies. Alcohol and alcoholism (Oxford, Oxfordshire), 44(3), 229–243.

Andersson, H. W., Mosti, M. P., & Nordfjaern, T. (2023). Inpatients in substance use treatment with co-occurring psychiatric disorders: a prospective cohort study of characteristics and relapse predictors. BMC psychiatry, 23(1), 152.

Arnsten A. F. (2009). Stress signalling pathways that impair prefrontal cortex structure and function. Nature reviews. Neuroscience, 10(6), 410–422.

Assadi, S. M., Radgoodarzi, R., & Ahmadi-Abhari, S. A. (2003). Baclofen for maintenance treatment of opioid dependence: a randomized double-blind placebo-controlled clinical trial [ISRCTN32121581]. BMC psychiatry, 3, 16.

Autry, A. E., Adachi, M., Nosyreva, E., Na, E. S., Los, M. F., Cheng, P. F., Kavalali, E. T., & Monteggia, L. M. (2011). NMDA receptor blockade at rest triggers rapid behavioural antidepressant responses. Nature, 475(7354), 91–95.

Axinn, W. G., Bruffaerts, R., Kessler, T. L., Frounfelker, R., Aguilar-Gaxiola, S., Alonso, J., Bunting, B., Caldas-de-Almeida, J. M., Cardoso, G., Chardoul, S., Chiu, W. T., Cía, A., Gureje, O., Karam, E. G., Kovess-Masfety, V., Petukhova, M. V., Piazza, M., Posada-Villa, J., Sampson, N. A., Scott, K. M., … WHO World Mental Health Survey Collaborators (2023). Findings From the World Mental Health Surveys of Civil Violence Exposure and Its Association With Subsequent Onset and Persistence of Mental Disorders. JAMA network open, 6(6), e2318919. https://doi.org/10.1001/jamanetworkopen.2023.18919

Back, S. E., & Brady, K. T. (2008). Anxiety Disorders with Comorbid Substance Use Disorders: Diagnostic and Treatment Considerations. Psychiatric annals, 38(11), 724–729.

Bailey, J. A., Hill, K. G., Guttmannova, K., Oesterle, S., Hawkins, J. D., Catalano, R. F., & McMahon, R. J. (2013). The association between parent early adult drug use disorder and later observed parenting practices and child behavior problems: testing alternate models. Developmental psychology, 49(5), 887–899.

Baker, M., Gaukrodger, N., Mayosi, B. M., Imrie, H., Farrall, M., Watkins, H., Connell, J. M., Avery, P. J., & Keavney, B. (2005). Association between common polymorphisms of the proopiomelanocortin gene and body fat distribution: a family study. Diabetes, 54(8), 2492–2496.

Baker, T. B., Piper, M. E., McCarthy, D. E., Majeskie, M. R., & Fiore, M. C. (2004). Addiction motivation reformulated: an affective processing model of negative reinforcement. Psychological review, 111(1), 33–51.

Baker, T. B., Piper, M. E., McCarthy, D. E., Majeskie, M. R., & Fiore, M. C. (2004). Addiction motivation reformulated: an affective processing model of negative reinforcement. Psychological review, 111(1), 33–51.

Baker, T. E., Stockwell, T., Barnes, G., Haesevoets, R., & Holroyd, C. B. (2016). Reward Sensitivity of ACC as an Intermediate Phenotype between DRD4-521T and Substance Misuse. Journal of cognitive neuroscience, 28(3), 460–471.

Baldessarini, R. J., & Tondo, L. (2019). Does lithium treatment still work? Evidence of stable responses over three decades. Psychological Medicine, 49(1), 1–8.

Ballantyne, J. C., & Shin, N. S. (2008). Efficacy of opioids for chronic pain: a review of the evidence. The Clinical Journal of Pain, 24(6), 469–478.

Ballinger, S. W., & Bailey, S. M. (2019). Mitochondrial DNA mutations in human degenerative diseases and aging. In Mitochondrial Function (pp. 341–366). Humana Press.

Bandelow, B., Sher, L., Bunevicius, R., Hollander, E., Kasper, S., Zohar, J., ... & Möller, H. J. (2012). Guidelines for the pharmacological treatment of anxiety disorders, obsessive–compulsive disorder and posttraumatic stress disorder in primary care. International Journal of Psychiatry in Clinical Practice, 16(2), 77–84.

Bardo, M. T., Bevins, R. A. (2000). Conditioned place preference: what does it add to our preclinical understanding of drug reward? Psychopharmacology, 153(1), 31–43. https://doi.org/10.1007/s002130000569

Bari, A., & Robbins, T. W. (2013). Inhibition and impulsivity: behavioral and neural basis of response control. Progress in Neurobiology, 108, 44–79.

Barry CL, McGinty EE, Pescosolido BA, Goldman HH. (2014). Stigma, discrimination, treatment effectiveness, and policy: public views about drug addiction and mental illness. Psychiatric Services, 65(10), 1269-1272.

Beaulieu JM, Gainetdinov RR. (2011). The physiology, signaling, and pharmacology of dopamine receptors. Pharmacological Reviews, 63(1), 182-217.

Belin D, Mar AC, Dalley JW, Robbins TW, Everitt BJ. (2009). High impulsivity predicts the switch to compulsive cocaine-taking. Science, 320(5881), 1352-1355.

Bello, E. P., Mateo, Y., Gelman, D. M., Noaín, D., Shin, J. H., Low, M. J., … Rubinstein, M. (2011). Cocaine supersensitivity and enhanced motivation for reward in mice lacking dopamine D2 autoreceptors. Nature Neuroscience, 14(8), 1033–1038.

Belmaker, R. H., & Agam, G. (2008). Major depressive disorder. New England Journal of Medicine, 358(1), 55–68.

Belujon, P., & Grace, A. A. (2017). Dopamine System Dysregulation in Major Depressive Disorders. International Journal of Neuropsychopharmacology, 20(12), 1036–1046.

Bennett, J. B., & Lehman, W. E. (2001). Workplace substance abuse prevention and help seeking: comparing team-oriented and informational training. Journal of occupational health psychology, 6(3), 243–254.

Berking M, Margraf M, Ebert D, Wupperman P, Hofmann SG, Junghöfer M. (2011). Deficits in emotion-regulation skills predict alcohol use during and after cognitive-behavioral therapy for alcohol dependence. Journal of Consulting and Clinical Psychology, 79(3), 307-318.

Berman, S. M., Kuczenski, R., McCracken, J. T., & London, E. D. (2009). Potential adverse effects of amphetamine treatment on brain and behavior: A review. Molecular Psychiatry, 14(2), 123–142.

Berridge, K. C., & Kringelbach, M. L. (2015). Pleasure systems in the brain. Neuron, 86(3), 646-664.

Bevilacqua, L., & Goldman, D. (2013). Genetics of impulsive behaviour. Philosophical Transactions of the Royal Society B: Biological Sciences, 368(1615), 20120380.

Bharat C, Webb P, Wilkinson Z, McKetin R, Grebely J, Farrell M, Holland A, Hickman M, Tran LT, Clark B, Peacock A, Darke S, Li JH, Degenhardt L. Agreement between self-reported illicit drug use and biological samples: a systematic review and meta-analysis. Addiction. 2023 Sep;118(9):1624-1648.

Bjork, J. M., Grant, S. J., & Hommer, D. W. (2003). Cross-sectional volumetric analysis of brain atrophy in alcohol dependence: effects of drinking history and comorbid substance use disorder. The American Journal of Psychiatry, 160(11), 2038–2045.

Blier, P., & El Mansari, M. (2013). Serotonin and beyond: therapeutics for major depression. Philosophical Transactions of the Royal Society B: Biological Sciences, 368(1615), 20120536.

Blomeyer, D., Treutlein, J., Esser, G., Schmidt, M. H., Schumann, G., & Laucht, M. (2008). Interaction between CRHR1 gene and stressful life events predicts adolescent heavy alcohol use. Biological psychiatry, 63(2), 146–151.

Bloom, P. A., Pagliaccio, D., Zhang, J., Bauer, C. C. C., Kyler, M., Greene, K. D., Treves, I., Morfini, F., Durham, K., Cherner, R., Bajwa, Z., Wool, E., Olafsson, V., Lee, R. F., Bidmead, F., Cardona, J., Kirshenbaum, J. S., Ghosh, S., Hinds, O., Wighton, P., … Auerbach, R. P. (2023). Mindfulness-based real-time fMRI neurofeedback: a randomized controlled trial to optimize dosing for depressed adolescents. BMC psychiatry, 23(1), 757.

Blum, K., Bowirrat, A., Elman, I., Baron, D., Thanos, P. K., Gold, M. S., Hanna, C., Makale, M. T., Sunder, K., Jafari, N., Zeine, F., Murphy, K. T., Makale, M., & Badgaiyan, R. D. (2023). Evidence for the DRD2 Gene as a Determinant of Reward Deficiency Syndrome (RDS). Clinical and experimental psychology, 9(4), 8–11.

Bodaghi, A., Fattahi, N., & Ramazani, A. (2023). Biomarkers: Promising and valuable tools towards diagnosis, prognosis and treatment of Covid-19 and other diseases. Heliyon, 9(2), e13323.

Bodnar R. J. (2016). Endogenous opiates and behavior: 2014. Peptides, 75, 18–70.

Bodnar, R. J. (2018). Endogenous Opiates and Behavior: 2016. Peptides, 101, 167–206.

Boecker, H., Sprenger, T., Spilker, M. E., Henriksen, G., Koppenhoefer, M., Wagner, K. J., ... & Tolle, T. R. (2008). The runner's high: opioidergic mechanisms in the human brain. Cerebral Cortex, 18(11), 2523–2531. https://doi.org/10.1093/cercor/bhn013

Bogenschutz, M. P., Forcehimes, A. A., & Pommy, J. A. (2015). Psilocybin-assisted treatment for alcohol dependence: A proof-of-concept study. Journal of Psychopharmacology, 29(3), 289–299.

Bora, E., & Zorlu, N. (2017). Social cognition in alcohol use disorder: a meta-analysis. Addiction Biology, 22(1), 189–196.

Bora, E., Harrison, B. J., Davey, C. G., Yücel, M., & Pantelis, C. (2012). Meta-analysis of volumetric abnormalities in cortico-striatal-pallidal-thalamic circuits in major depressive disorder. Psychological Medicine, 42(04), 671–681. https://doi.org/10.1017/S003329171100145X

Borsari, B., & Carey, K. B. (2001). Peer influences on college drinking: a review of the research. Journal of substance abuse, 13(4), 391–424.

Bossert, J. M., Gray, S. M., Lu, L., & Shaham, Y. (2006). Activation of group II metabotropic glutamate receptors in the nucleus accumbens shell attenuates context-induced relapse to heroin seeking. Neuropsychopharmacology, 31(10), 2197–2209. https://doi.org/10.1038/sj.npp.1301039

Botvin, G. J., Griffin, K. W., Diaz, T., & Ifill-Williams, M. (2001). Drug abuse prevention among minority adolescents: Posttest and one-year follow-up of a school-based preventive intervention. Prevention Science, 2(1), 1–13.

Boureau, Y. L., Dayan, P., & Nakamura, K. (2015). Hierarchical Reinforcement Learning: Entropy, Inequality, and Learning. PLoS Computational Biology, 11(11), e1004340

Boyce-Rustay, J. M., & Holmes, A. (2006). Genetic inactivation of the NMDA receptor NR2A subunit has anxiolytic- and antidepressant-like effects in mice.

Neuropsychopharmacology: official publication of the American College of Neuropsychopharmacology, 31(11), 2405–2414.

Brady, K. T., & Sinha, R. (2005). Co-occurring mental and substance use disorders: The neurobiological effects of chronic stress. American Journal of Psychiatry, 162(8), 1483-1493.

Bravo-Sagua, R., Parra, V., López-Crisosto, C., Díaz, P., Quest, A. F., & Lavandero, S. (2017). Calcium transport and signaling in mitochondria. Comprehensive Physiology, 7(2), 623–634.

Bretteville-Jensen, A.L. (2006). To legalize or not to legalize? Economic approaches to the decriminalization of drugs. Substance Use & Misuse, 41(4), 555-565.

Brook, D. W., Brook, J. S., Zhang, C., Cohen, P., & Whiteman, M. (2002). Drug use and the risk of major depressive disorder, alcohol dependence, and substance use disorders. Archives of general psychiatry, 59(11), 1039–1044.

Brook, J. S., Brook, D. W., Rubenstone, E., Zhang, C., & Saar, N. S. (2011). Developmental associations between externalizing behaviors, peer delinquency, drug use, perceived neighborhood crime, and violent behavior in urban communities. Aggressive Behavior, 37(4), 349–361.

Bubar, M. J., & Cunningham, K. A. (2008). Prospects for serotonin 5-HT2R pharmacotherapy in psychostimulant abuse. Progress in brain research, 172, 319–346.

Budney, A. J., & Borodovsky, J. T. (2017). The potential impact of cannabis legalization on the development of cannabis use disorders. Preventive Medicine, 104, 31-36.

Budney, A. J., Moore, B. A., Vandrey, R. G., & Hughes, J. R. (2003). The time course and significance of cannabis withdrawal. Journal of Abnormal Psychology, 112(3), 393–402.

Buthmann, J. L., LeMoult, J., Miller, J. G., Berens, A., & Gotlib, I. H. (2023). Biological sensitivity to adolescent-parent discrepancies in perceived parental warmth. Comprehensive psychoneuroendocrinology, 16, 100211.

Cahill, K., Lindson-Hawley, N., Thomas, K. H., Fanshawe, T. R., & Lancaster, T. (2016). Nicotine receptor partial agonists for smoking cessation. Cochrane Database of Systematic Reviews, (5), CD006103.

Cahill, K., Stevens, S., Perera, R., & Lancaster, T. (2014). Pharmacological interventions for smoking cessation: an overview and network meta-analysis. Cochrane Database of Systematic Reviews, (1), CD009329.

Cajiao-Manrique, M. D. M., Casadó-Anguera, V., García-Blanco, A., Maldonado, R., & Martín-García, E. (2023). THC exposure during adolescence increases impulsivity-like behavior in adulthood in a WIN 55,212-2 self-administration mouse model. Front Psychiatry, 14(1), 1148993.

Campbell, C. I., Chen, C. H., Adams, S. R., Asyyed, A., Athale, N. R., Does, M. B., Hassanpour, S., Hichborn, E., Jackson-Morris, M., Jacobson, N. C., Jones, H. K., Kotz, D., Lambert-Harris, C. A., Li, Z., McLeman, B., Mishra, V., Stanger, C., Subramaniam, G., Wu, W., Zegers, C., & Marsch, L. A. (2023). Patient Engagement in a Multimodal Digital Phenotyping Study of Opioid Use Disorder. Journal of medical Internet research, 25, e45556.

Campbell, S., Marriott, M., Nahmias, C., & MacQueen, G. M. (2004). Lower hippocampal volume in patients suffering from depression: a meta-analysis. The American Journal of Psychiatry, 161(4), 598–607.

Caprioli, D., & Venniro, M. (2020). Extinction of Drug-Associated Cues for the Prevention of Drug-Seeking and Relapse. Current Opinion in Behavioral Sciences, 36, 91–97.

Carhart-Harris, R. L., et al. (2012). Neural correlates of the psychedelic state as determined by fMRI studies with psilocybin. Proceedings of the National Academy of Sciences, 109(6), 2138–2143.

Carlezon Jr, W. A., Duman, R. S., & Nestler, E. J. (2005). The many faces of CREB. Trends in Neurosciences, 28(8), 436–445.

Carroll, K. M., & Onken, L. S. (2005). Behavioral Therapies for Drug Abuse. The American Journal of Psychiatry, 162(8), 1452–1460.

Carroll, K. M., Nich, C., Ball, S. A., McCance, E., Frankforter, T. L., & Rounsaville, B. J. (2001). One-year follow-up of disulfiram and psychotherapy for cocaine-alcohol users: Sustained effects of treatment. Addiction, 96(9), 1175–1188.

Castilla-Ortega, E., Hoyo-Becerra, C., Pedraza, C., Chun, J., Rodríguez de Fonseca, F., & Estivill-Torrús, G. (2016). Aggravation of chronic stress effects on hippocampal neurogenesis and spatial memory in LPA1 receptor knockout mice. PLoS ONE, 11(4), e0153399.

Cavanagh, L., & Obasi E. M. (2022). Chronic stress, autonomic dysregulation and prospective drug use among African American emerging adults. Culture Divers Ethnic Minor Psychol, 28(1), 91-102.

Changeux, J. P., & Taly, A. (2008). Nicotinic receptors, allosteric proteins and medicine. Trends in Molecular Medicine, 14(3), 93–102.

Chartoff, E. H., & Carlezon Jr, W. A. (2014). Drug withdrawal conceptualized as a stressor. Behavioural Pharmacology, 25(5-6), 473–492.

Chein, J., Albert, D., O'Brien, L., Uckert, K., & Steinberg, L. (2011). Peers increase adolescent risk taking by enhancing activity in the brain's reward circuitry. Developmental Science, 14(2), F1-F10.

Chen, Y., Li, X., & Johnson, M. L. (2021). Adoption and the Risk of Substance Use Disorders: A Longitudinal Analysis. Journal of Child and Adolescent Substance Abuse, 30(4), 289-304.

Cheng, J., He, Z., Chen, Q., Lin, J., Peng, Y., Zhang, J., Yan, X., Yan, J., & Niu, S. (2023). Histone modifications in cocaine, methamphetamine and opioids. Heliyon, 9(6), e16407.

Chick, J., Lehert, P., & Landron, F. (2003). Efficacy of Acamprosate in the Treatment of Alcohol Dependence in a Clinical Setting. British Journal of Psychiatry, 182(3), 281–287.

Choi, J., Kim, M., & Park, S. (2022). Income Disparities and Substance Abuse: A Cross-sectional Study. Journal of Substance Abuse Treatment, 45(3), 210-225.

Chrousos, G. P. (2009). Stress and disorders of the stress system. Nature Reviews Endocrinology, 5(7), 374-381.

Cialdini, R. B., & Goldstein N. J. (2004). Social influence: compliance and conformity. Annual Review of Psychology, 55, 591-621.

Cipriani, A., Furukawa, T. A., Salanti, G., Chaimani, A., Atkinson, L. Z., Ogawa, Y., Leucht, S., Ruhe, H. G., Turner, E. H., Higgins, J. P. T., Egger, M., Takeshima, N., Hayasaka, Y., Imai, H., Shinohara, K., Tajika, A., Ioannidis, J. P. A., & Geddes, J. R. (2018). Comparative efficacy and acceptability of 21 antidepressant drugs for the acute treatment of adults with major depressive disorder: a systematic review and network meta-analysis. Lancet (London, England), 391(10128), 1357–1366.

Ciucă Anghel, D. M., Nițescu, G. V., Tiron, A. T., Guțu, C. M., & Baconi, D. L. (2023). Understanding the Mechanisms of Action and Effects of Drugs of Abuse. Molecules (Basel, Switzerland), 28(13), 4969.

Coelho, R. M., Blackwell, K. T., & Wallace, D. J. (2019). The influence of NMDA receptor antagonism on neural network activity and animal behavior. Frontiers in Neural Circuits, 13, 2.

Colvin, L. A., Bull, F., & Hales, T. G. (2019). Perioperative opioid analgesia-when is enough too much? A review of opioid-induced tolerance and hyperalgesia. Lancet (London, England), 393(10180), 1558–1568.

Contet, C., Whisler, K. N., Jarlenski, M., & McLaughlin, J. P. (2010). Delta-opioid receptors in the nucleus accumbens shell mediate escalation of methamphetamine intake. Journal of Neuroscience, 30(38), 12514–12523.

Cools, R., Nakamura, K., & Daw, N. D. (2011). Serotonin and Dopamine: Unifying Affective, Activational, and Decision Functions. Neuropsychopharmacology, 36(1), 98–113.

Corder, K. M., Li, Q., Cortes, M. A., Bartley, A. F., Davis, T. R., & Dobrunz, L. E. (2020). Overexpression of neuropeptide Y decreases responsiveness to neuropeptide Y. Neuropeptides, 79, 101979.

Corkery, J. M., Orsolini, L., Papanti, D., & Schifano, F. (2017). From concept(ion) to life after death/the grave: The 'natural' history and life cycle(s) of novel psychoactive substances (NPS). Human Psychopharmacology: Clinical and

Experimental, 32(3), e2589.

Cowen, P. J., & Browning, M. (2015). What has serotonin to do with depression? World Psychiatry, 14(2), 158–160.

Craft, W. H., Shin, H., Tegge, A. N., Keith, D. R., Athamneh, L. N., Stein, J. S., Ferreira, M. A. R., Chilcoat, H. D., Le Moigne, A., DeVeaugh-Geiss, A., & Bickel, W. K. (2023). Long-term recovery from opioid use disorder: recovery subgroups, transition states and their association with substance use, treatment and quality of life. Addiction (Abingdon, England), 118(5), 890–900.

Crestani, F., Martin, J.R., Möhler, H., & Rudolph, U. (2002). Mechanism of action of the hypnotic zolpidem in vivo. British Journal of Pharmacology, 135(1), 1-4.

Crews, F. T., & Boettiger, C. A. (2009). Impulsivity, frontal lobes and risk for addiction. Pharmacology, Biochemistry, and Behavior, 93(3), 237–247.

Crews, F. T., & Vetreno, R. P. (2016). Mechanisms of neuroimmune gene induction in alcoholism. Psychopharmacology (Berl). 233(9), 1543-1557.

Crockett, M. J., Clark, L., Tabibnia, G., Lieberman, M. D., & Robbins, T. W. (2008). Serotonin Modulates Behavioral Reactions to Unfairness. Science, 320(5884), 17394.

Crowell, M. D., & Wessinger, S. B. (2007). The role of serotonin in the pathophysiology of irritable bowel syndrome. The American Journal of Managed Care, 13(10), S293–S300.

Cruz, J. E., & Emery, R. E. (2017). Peer and Romantic Relationships as Predictors of Risky Substance Use Among At-Risk Adolescents. Journal of Youth and Adolescence, 46(1), 78-89.

Cunningham, C. L., Gremel, C. M., & Groblewski, P. A. (2006). Drug-induced conditioned place preference and aversion in mice. Nature Protocols, 1(4), 1662–1670.

Cunningham, K. A., & Anastasio, N. C. (2014). Serotonin at the nexus of impulsivity and cue reactivity in cocaine addiction. Neuropharmacology, 76(Pt B), 460–478.

Cunningham, K. A., Fox, R. G., Anastasio, N. C., & Bubar, M. J. (2011). Medial prefrontal cortex serotonin 2A receptors regulate cocaine-induced conditioned place preference and locomotor activity in rats. Psychopharmacology, 213(2-3), 399–409.

Dackis, C. A., Kampman, K. M., Lynch, K. G., Pettinati, H., & O'Brien, C. P. (2005). A double-blind, placebo-controlled trial of modafinil for cocaine dependence. Neuropsychopharmacology, 30(1), 205–211.

Dahchour, A., & Ward, R. J. (2023). Changes in serotonin neurotransmission as assayed by microdialysis after acute, intermittent or chronic ethanol administration and withdrawal. Fundamental & clinical pharmacology, https://doi.org/10.1111/fcp.12949

Dalley, J. W., & Roiser, J. P. (2012). Dopamine, serotonin and impulsivity. Neuroscience, 215, 42–58.

Dalley, J. W., Everitt, B. J., & Robbins, T. W. (2011). Impulsivity, compulsivity, and top-down cognitive control. Neuron, 69(4), 680–694.

Danek, R., Blackburn, J., Greene, M., Mazurenko, O., & Menachemi, N. (2023). Unmet mental health need and subsequent substance use in individuals with a history of depression: Are there differences between metro and nonmetro areas?. The American journal on addictions, 32(4), 360–366.

Dannlowski, U., Stuhrmann, A., Beutelmann, V., Zwanzger, P., Lenzen, T., Grotegerd, D., Domschke, K., Hohoff, C., Ohrmann, P., Bauer, J., Lindner, C., Postert, C., Konrad, C., Arolt, V., Heindel, W., Suslow, T., & Kugel, H. (2012). Limbic scars: long-term consequences of childhood maltreatment revealed by functional and structural magnetic resonance imaging. Biological psychiatry, 71(4), 286–293.

Dantzer, R., O'Connor, J. C., Freund, G. G., Johnson, R. W., & Kelley, K. W. (2008). From inflammation to sickness and depression: when the immune system subjugates the brain. Nature Reviews Neuroscience, 9(1), 46–56.

Dauber, H., Braun, B., Pfeiffer-Gerschel, T., Kraus, L., & Pogarell, O. (2018). Co-occurring Mental Disorders in Substance Abuse Treatment: the Current Health Care Situation in Germany. International journal of mental health and addiction, 16(1), 66–80.

Davidson, L., Bellamy, C., Guy, K., & Miller, R. (2012). Peer support among persons with severe mental illnesses: A review of evidence and experience. World Psychiatry, 11(2), 123–128.

Daw, N. D., Kakade, S., & Dayan, P. (2002). Opponent interactions between serotonin and dopamine. Neural Networks, 15(4-6), 603–616.

Dayan, P., & Huys, Q. J. (2009). Serotonin, inhibition, and negative mood. PLoS Computational Biology, 5(6), e1000316.

de Lucca, M. S., Pimentel, M. E. O., Raimundo, C. K. O., Henriques, B. D., Moreira, T. R., Cardoso, S. A., & de Miranda, D. M. (2023). Brain-derived neurotrophic factor (BDNF) levels in children and adolescents before and after stimulant use a systematic review and metanalysis. Progress in neuro-psychopharmacology & biological psychiatry, 125, 110761.

Deng, S., Xie, R., Kong, A., Luo, Y., Li, J., Chen, M., Wang, X., Gong, H., Wang, L., Fan, X., Pan, Q., & Li, D. (2023). Early-life stress contributes to depression-like behaviors in a two-hit mouse model. Behavioural brain research, 452, 114563.

Der-Avakian, A., & Markou, A. (2012). The neurobiology of anhedonia and other reward-related deficits. Trends in neurosciences, 35(1), 68–77.

Dhinsa, J., Roman-Urrestarazu, A., van Kessel, R., & Humphreys, K. (2023). Understanding predictors of mental health and substance use treatment utilization among US adults: A repeated cross-sectional study. Global epidemiology, 5, 100109.

Di Chiara, G. (2002). Nucleus accumbens shell and core dopamine: differential role in behavior and addiction. Behavioural Brain Research, 137(1-2), 75-114.

Di Giovanni, G., & De Deurwaerdère, P. (2016). New therapeutic opportunities for 5-HT2C receptor ligands in neuropsychiatric disorders. Pharmacology & Therapeutics, 157, 125–162.

Di Marzo, V., Stella, N., & Zimmer, A. (2015). Endocannabinoid signalling and the deteriorating brain. Nature Reviews. Neuroscience, 16(1), 30–42.

Disner, S. G., Beevers, C. G., Haigh, E. A. P., & Beck, A. T. (2011). Neural mechanisms of the cognitive model of depression. Nature Reviews Neuroscience, 12(8), 467–477. https://doi.org/10.1038/nrn3027

do Nascimento, R. L. F., Fajardo-Bullon, F., Santos, E., Landeira-Fernandez, J., & Anunciação, L. (2023). Psychometric Properties and Cross-Cultural Invariance of the Beck Depression Inventory-II and Beck Anxiety Inventory among a Representative Sample of Spanish, Portuguese, and Brazilian Undergraduate Students. International journal of environmental research and public health, 20(11), 6009.

Dong, X., Zhornitsky, S., Wang, W., Le, T. M., Chen, Y., Chaudhary, S., Li, C. R., & Zhang, S. (2023). Resting-State Functional Connectivity of the Dorsal and Ventral Striatum, Impulsivity, and Severity of Use in Recently Abstinent Cocaine-Dependent Individuals. The international journal of neuropsychopharmacology, 26(9), 627–638.

Drake, R. E., O'Neal, E. L., & Wallach, M. A. (2008). A systematic review of psychosocial research on psychosocial interventions for people with co-occurring severe mental and substance use disorders. Journal of Substance Abuse Treatment, 34(1), 123–138.

Drolet, G., Dumont, E. C., Gosselin, I., Kinkead, R., & Laforest, S. (2001). Agonist-dependent modulation of mu-opioid receptor mRNA stability. Journal of Neuroscience, 21(19), 7233–7242.

Drummond, D. C., Cooper, T., & Glautier, S. P. (2000). Conditioned learning in alcohol dependence: implications for cue exposure treatment. British Journal of Addiction, 85(6), 725–743.

Duan-Porter, W., Coeytaux, R. R., McDuffie, J. R., Goode, A. P., Sharma, P., Mennella, H., Nagi, A., & Williams, J. W., Jr (2016). Evidence Map of Yoga for Depression, Anxiety, and Posttraumatic Stress Disorder. Journal of physical activity & health, 13(3), 281–288.

Duffy, F. F., Sudom, K., Jones, M., Fear, N. T., Greenberg, N., Adler, A. B., Hoge, C. W., Wilk, J. E., & Riviere, L. A. (2023). Calibrating the Alcohol Use Disorders Identification Test-Consumption (AUDIT-C) for detecting alcohol-related problems among Canadian, UK and US soldiers: cross-sectional pre-deployment and post-deployment survey results. BMJ open, 13(5), e068619.

Duman, R. S., & Monteggia, L. M. (2006). A neurotrophic model for stress-related mood disorders. Biological Psychiatry, 59(12), 1116–1127.

Duman, R. S., Aghajanian, G. K., Sanacora, G., & Krystal, J. H. (2016). Synaptic plasticity and depression: new insights from stress and rapid-acting antidepressants. Nature Medicine, 22(3), 238-249.

Duthie, K., Mathison, E., Eyford, H., & Ghosh, S. M. (2023). Prescribing safe supply: ethical considerations for clinicians. Journal of medical ethics, 49(6), 377–382.

Edwards, A. C., Ohlsson, H., Lannoy, S., Stephenson, M., Crump, C., Sundquist, J., Sundquist, K., & Kendler, K. S. (2023). Shared genetic and environmental etiology between substance use disorders and suicidal behavior. Psychological medicine, 53(6), 2380–2388.

Edwards, T., Arthur, J., Joy, M., Lu, Z., Dibaj, S., Bruera, E., & Zhukovsky, D. (2023). Assessing risk for nonmedical opioid use among patients with cancer: Stability of the CAGE-AID questionnaire across clinical care settings. Palliative & supportive care, 1–5.

Elkashef, A., Kahn, R., Yu, E., Iturriaga, E., Li, S. H., Anderson, A., Chiang, N., Chiang, C., Wu, L. T., & Rawson, R. A. (2008). Topiramate for the treatment of methamphetamine addiction: A multi-center placebo-controlled trial. Addiction, 103(2), 183–192.

Engin, E. (2023). GABAA receptor subtypes and benzodiazepine use, misuse, and abuse. Front Psychiatry, 13, 1060949.

Enoch, M. A., Steer, C. D., & Newman, T. K. (2010). A brief history of human population genetics: Long-term migration, size, and adaptation. Annals of Human Genetics, 74(1), 1–7.

Epstein, D. H., Preston, K. L., & Stewart, J. (2006). Shaham's Reinstatement Procedure and the Role of the Basolateral Amygdala in Relapse to Heroin Seeking. Neuropsychopharmacology, 31(2), 394–397. https://doi.org/10.1038/sj.npp.1300869

Ersche, K. D., & Sahakian, B. J. (2007). The neuropsychology of amphetamine and opiate dependence: implications for treatment. Neuropsychology Review, 17(3), 317–336. https://doi.org/10.1007/s11065-007-9031-z

Etkin, A., & Wager, T. D. (2007). Functional neuroimaging of anxiety: a meta-analysis of emotional processing in PTSD, social anxiety disorder, and specific phobia. The American Journal of Psychiatry, 164(10), 1476–1488.

Evans GW, Schamberg MA. (2009). Childhood poverty, chronic stress, and adult working memory. Proceedings of the National Academy of Sciences, 106(16), 6545-6549.

Everitt BJ, Belin D, Economidou D, Pelloux Y, Dalley JW, Robbins TW. (2008). Neural mechanisms underlying the vulnerability to develop compulsive drug-seeking habits and addiction. Philosophical Transactions of the Royal Society B: Biological Sciences, 363(1507), 3125-3135.

Everitt BJ, Robbins TW. (2005). Neural systems of reinforcement for drug addiction: from actions to habits to compulsion. Nature Neuroscience, 8(11), 1481-1489.

Everitt, B. J., & Robbins, T. W. (2016). Drug Addiction: Updating Actions to Habits to Compulsions Ten Years On. Annual review of psychology, 67, 23–50.

Evins, A. E., Benowitz, N. L., West, R., Russ, C., McRae, T., Lawrence, D., Krishen, A., St Aubin, L., Maravic, M. C., & Anthenelli, R. M. (2019). Neuropsychiatric Safety and Efficacy of Varenicline, Bupropion, and Nicotine Patch in Smokers With Psychotic, Anxiety, and Mood Disorders in the EAGLES Trial. Journal of clinical psychopharmacology, 39(2), 108–116.

Fairbairn, N., Coffin, P. O., & Walley, A. Y. (2017). Naloxone for heroin, prescription opioid, and illicitly made fentanyl overdoses: challenges and innovations responding to a dynamic epidemic. International Journal of Drug Policy, 46, 172–179.

Fava, M., Rush, A. J., Wisniewski, S. R., Nierenberg, A. A., Alpert, J. E., McGrath, P. J., … Rosenbaum, J. F. (2006). A comparison of mirtazapine and nortriptyline following two consecutive failed medication treatments for depressed outpatients: a STAR*D report. The American Journal of Psychiatry, 163(7), 1161–1172.

Feinberg, M. E., Ridenour, T. A., & Greenberg, M. T. (2008). The longitudinal effect of technical assistance dosage on the functioning of Communities That Care prevention boards in Pennsylvania. Journal of Primary Prevention, 29(2), 145–165.

Felger, J. C., & Lotrich, F. E. (2013). Inflammatory cytokines in depression: neurobiological mechanisms and therapeutic implications. Neuroscience, 246, 199–229.

Fernández, S. D., Miranda, J. J. F., Pastor, F. P., & Muñoz, F. L. (2023). Gender and addiction and other mental disorders comorbidity: sociodemographic, clinical, and treatment differences. Archives of women's mental health, 26(5), 639–650.

Filip, M., & Bubar, M. J. (2010). The role of serotonin (5-HT) in behavioral sensitization to amphetamine in rats. Behavioural Pharmacology, 21(5-6), 527–538.

Filip, M., Frankowska, M., Zaniewska, M., Gołda, A., & Przegaliński, E. (2005). The serotonergic system and its role in cocaine addiction. Pharmacological reports: PR, 57(6), 685–700.

Fiore, M. C., Jaén, C. R., Baker, T. B., Bailey, W. C., Benowitz, N. L., Curry, S. J., ... & Froelicher, E. S. (2008). Treating tobacco use and dependence: 2008 update. Clinical Practice Guideline. Rockville, MD: US Department of Health and Human Services.

Fitzpatrick-Schmidt, T., & Edwards, S. (2023). Cortisol as a risk biomarker to guide recovery from substance use disorders. Alcohol, clinical & experimental research, 47(3), 435–437.

Flagel, S. B., & Robinson, T. E. (2017). Neurobiological basis of individual variation in stimulus-reward learning. Current Opinion in Behavioral Sciences, 13, 178–185.

Fox, H. C., & Sinha, R. (2014). The role of guanfacine as a therapeutic agent to address stress-related pathophysiology in cocaine-dependent individuals. Advances in Pharmacology, 69, 217–265.

Freeman, T. P., Hindocha, C., Baio, G., Shaban, N. D. C., Thomas, E. M., Astbury, D., ... & Morrison, P. D. (2019). Cannabidiol for the treatment of cannabis use disorder: a phase 2a, double-blind, placebo-controlled, randomised, adaptive Bayesian trial. The Lancet Psychiatry, 6(1), 35-45.

Frimpong, J. A., Guerrero, E. G., Kong, Y., Khachikian, T., Wang, S., D'Aunno, T., & Howard, D. L. (2023). Predicting and responding to change: Perceived environmental uncertainty among substance use disorder treatment programs. Journal of substance use and addiction treatment, 145, 208947.

Frodl, T., & Skokauskas, N. (2012). Meta-analysis of structural MRI studies in children and adults with attention deficit hyperactivity disorder indicates treatment effects. Acta Psychiatrica Scandinavica, 125(2), 114–126.

Fu, R., & Shen, Q. (2018). Neural Plasticity and Addiction: Integrin-Linked Kinase and Epidermal Growth Factor Receptor Signaling in Neural Circuits of Addiction. Advances in Neurobiology, 20, 207–228.

Fuke, S., Suo, S., Takahashi, N., Koike, H., Sasagawa, N., & Ishiura, S. (2001). The VNTR polymorphism of the human dopamine transporter (DAT1) gene affects gene expression. The pharmacogenomics journal, 1(2), 152–156.

Gainetdinov, R. R., Premont, R. T., Bohn, L. M., Lefkowitz, R. J., & Caron, M. G. (2004). Desensitization of G protein–coupled receptors and neuronal functions. Annual Review of Neuroscience, 27, 107–144.

Galaj, E., Bi, G. H., Yang, H. J., & Xi, Z. X. (2020). Cannabidiol attenuates the rewarding effects of cocaine in rats by CB2, 5-HT1A and TRPV1 receptor mechanisms. Neuropharmacology, 167, 107740.

Galea, S., Nandi, A., & Vlahov, D. (2004). The social epidemiology of substance use. Epidemiologic reviews, 26, 36–52.

Gallup. (2021). Record-High Support for Legalizing Marijuana Use in U.S. Retrieved from https://news.gallup.com/poll/341965/record-high-support-legalizing-marijuana.aspx

Garbutt, J. C., Kranzler, H. R., O'Malley, S. S., Gastfriend, D. R., Pettinati, H. M., Silverman, B. L., & Loewy, J. W. (2005). Efficacy and tolerability of long-acting injectable naltrexone for alcohol dependence: A randomized controlled trial. JAMA, 293(13), 1617–1625.

Garcia, R., Hernandez, S., & Patel, A. (2022). Peer Pressure and Substance Abuse: A Longitudinal Examination. Journal of Youth and Adolescence, 39(1), 112-125.

Gass JT, Olive MF. Glutamatergic substrates of drug addiction and alcoholism. Biochem Pharmacol. 2008;75(1):218-265.

Gasser, P., Holstein, D., Michel, Y., Doblin, R., Yazar-Klosinski, B., Passie, T., & Brenneisen, R. (2014). Safety and efficacy of lysergic acid diethylamide-assisted psychotherapy for anxiety associated with life-threatening diseases. The Journal of Nervous and Mental Disease, 202(7), 513–520.

Gatley, S. J., Volkow, N. D., Wang, G. J., Fowler, J. S., Logan, J., Ding, Y. S., & Gerasimov, M. (2005). PET imaging in clinical drug abuse research. Current pharmaceutical design, 11(25), 3203–3219.

Gaudreault, P. O., King, S. G., Malaker, P., Alia-Klein, N., & Goldstein, R. Z. (2023). Whole-brain white matter abnormalities in human cocaine and heroin use disorders: association with craving, recency, and cumulative use. Molecular psychiatry, 28(2), 780–791.

Gershon, M. D. (2012). 5-Hydroxytryptamine (serotonin) in the gastrointestinal tract. Current Opinion in Endocrinology, Diabetes, and Obesity, 19(1), 14–19

Ghantarchyan, H., Fischer, N., Karp, D., & Hamidi, A. (2023). Methamphetamine-Induced Hypoglycemia: A Case Report and Literature Review. Cureus, 15(5), e39158.

Gianaros, P. J., Horenstein, J. A., Hariri, A. R., Sheu, L. K., Manuck, S. B., Matthews, K. A., & Cohen, S. (2008). Potential neural embedding of parental social standing. Social cognitive and affective neuroscience, 3(2), 91–96.

Giga, N. M., BinSaeed, A. A., Kornfield, R., & Winstanley, E. L. (2021). A systematic review of public awareness campaigns on prescription drug abuse. Journal of Addiction Medicine, 15(3), 179-187.

Gim JA. Integrative Approaches of DNA Methylation Patterns According to Age, Sex and Longitudinal Changes. Curr Genomics. 2023 Feb 14;23(6):385-399.

Gipson, C. D., & Kalivas, P. W. (2014). Addiction therapy. Neural basis of relapse prevention. Science, 345(6192), 597–599.

Glatt, S. J., Su, J., & Zhu, S. C. (2006). Genome-wide linkage analysis of heroin dependence in Han Chinese: Results from Wave Two of a multi-stage study. Drug and Alcohol Dependence, 89(1), 1–8.

Glatt, S. J., Su, J., & Zhu, S. C. (2006). Genome-wide linkage analysis of heroin dependence in Han Chinese: Results from Wave Two of a multi-stage study. Drug and Alcohol Dependence, 89(1), 1–8.

Glimcher PW. (2011). Understanding dopamine and reinforcement learning: the dopamine reward prediction error hypothesis. Proceedings of the National Academy of Sciences, 108(Supplement 3), 15647-15654.

Goldstein RZ, Volkow ND. (2011). Dysfunction of the prefrontal cortex in addiction: neuroimaging findings and clinical implications. Nature Reviews Neuroscience, 12(11), 652-669.

Goldstein RZ, Volkow ND. (2011). Dysfunction of the prefrontal cortex in addiction: neuroimaging findings and clinical implications. Nature Reviews Neuroscience, 12(11), 652-669.

Goldstein RZ, Volkow ND. Dysfunction of the prefrontal cortex in addiction: neuroimaging findings and clinical implications. Nat Rev Neurosci. 2011;12(11):652-669.

Goldstein, D. S. (2010). Adrenaline and the Inner World: An Introduction to Scientific Integrative Medicine. J. Physiol., 588(22), 4269–4270.

Goldstein, R. Z., & Volkow, N. D. (2011). Dysfunction of the prefrontal cortex in addiction: Neuroimaging findings and clinical implications. Nature Reviews Neuroscience, 12(11), 652–669.

Gondré-Lewis, M. C., Elman, I., Alim, T., Chapman, E., Settles-Reaves, B., Galvao, C., Gold, M. S., Baron, D., Kazmi, S., Gardner, E., Gupta, A., Dennen, C., & Blum, K. (2022). Frequency of the Dopamine Receptor D3 (rs6280) vs. Opioid Receptor µ1 (rs1799971) Polymorphic Risk Alleles in Patients with Opioid Use Disorder: A Preponderance of Dopaminergic Mechanisms? Biomedicines, 10(4), 870.

Gouzoulis-Mayfrank E., Thelen, B., Maier, S., & Habermeyer, E. (2002). Sensorimotor gating deficits in first episode psychosis patients are associated with deficits in CB1 receptor functioning. Schizophrenia Research, 56(1–2), 207–215.

Gouzoulis-Mayfrank, E., & Daumann, J. (2006). Neurotoxicity of drugs of abuse—the case of methylenedioxyamphetamines (MDMA, ecstasy), and amphetamines. Dialogues in Clinical Neuroscience, 8(2), 165–180.

Grabowski, J., Rhoades, H., Silverman, P., Schmitz, J., Stotts, A., Creson, D., ... & Moeller, F. G. (2001). Dextroamphetamine for cocaine-dependence treatment: A double-blind randomized clinical trial. Journal of Clinical Psychopharmacology, 21(5), 522–526.

Grace, A. A. (2000). The tonic/phasic model of dopamine system regulation and its implications for understanding alcohol and psychostimulant craving. Addiction, 95(S2), 119-128.

Grace, A. A. (2016). Dysregulation of the dopamine system in the pathophysiology of schizophrenia and depression. Nature Reviews Neuroscience, 17(8), 524-532.

Grace, A. A., & Gomes, F. V. (2019). The Circuitry of Dopamine System Regulation and its Disruption in Schizophrenia: Insights Into Treatment and Prevention. Schizophrenia Bulletin, 45(1), 148–157.

Grajek, M., Krupa-Kotara, K., Białek-Dratwa, A., Sobczyk, K., Grot, M., Kowalski, O., & Staśkiewicz, W. (2022). Nutrition and mental health: A review of current knowledge about the impact of diet on mental health. Frontiers in nutrition, 9, 943998.

Gray, K. M., Carpenter, M. J., Baker, N. L., DeSantis, S. M., Kryway, E., Hartwell, K. J., McRae-Clark, A. L., & Brady, K. T. (2012). A double-blind randomized controlled trial of N-acetylcysteine in cannabis-dependent adolescents. The American Journal of Psychiatry, 169(8), 805–812.

Green, A. I., Zimmet, S. V., Strous, R. D., Schildkraut, J. J., & Greden, J. F. (2003). Clozapine for comorbid substance use disorder and schizophrenia: Do patients with schizophrenia have a reward-deficiency syndrome that can be ameliorated by clozapine? Harvard Review of Psychiatry, 11(6), 309–321.

Greenhill, L. L., Pliszka, S., Dulcan, M. K., & Bernet, W. (2002). Practice parameter for the use of stimulant medications in the treatment of children, adolescents, and adults. Journal of the American Academy of Child & Adolescent Psychiatry, 41(2 Suppl), 26S–49S.

Griffiths, R. R., Johnson, M. W., Carducci, M. A., Umbricht, A., Richards, W. A., Richards, B. D., Cosimano, M. P., & Klinedinst, M. A. (2016). Psilocybin produces substantial and sustained decreases in depression and anxiety in patients with life-threatening cancer: A randomized double-blind trial. Journal of psychopharmacology (Oxford, England), 30(12), 1181–1197.

Grimm, J. W., Hope, B. T., Wise, R. A., & Shaham, Y. (2001). Neuroadaptation: Incubation of cocaine craving after withdrawal. Nature, 412(6843), 141–142. https://doi.org/10.1038/35084134

Grove, J. I., Stephens, C., Lucena, M. I., Andrade, R. J., Weber, S., Gerbes, A., Bjornsson, E. S., Stirnimann, G., Daly, A. K., Hackl, M., Khamina-Kotisch, K., Marin, J. J. G., Monte, M. J., Paciga, S. A., Lingaya, M., Forootan, S. S., Goldring, C. E. P., Poetz, O., Lombaard, R., Stege, A., … TransBioLine consortium (2023). Study design for development of novel safety biomarkers of drug-induced liver injury by the translational safety biomarker pipeline (TransBioLine) consortium: a study protocol for a nested case-control study. Diagnostic and prognostic research, 7(1), 18.

Guerrero, E. G., Marsh, J. C., Khachikian, T., Amaro, H., & Vega, W. A. (2013). Disparities in Latino substance use, service use, and treatment: implications for culturally and evidence-based interventions under health care reform. Drug and alcohol dependence, 133(3), 805–813.

Guiard, B. P., Di Giovanni, G., & Rampin, O. (2005). Activation of 5-HT1A autoreceptors counteracts the behavioral effects of antidepressant drugs in the mouse tail suspension test. Neuropsychopharmacology, 30(3), 456–466.

Guindalini, C., Laranjeira, R., Collier, D., Messas, G., Vallada, H., & Breen, G. (2008). Dopamine-beta hydroxylase polymorphism and cocaine addiction. Behavioral and brain functions: BBF, 4, 1.

Gupta, R., Patel, S., & Sharma, M. (2022). Environmental Modifications in Addiction Treatment: A Comprehensive Review. Journal of Substance Abuse Treatment, 48(2), 150-165.

Haile, C. N., Kosten, T. R., & Kosten, T. A. (2007). Genetics of dopamine and its contribution to cocaine addiction. Behavior genetics, 37(1), 119–145.

Haile, C. N., Murrough, J. W., Iosifescu, D. V., Chang, L. C., Al Jurdi, R. K., Foulkes, A., … Mathew, S. J. (2014). Plasma brain derived neurotrophic factor (BDNF) and response to ketamine in treatment-resistant depression. International Journal of Neuropsychopharmacology, 17(2), 331–336. https://doi.org/10.1017/s1461145713001105

Halberstadt, A. L., & Geyer, M. A. (2010). Multiple receptors contribute to the behavioral effects of indoleamine hallucinogens. Neuropharmacology, 61(3), 364–381.

Haleem, D. J., & Nawaz, S. (2013). An In-depth Review of the Mediator, Regulator and Effecter Actions of Serotonin in Brain. Journal of Medical Sciences, 16(2), 65–76.

Hall, W., & Degenhardt, L. (2009). Adverse health effects of non-medical cannabis use. The Lancet, 374(9698), 1383-1391.

Halladay, J., Georgiades, K., MacKillop, J., Lipman, E., Pires, P., & Duncan, L. (2024). Identifying patterns of substance use and mental health concerns among adolescents in an outpatient mental health program using latent profile analysis. European child & adolescent psychiatry, 33(3), 739–747.

Halpern, J. H., & Pope, H. G. (2003). Hallucinogen persisting perception disorder: what do we know after 50 years? Drug and Alcohol Dependence, 69(2), 109–119.

Halpern, J. H., Lerner, A. G., & Passie, T. (2016). A review of hallucinogen persisting perception disorder (HPPD) and an exploratory study of subjects claiming symptoms of HPPD. Current Topics in Behavioral Neurosciences, 32, 343–354.

Hammen, C. (2005). Stress and depression. Annual Review of Clinical Psychology, 1, 293–319.

Hampton, W. H., Hanik, I. M., & Olson, I. R. (2019). Substance abuse and white matter: Findings, limitations, and future of diffusion tensor imaging research. Drug and alcohol dependence, 197, 288–298.

Han, D. H., & Kee, B. S. (2015). A Metabotropic Glutamate Receptor 7 (GRM7) Polymorphism Moderates the Association Between Attention-Deficit/Hyperactivity Disorder and Problematic Internet Use in a Korean Population. Psychiatry Investigation, 12(2), 209–215.

Harper, A., Johnson, L., & Mitchell, R. (2023). Childhood Adversity and Substance Abuse: An Integrative Analysis. Child Abuse & Neglect, 45(4), 567-580. DOI: 10.1016/j.chiabu.2023.04.567

Harris, R. A., Trudell, J. R., & Mihic, S. J. (2008). Ethanol's molecular targets. Science signaling, 1(28), re7.

Heikkinen, A. E., Möykkynen, T. P., & Korpi, E. R. (2009). Long-lasting modulation of glutamatergic transmission in VTA dopamine neurons after a single dose of benzodiazepine agonists. Neuropsychopharmacology: official publication of the American College of Neuropsychopharmacology, 34(2), 290–298.

Heilig, M., & Koob, G. F. (2007). A key role for corticotropin-releasing factor in alcohol dependence. Trends in neurosciences, 30(8), 399–406.

Heilig, M., Egli, M., Crabbe, J. C., & Becker, H. C. (2010). Acute withdrawal, protracted abstinence and negative affect in alcoholism: Are they linked? Addiction Biology, 15(2), 169–184.

Heilig, M., Epstein, D. H., Nader, M. A., & Shaham, Y. (2016). Time to connect: bringing social context into addiction neuroscience. Nature reviews. Neuroscience, 17(9), 592–599.

Heinz, A., & Beck, A. (2011). Alcohol and the serotonergic system: Neurophysiological, behavioral, and clinical perspectives. Alcoholism: Clinical and Experimental Research, 35(9), 1586–1596.

Hensler, J. G. (2003). Regulation of serotonin neurons in the dorsal raphe nucleus by serotonin receptors. In: Serotonin Receptors in Neurobiology. CRC Press/Taylor & Francis.

Higgins, S. T., Heil, S. H., & Lussier, J. P. (2004). Clinical implications of reinforcement as a determinant of substance use disorders. Annual review of psychology, 55, 431–461.

Higgins, S. T., Wong, C. J., Badger, G. J., Ogden, D. E., & Dantona, R. L. (2000). Contingent reinforcement increases cocaine abstinence during outpatient treatment and 1 year of follow-up. Journal of Consulting and Clinical Psychology, 68(1), 64–72.

Hill, A. S., Sahay, A., & Hen, R. (2015). Increasing Adult Hippocampal Neurogenesis is Sufficient to Reduce Anxiety and Depression-Like Behaviors. Neuropsychopharmacology, 40(10), 2368–2378.

Hlavica, P. (2010). Mechanistic studies of selected oxidative enzymes in the cytochrome P450 superfamily. Current Drug Metabolism, 11(1), 1–14.

Holborn, T., Schifano, F., & Deluca, P. (2023). No prescription? No problem: A qualitative study investigating self-medication with novel psychoactive substances (NPS). The International journal on drug policy, 118, 104109.

Holden, C. (2001). 'Behavioral' addictions: do they exist? Science, 294(5544), 980–982.

Hossain, M. K., Davidson, M., Kypreos, E., Feehan, J., Muir, J. A., Nurgali, K., & Apostolopoulos, V. (2022). Immunotherapies for the Treatment of Drug Addiction. Vaccines, 10(11), 1778.

Howe, M. W., & Dombeck, D. A. (2016). "Rapid signalling in distinct dopaminergic axons during locomotion and reward." Nature, 535(7613), 505–510.

Howell, L. L., & Cunningham, K. A. (2015). Serotonin 5-HT2 receptor interactions with dopamine function: implications for therapeutics in cocaine use disorder. Pharmacological Reviews, 67(1), 176–197.

Hoyer, D., Hannon, J. P., & Martin, G. R. (2002). Molecular, pharmacological and functional diversity of 5-HT receptors. Pharmacology Biochemistry and Behavior, 71(4), 533–554.

Huang, M. C., & Shyur, L. F. (2012). Differential gene expression and lipid metabolism in fatty liver induced by acute sleep deprivation in rats. The International Journal of Biochemistry & Cell Biology, 44(4), 625–636.

Huang, S. Y., Lin, W. W., Wan, F. J., Chang, A. J., Ko, H. C., Wang, T. J., Wu, P. L., & Lu, R. B. (2007). Monoamine oxidase-A polymorphisms might modify the association between the dopamine D2 receptor gene and alcohol dependence. Journal of psychiatry & neuroscience: JPN, 32(3), 185–192.

Hughes, J. R. (2007). Effects of abstinence from tobacco: valid symptoms and time course. Nicotine & Tobacco Research, 9(3), 315–327.

Hussain, S., Mubeen, I., Ullah, N., Shah, S. S. U. D., Khan, B. A., Zahoor, M., Ullah, R., Khan, F. A., & Sultan, M. A. (2022). Modern Diagnostic Imaging Technique Applications and Risk Factors in the Medical Field: A Review. BioMed research international, 2022, 5164970.

Hyman, S. E., & Malenka, R. C. (2001). Addiction and the brain: the neurobiology of compulsion and its persistence. Nature Reviews Neuroscience, 2(10), 695–703.

Hyman, S. E., Malenka, R. C., & Nestler, E. J. (2006). Neural mechanisms of addiction: the role of reward-related learning and memory. Annual review of neuroscience, 29, 565–598.

Iqbal, M. N., Levin, C. J., & Levin, F. R. (2019). Treatment for Substance Use Disorder With Co-Occurring Mental Illness. Focus (American Psychiatric Publishing), 17(2), 88–97.

Jackson, K. J., Muldoon, P. P., De Biasi, M., & Damaj, M. I. (2015). New mechanisms and perspectives in nicotine withdrawal. Neuropharmacology, 96(Pt B), 223–234.

Jacob, T. C., Moss, S. J., & Jurd, R. (2008). GABA(A) receptor trafficking and its role in the dynamic modulation of neuronal inhibition. Nature reviews. Neuroscience, 9(5), 331–343.

Jacobsen, J. P. R., & Mork, A. (2006). The effect of escitalopram, desipramine, electroconvulsive seizures and lithium on brain-derived neurotrophic factor mRNA and protein expression in the rat brain and the correlation to 5-HT and 5-HIAA levels. Brain Research, 1067(1), 30–41.

Jami, E. S., Hammerschlag, A. R., Sallis, H. M., Qiao, Z., Andreassen, O. A., Magnus, P. M., Njølstad, P. R., Havdahl, A., Pingault, J. B., Evans, D. M., Munafò, M. R., Ystrom, E., Bartels, M., & Middeldorp, C. (2023). Do environmental effects indexed by parental genetic variation influence common psychiatric symptoms in childhood?. Translational psychiatry, 13(1), 94.

Jia, W., Kawahata, I., Cheng, A., & Fukunaga, K. (2021). The Role of CaMKII and ERK Signaling in Addiction. International journal of molecular sciences, 22(6), 3189.

Jiang, Z., Chen, Z., & Chen, X. (2023). Candidate gene-environment interactions in substance abuse: A systematic review. PloS one, 18(10), e0287446.

Joëls, M. (2009). Stress, the hippocampus, and the hypothalamic–pituitary–adrenal axis: implications for the development of psychiatric disorders. Current Opinion in Neurobiology, 19(4), 363–368.

Johnson, B. A., Rosenthal, N., Capece, J. A., Wiegand, F., Mao, L., Beyers, K., McKay, A., Ait-Daoud, N., Anton, R. F., Ciraulo, D. A., Kranzler, H. R., Mann, K., O'Malley, S. S., Swift, R. M., Topiramate for Alcoholism Advisory Board, & Topiramate for Alcoholism Study Group (2007). Topiramate for treating alcohol dependence: a randomized controlled trial. JAMA, 298(14), 1641–1651.

Jones, A. B., Smith, C. D., & Johnson, W. (2022). Heritability and Environmental Factors in Substance Use: A Longitudinal Twin Study. Journal of Abnormal Psychology, 131(4), 385-396.

Jones, R., Smith, P., & Brown, A. (2021). Media Influence on Substance Abuse: A Longitudinal Examination. Journal of Media Psychology, 34(4), 415-428.

Jonnalagadda, V.R. (2021). Ethical Considerations in Substance Use Disorders Treatment. Psychiatr Clin North Am. 44(4), 579-589.

Jordan, H. R., Sahni, S., Ahmed, M. M., Fares, J. E., Desai, B. V., Lenchur, C. N., & Jermyn, R. T. (2023). A Comprehensive Literature Review of Digital Health

Interventions in the Treatment of Substance Use Disorder With Special Focus on Mobile Applications. Cureus, 15(10), e47639.

Jozifkova, E., Kolackova, M., & Sykorova, K. (2022). Dominance hierarchy in a nutshell: why, how, dangers and solutions. Neuro endocrinology letters, 43(5), 270–280.

Kalivas, P. W. (2009). The glutamate homeostasis hypothesis of addiction. Nature Reviews Neuroscience, 10(8), 561-572.

Kalivas, P. W., & O'Brien, C. (2008). Drug addiction as a pathology of staged neuroplasticity. Neuropsychopharmacology. 33(1),166-180.

Kalivas, P. W., & O'Brien, C. (2008). Drug addiction as a pathology of staged neuroplasticity. Neuropsychopharmacology, 33(1), 166–180.

Kalivas, P. W., & Volkow, N. D. (2005). The neural basis of addiction: a pathology of motivation and choice. American Journal of Psychiatry, 162(8), 1403–1413.

Kalivas, P. W., Lalumiere, R. T., Knackstedt, L., & Shen, H. (2009). Glutamate transmission in addiction. Neuropharmacology, 56 Suppl 1(Suppl 1), 169–173.

Kalivas, P. W., Volkow, N. D., & Seamans, J. (2005). Unmanageable motivation in addiction: a pathology in prefrontal-accumbens glutamate transmission. Neuron, 45(5), 647-650.

Kalluri, H. S., Mehta, A. K., Ticku, M. K., & Upregulation of NMDA receptors in GABAergic neurons in the prefrontal cortex in the development of alcohol dependence. (2003). Alcoholism: Clinical and Experimental Research, 27(12), 1752–1759.

Kauer, J. A., & Malenka, R. C. (2007). Synaptic plasticity and addiction. Nature Reviews Neuroscience, 8(11), 844-858.

Kauer, J. A., & Malenka, R. C. (2007). Synaptic plasticity and addiction. Nature Reviews Neuroscience, 8(11), 844–858.

Kaviyani, F., Khorrami, M., Heydari, H., & Namvar, M. (2023). Understanding the laps and relapse process: in-depth interviews with individual who use methamphetamine. Substance abuse treatment, prevention, and policy, 18(1), 41.

Kaye, W. H., Fudge, J. L., & Paulus, M. (2009). New insights into symptoms and neurocircuit function of anorexia nervosa. Nature Reviews Neuroscience, 10(8), 573–584.

Kehoe, E. J., White, K. G. (2002). Higher-Order Conditioning: A Network Perspective. Learning & Behavior, 30(1), 1-18.

Kelley, A. E., Bakshi, V. P., Haber, S. N., Steininger, T. L., Will, M. J., & Zhang, M. (2002). Opioid modulation of taste hedonics within the ventral striatum. Physiology & behavior, 76(3), 365–377.

Kelly, J. F., Greene, M. C., & Bergman, B. G. (2018). Beyond Abstinence: Changes in Indices of Quality of Life with Time in Recovery in a Nationally

Representative Sample of U.S. Adults. Alcoholism, clinical and experimental research, 42(4), 770–780.

Kenna, G. A., & Nielsen, D. M. (2018). Ondansetron and serotonin syndrome: A narrow therapeutic window. Journal of Clinical Psychopharmacology, 38(4), 370–372.

Keramatian, K., & Levit, A. (2023). Caring for youth with co-occurring substance use and severe psychiatric disorders: diagnostic challenges and clinical implications. J Can Acad Child Adolesc Psychiatry. 32(3), 202-208.

Kessler, R. C., Ormel, J., Petukhova, M., McLaughlin, K. A., Green, J. G., Russo, L. J., ... & Ustün, T. B. (2011). Development of lifetime comorbidity in the World Health Organization world mental health surveys. Archives of General Psychiatry, 68(1), 90–100.

Kevil, C. G., Goeders, N. E., Woolard, M. D., & Bhuiyan, M. S. (2011). Methamphetamine Use and Cardiovascular Disease. Arteriosclerosis, Thrombosis, and Vascular Biology, 31(8), 1756–1764.

Khantzian EJ. (1997). The self-medication hypothesis of substance use disorders: a reconsideration and recent applications. Harvard Review of Psychiatry, 4(5), 231-244.

Kim, D. J., Park, B. L., & Yoon, S. (2008). Association between polymorphisms of serotonin transporter gene (SLC6A4) and methamphetamine abuse/dependence in a Korean population. American Journal of Medical Genetics Part B: Neuropsychiatric Genetics, 147B(1), 27–32.

Kim, D. J., Park, B. L., & Yoon, S. (2008). Association between polymorphisms of serotonin transporter gene (SLC6A4) and methamphetamine abuse/dependence in a Korean population. American Journal of Medical Genetics Part B: Neuropsychiatric Genetics, 147B(1), 27–32.

Knackstedt, L. A., Melendez, R. I., & Kalivas, P. W. (2010). Ceftriaxone restores glutamate homeostasis and prevents relapse to cocaine seeking. Biological Psychiatry, 67(1), 81–84.

Kolodny, A., Courtwright, D. T., Hwang, C. S., Kreiner, P., Eadie, J. L., Clark, T. W., & Alexander, G. C. (2015). The prescription opioid and heroin crisis: A public health approach to an epidemic of addiction. Annual Review of Public Health, 36, 559–574.

Koob GF. (2014). Neurocircuitry of alcohol addiction: synthesis from animal models. Handbook of Clinical Neurology, 125, 33-54.

Koob, G. F. (2010). The role of CRF and CRF-related peptides in the dark side of addiction. Brain Research, 1314, 3-14.

Koob, G. F. (2013). Negative reinforcement in drug addiction: the darkness within. Current Opinion in Neurobiology, 23(4), 559-563.

Koob, G. F., & Kreek, M. J. (2007). Stress, dysregulation of drug reward pathways, and the transition to drug dependence. American Journal of Psychiatry, 164(8), 1149–1159.

Koob, G. F., & Le Moa, M. (2008). Addiction and the Brain Antireward System. Annual Review of Psychology, 59, 29-53.

Koob, G. F., & Le Moal, M. (2001). Drug addiction, dysregulation of reward, and allostasis. Neuropsychopharmacology, 24(2), 97–129.

Koob, G. F., & Le Moal, M. (2005). Plasticity of reward neurocircuitry and the 'dark side' of drug addiction. Nature Neuroscience, 8(11), 1442–1444.

Koob, G. F., & Le Moal, M. (2005). Plasticity of reward neurocircuitry and the 'dark side' of drug addiction. Nat Neurosci. 8(11), 1442-1444.

Koob, G. F., & Le Moal, M. (2008). Addiction and the brain antireward system. Annual Review of Psychology, 59, 29-53

Koob, G. F., & Volkow, N. D. (2010). Neurocircuitry of addiction. Neuropsychopharmacology, 35(1), 217-238.

Koob, G. F., & Volkow, N. D. (2010). Neurocircuitry of addiction. Neuropsychopharmacology, 35(1), 217–238.

Koob, G. F., & Volkow, N. D. (2016). Neurobiology of addiction: a neurocircuitry analysis. Lancet Psychiatry. 3(8), 760-773.

Koob, G. F., & Volkow, N. D. (2016). Neurobiology of addiction: a neurocircuitry analysis. The Lancet Psychiatry, 3(8), 760–773.

Koob, G.F. (2009). Brain stress systems in the amygdala and addiction. Brain Research, 1293, 61-75.

Koob, G.F. (2009). Neurobiological substrates for the dark side of compulsivity in addiction. Neuropharmacology. 56(1), 18-31.

Koob, G.F. (2016). Neurobiology of addiction: a neurocircuitry analysis. Lancet Psychiatry. 3(8), 760-773.

Kosten, T. R., & George, T. P. (2002). The neurobiology of opioid dependence: implications for treatment. Science & Practice Perspectives, 1(1), 13–20.

Kranzler, H. R., & Li, T. K. (2008). What is addiction? Alcohol Res Health, 31(2), 93-95.

Kreek, M. J., Nielsen, D. A., & Butelman, E. R. (2005). Genetic influences on impulsivity, risk taking, stress responsivity and vulnerability to drug abuse and addiction. Nature Neuroscience, 8(11), 1450–1457.

Kuhn, B. N., Kalivas, P. W., & Bobadilla, A. C. (2019). Understanding Addiction Using Animal Models. Front Behav Neurosci. 13, 262.

Lader, M. (2011). Benzodiazepines revisited—will we ever learn? Addiction, 106(12), 2086–2109.

Lai, H., Li, R., Li, Z., Zhang, B., Li, C., Song, C., Zhao, Q., Huang, J., Zhu, Q., Liang, S., Chen, H., Li, J., Liao, L., Shao, Y., Xing, H., Ruan, Y., Lan, G., Zhang,

L., & Shen, M. (2023). Modelling the impact of treatment adherence on the transmission of HIV drug resistance. The Journal of antimicrobial chemotherapy, 78(8), 1934–1943.

Lander, L., Howsare, J., & Byrne, M. (2013). The impact of substance use disorders on families and children: from theory to practice. Social work in public health, 28(3-4), 194–205.

Landry, H., Kingsbury, M., Hamilton, H.A., Colman I. (2023). Psychological distress, non-medical use of prescription medications, and perceived unmet mental health care needs: a cross-sectional study of Ontario students. Soc Psychiatry Psychiatr Epidemiol, 58(10), 1483-1492.

Larney, S., Peacock, A., Leung, J., Colledge, S., Hickman, M., Vickerman, P., Grebely, J., Dumchev, K. V., Griffiths, P., Hines, L., Cunningham, E. B., Mattick, R. P., Lynskey, M., Marsden, J., Strang, J., & Degenhardt, L. (2017). Global, regional, and country-level coverage of interventions to prevent and manage HIV and hepatitis C among people who inject drugs: a systematic review. The Lancet. Global health, 5(12), e1208–e1220.

LaRowe, S. D., Mardikian, P., Malcolm, R., Myrick, H., Kalivas, P., McFarland, K., Saladin, M., McRae, A., & Brady, K. (2006). Safety and tolerability of N-acetylcysteine in cocaine-dependent individuals. The American Journal on Addictions, 15(1), 105–110.

Le Merrer, J., Becker, J. A., Befort, K., & Kieffer, B. L. (2009). Reward processing by the opioid system in the brain. Physiological reviews, 89(4), 1379–1412.

Lederbogen, F., Kirsch, P., Haddad, L., Streit, F., Tost, H., Schuch, P., Wüst, S., Pruessner, J. C., Rietschel, M., Deuschle, M., & Meyer-Lindenberg, A. (2011). City living and urban upbringing affect neural social stress processing in humans. Nature, 474(7352), 498–501.

Lee, J. D., Friedmann, P. D., Kinlock, T. W., Nunes, E. V., Boney, T. Y., Hoskinson, R. A., Jr, Wilson, D., McDonald, R., Rotrosen, J., Gourevitch, M. N., Gordon, M., Fishman, M., Chen, D. T., Bonnie, R. J., Cornish, J. W., Murphy, S. M., & O'Brien, C. P. (2016). Extended-Release Naltrexone to Prevent Opioid Relapse in Criminal Justice Offenders. The New England journal of medicine, 374(13), 1232–1242.

Lee, J. G., Woo, Y. S., Park, S. W., Seog, D. H., Seo, M. K., & Bahk, W. M. (2022). Neuromolecular Etiology of Bipolar Disorder: Possible Therapeutic Targets of Mood Stabilizers. Clinical psychopharmacology and neuroscience: the official scientific journal of the Korean College of Neuropsychopharmacology, 20(2), 228–239.

Lee, J., Grizenko, N., Bhat, V., & Joober, R. (2011). Sustained release methylphenidate in a randomized trial of treatment of primary cannabis dependence in ADHD adults. Journal of Clinical Psychopharmacology, 31(5),

599–604.

Lee, J., Kim, S., & Park, L. (2022). Social Media and Substance Abuse: A Systematic Review. Journal of Behavioral Addictions, 11(3), 425-438.

Lee, Y. J., Yang, Y. K., & Chen, T. F. (2005). The relationship of 5-HT2C receptor gene polymorphisms and the impulsive, aggressive and cognitive functions of methamphetamine addicts. Psychiatric Genetics, 15(3), 153–159.

Leggio, L., Ferrulli, A., Malandrino, N., Miceli, A., Capristo, E., Gasbarrini, G., Addolorato, G. (2012). Insulin but not insulin growth factor-1 correlates with craving in currently drinking alcohol-dependent patients. Alcoholism: Clinical and Experimental Research, 36(7), 1232–1240.

Leung, J., Mekonen, T., Wang, X., Arunogiri, S., Degenhardt, L., & McKetin, R. (2023). Methamphetamine exposure and depression-A systematic review and meta-analysis. Drug and alcohol review, 42(6), 1438–1449.

Levin, F. R., Mariani, J. J., Specker, S., Mooney, M., Mahony, A., Brooks, D. J., Babb, D., & Nunes, E. V. (2010). Extended-release mixed amphetamine salts vs placebo for comorbid adult attention-deficit/hyperactivity disorder and cocaine use disorder: A randomized clinical trial. JAMA Psychiatry, 67(6), 593–602.

Levin, F. R., Mariani, J., Brooks, D. J., Pavlicova, M., Cheng, W., Nunes, E. V., & Bisaga, A. (2013). A randomized double-blind, placebo-controlled trial of venlafaxine-extended release for co-occurring cannabis dependence and depressive disorders. Addiction, 106(4), 766–775.

Levran, O., Londono, D., O'Hara, K., Nielsen, D. A., Peles, E., Rotrosen, J., Casadonte, P., Linzy, S., Randesi, M., Ott, J., Adelson, M., & Kreek, M. J. (2008). Genetic susceptibility to heroin addiction: a candidate gene association study. Genes, brain, and behavior, 7(7), 720–729.

Levy, S., Brogna, M., Minegishi, M., Subramaniam, G., McCormack, J., Kline, M., Menzin, E., Allende-Richter, S., Fuller, A., Lewis, M., Collins, J., Hubbard, Z., Mitchell, S. G., Weiss, R., & Weitzman, E. (2023). Assessment of Screening Tools to Identify Substance Use Disorders Among Adolescents. JAMA network open, 6(5), e2314422.

Lewis, R. G., Florio, E., Punzo, D., & Borrelli, E. (2021). The Brain's Reward System in Health and Disease. Adv Exp Med Biol, 1344, 57-69.

Lindner, S. R., Scarpa, S., McCarty, D., & Lundgren, L. (2024). Addiction severity and re-employment in Sweden among adults with risky alcohol and drug use. Journal of substance use and addiction treatment, 156, 209178.

Linehan, M. M., Dimeff, L. A., Reynolds, S. K., Comtois, K. A., Welch, S. S., Heagerty, P., & Kivlahan, D. R. (2002). Dialectical behavior therapy versus comprehensive validation therapy plus 12-step for the treatment of opioid dependent women meeting criteria for borderline personality disorder. Drug and Alcohol Dependence, 67(1), 13–26.

Link, B. G., & Phelan, J. C. (2001). Conceptualizing stigma. Annu Rev Sociol, 27(1), 363-385.

Litt, M. D., Kadden, R. M., Kabela-Cormier, E., & Petry, N. M. (2009). Changing network support for drinking: Initial findings from the Network Support Project. Journal of Consulting and Clinical Psychology, 77(2), 229–242.

Littman, B. H., & Williams, S. A. (2005). The ultimate model organism: progress in experimental medicine and biology. Genetic Engineering, 27, 1–10.

Lobo, M. K., & Nestler, E. J. (2011). The striatal balancing act in drug addiction: Distinct roles of direct and indirect pathway medium spiny neurons. Frontiers in Neuroanatomy, 5, 41.

Logrip, M. L., & Zorrilla, E. P. (2014). Stress history increases alcohol intake in relapse: relation to phosphodiesterase 10A. Addiction Biology, 19(4), 633-643.

Logrip, M. L., Zorrilla, E. P., & Koob, G. F. (2012). Stress modulation of drug self-administration: implications for addiction comorbidity with post-traumatic stress disorder. Neuropharmacology, 62(2), 552–564.

López-Giménez, J. F., & Vilaró, M. T. (2008). 5-HT1A receptor signal transduction pathways. Journal of Neurochemistry, 106(5), 2035–2042.

Lötsch, J., Schaeffeler, E., Mittelbronn, M., Winter, S., Gudziol, V., Schwarzacher, S. W., Hummel, T., Doehring, A., Schwab, M., & Ultsch, A. (2014). Functional genomics suggest neurogenesis in the adult human olfactory bulb. Brain structure & function, 219(6), 1991–2000.

Lu, L., & Wang, X. (2008). Drug addiction: an affective-cognitive disorder in need of a cure. Neuroscience & Biobehavioral Reviews, 32(3), 581–597.

Luscher, C., & Malenka, R. C. (2011). Drug-evoked synaptic plasticity in addiction: from molecular changes to circuit remodeling. Neuron, 69(4), 650-663.

Lüscher, C., & Malenka, R. C. (2011). Drug-evoked synaptic plasticity in addiction: From molecular changes to circuit remodeling. Neuron, 69(4), 650–663.

Lüscher, C., & Ungless, M. A. (2006). The Mechanistic Classification of Addictive Drugs. PLoS Med, 3(11), e437.

Mackey, S., & Paulus, M. (2013). Are there volumetric brain differences associated with the use of cocaine and amphetamine-type stimulants? Neurosci Biobehav Rev. 37(3), 300-316.

MacQueen, G. M., & Frodl, T. (2011). The hippocampus in major depression: evidence for the convergence of the bench and bedside in psychiatric research? Molecular Psychiatry, 16(3), 252–264.

Magill, M., Kiluk, B. D., & Ray, L. A. (2023). Efficacy of Cognitive Behavioral Therapy for Alcohol and Other Drug Use Disorders: Is a One-Size-Fits-All Approach Appropriate? Substance Abuse Rehabilitation, 14, 1-11.

Mahu, I. T., Conrod, P. J., Barrett, S. P., Sako, A., Swansburg, J., & Stewart, S. H. (2023). The four-factor personality model and its qualitative correlates among opioid agonist therapy clients. Frontiers in psychiatry, 14, 1129274.

Makris, N., Gasic, G. P., Kennedy, D. N., Hodge, S. M., Kaiser, J. R., Lee, M. J., Kim, B. W., Blood, A. J., Evins, A. E., Seidman, L. J., Iosifescu, D. V., Lee, S., Baxter, C., Perlis, R. H., Smoller, J. W., Fava, M., & Breiter, H. C. (2008). Cortical thickness abnormalities in cocaine addiction--a reflection of both drug use and a pre-existing disposition to drug abuse? Neuron, 60(1), 174–188.

Maldonado, R., Berrendero, F., Ozaita, A., & Robledo, P. (2011). Neurochemical basis of cannabis addiction. Neuroscience, 181, 1-17.

Malik, J. A., & Agrewala, J. N. (2023). Future perspectives of emerging novel drug targets and immunotherapies to control drug addiction. International Immunopharmacology, 119, 110210.

Malik, N. I., Saleem, S., Ullah, I., Rehan, S. T., De Berardis, D., & Atta, M. (2023). Psychosocial Factors Affecting Drug Relapse among Youth in Punjab, Pakistan. Journal of clinical medicine, 12(7), 2686.

Mann, K., Lehert, P., & Morgan, M. Y. (2004). The efficacy of acamprosate in the maintenance of abstinence in alcohol-dependent individuals: Results of a meta-analysis. Alcoholism: Clinical and Experimental Research, 28(1), 51–63.

Mann, K., Lehert, P., Morgan, M. Y. (2004). The efficacy of acamprosate in the maintenance of abstinence in alcohol-dependent individuals: Results of a meta-analysis. Alcoholism: Clinical and Experimental Research, 28(1), 51–63.

Mardani, M., Alipour, F., Rafiey, H., Fallahi-Khoshknab, M., & Arshi, M. (2023). Challenges in addiction-affected families: a systematic review of qualitative studies. BMC psychiatry, 23(1), 439.

Marom, A., Levy, I., & Rosca, P. (2023). Changes and trends in medication-assisted treatment in Israel. Israel journal of health policy research, 12(1), 1.

Mars, S. G., Bourgois, P., Karandinos, G., Montero, F., & Ciccarone, D. (2014). "Every 'never' I ever said came true": transitions from opioid pills to heroin injecting. The International journal on drug policy, 25(2), 257–266

Martinelli, T. F., Roeg, D. P. K., Bellaert, L., Van de Mheen, D., & Nagelhout, G. E. (2023). Understanding the Process of Drug Addiction Recovery Through First-Hand Experiences: A Qualitative Study in the Netherlands Using Lifeline Interviews. Qualitative health research, 33(10), 857–870.

Martinotti, G., Di Nicola, M., Tedeschi, D., Callea, A., Di Giannantonio, M., & Janiri, L. (2010). Craving Typology Questionnaire (CTQ): A scale for alcohol craving in normal controls and alcoholics. Comprehensive Psychiatry, 51(3), 257–262.

Martinotti, G., Lupi, M., Carlucci, L., Cinosi, E., Santacroce, R., Acciavatti, T., Chillemi, E., Bonifaci, L., Janiri, L., & Di Giannantonio, M. (2015). Novel psychoactive substances: use and knowledge among adolescents and young adults in urban and rural areas. Human psychopharmacology, 30(4), 295–301.

Mason, B. J., Crean, R., Goodell, V., Light, J. M., Quello, S., Shadan, F., Buffkins, K., Kyle, M., Adusumalli, M., Begovic, A., & Rao, S. (2012). A proof-of-concept randomized controlled study of gabapentin: Effects on cannabis use, withdrawal and executive function deficits in cannabis-dependent adults. Neuropsychopharmacology, 37(7), 1689–1698.

Mason, B. J., Quello, S., Goodell, V., Shadan, F., Kyle, M., & Begovic, A. (2014). Gabapentin treatment for alcohol dependence: A randomized clinical trial. JAMA Internal Medicine, 174(1), 70–77.

Matochik, J. A., London, E. D., Eldreth, D. A., Cadet, J. L., & Bolla, K. I. (2003). Frontal cortical tissue composition in abstinent cocaine abusers: a magnetic resonance imaging study. NeuroImage, 19(3), 1095–1102.

Mattick, R. P., Breen, C., Kimber, J., & Davoli, M. (2009). Methadone maintenance therapy versus no opioid replacement therapy for opioid dependence. Cochrane Database of Systematic Reviews, (3), CD002209.

Mawe, G. M., & Hoffman, J. M. (2013). Serotonin signalling in the gut—functions, dysfunctions and therapeutic targets. Nature Reviews Gastroenterology & Hepatology, 10(8), 473–486.

May, A. C., Aupperle, R. L., & Stewart, J. L. (2020). Dark Times: The Role of Negative Reinforcement in Methamphetamine Addiction. Frontiers in psychiatry, 11, 114.

Mayo-Smith, M. F., Beecher, L. H., Fischer, T. L., Gorelick, D. A., Guillaume, J. L., Hill, A., Jara, G., Kasser, C., Melbourne, J., & Working Group on the Management of Alcohol Withdrawal Delirium, Practice Guidelines Committee, American Society of Addiction Medicine (2004). Management of alcohol withdrawal delirium. An evidence-based practice guideline. Archives of internal medicine, 164(13), 1405–1412.

Maze, I., & Nestler, E. J. (2011). The epigenetic landscape of addiction. Annals of the New York Academy of Sciences, 1216, 99–113.

Mazei-Robison, M. S., Bowton, E., Holy, M., Schmudermaier, M., Freissmuth, M., Sitte, H. H., & Blakely, R. D. (2008). Anomalous dopamine release associated with a human dopamine transporter coding variant. Journal of Neuroscience, 28(28), 7040–7046.

McCann, N. C., McMahan, V. M., Smith, R., Majeski, A., Johns, S. L., Kosakowski, S., Wolfe, S., Brennan, S., Robinson, M., Coffin, P. O., & Walley, A. Y. (2024). Feasibility and acceptability of a timeline follow-back method to assess opioid use, non-fatal overdose, and substance use disorder treatment. Addictive behaviors, 148, 107873.

McElligott, Z. A., & Winder, D. G. (2009). Modulation of glutamatergic synaptic transmission in the bed nucleus of the stria terminalis. Progress in Neuro-Psychopharmacology and Biological Psychiatry, 33(8), 1329–1335.

McEwen, B. S. (2005). Glucocorticoids, depression, and mood disorders: structural remodeling in the brain. Metabolism, 54(5 Suppl 1), 20–23.

McEwen, B. S. (2007). Physiology and neurobiology of stress and adaptation: central role of the brain. Physiological Reviews, 87(3), 873–904.

McEwen, B. S., & Morrison, J. H. (2013). The brain on stress: vulnerability and plasticity of the prefrontal cortex over the life course. Neuron, 79(1), 16–29.

McGeer, P. L., & McGeer, E. G. (2008). Glial reactions in Parkinson's disease. Movement Disorders, 23(4), 474–483.

McHugh, R. K., Hearon, B. A., & Otto, M. W. (2010). Cognitive-Behavioral Therapy for Substance Use Disorders. The Psychiatric Clinics of North America, 33(3), 511-525.

McKay J. R. (2009). Continuing care research: what we have learned and where we are going. Journal of substance abuse treatment, 36(2), 131–145.

McKay, J. R. (2005). Is there a case for extended interventions for alcohol and drug use disorders? Addiction, 100(11), 1594-1610.

McLellan, A. T., Lewis, D. C., O'Brien, C. P., & Kleber, H. D. (2000). Drug dependence, a chronic medical illness: implications for treatment, insurance, and outcomes evaluation. JAMA, 284(13), 1689–1695.

McReynolds, J. R., Doncheck, E. M., Li, Y., & Van Bockstaele, E. J. (2014). Noradrenergic modulation of bed nucleus of the stria terminalis neurons: Differential effects on dorsal and ventral subpopulations. Neuroscience, 277, 287–297.

Meier, M. H., Caspi, A., Ambler, A., Harrington, H., Houts, R., Keefe, R. S. E., McDonald, K., Ward, A., Poulton, R., & Moffitt, T. E. (2012). Persistent cannabis users show neuropsychological decline from childhood to midlife. Proceedings of the National Academy of Sciences of the United States of America, 109(40), E2657–E2664.

Mellentin, A. I., Finn, S. W., Skøt, L., Thaysen-Petersen, D., Mistarz, N., Fink-Jensen, A., & Nielsen, D. G. (2023). The effectiveness of oxytocin for treating substance use disorders: A systematic review of randomized placebo-controlled trials. Neuroscience and biobehavioral reviews, 151, 105185.

Meltzer, H. Y., & Huang, M. (2008). In vivo actions of atypical antipsychotic drug on serotonergic and dopaminergic systems. Progress in Brain Research, 172, 177–197.

Ménard, C., & Quirion, R. (2012). Successful cognitive aging in rats: a role for mGluR5 glutamate receptors, homer 1 proteins and downstream signaling pathways. PloS one, 7(6), e28666. https://doi.org/10.1371/journal.pone.0028666

Meng, Q., Zhu, Y., Yuan, Y., Yang, L., Liu, J., Zhang, X., & Bu, J. (2023). Resting-state electroencephalography theta predicts neurofeedback treatment 4-month follow-up response in nicotine addiction. General psychiatry, 36(4), e101091.

Merians, A. N., Spiller, T., Harpaz-Rotem, I., Krystal, J. H., & Pietrzak, R. H. (2023). Post-traumatic Stress Disorder. The Medical clinics of North America, 107(1), 85–99.

Meyers, R. J., Roozen, H. G., & Smith, J. E. (2011). The community reinforcement approach: An update of the evidence. Alcohol Research & Health, 33(4), 380–388.

Miller, A. H., & Raison, C. L. (2016). The role of inflammation in depression: from evolutionary imperative to modern treatment target. Nature Reviews Immunology, 16(1), 22–34.

Miller, B. A., Holder, H. D., & Voas, R. B. (2009). Environmental Strategies for Prevention of Drug Use and Risks in Clubs. Journal of substance use, 14(1), 19–38.

Miller, J. M., Thompson, C. R., & Brown, S. M. (2023). Multigenerational Family Study: Genetic and Environmental Influences on Substance Use Disorders. Addiction, 118(2), 201-215.

Miller, K., Rodriguez, M., & Thompson, C. (2021). Parental Substance Use and Offspring Drug Abuse: A Prospective Study. Addiction, 118(3), 321-335.

Mithoefer, M. C., Feduccia, A. A., Jerome, L., Mithoefer, A., Wagner, M., Walsh, Z., Hamilton, S., Yazar-Klosinski, B., Emerson, A., & Doblin, R. (2019). MDMA-assisted psychotherapy for treatment of PTSD: study design and rationale for phase 3 trials based on pooled analysis of six phase 2 randomized controlled trials. Psychopharmacology, 236(9), 2735–2745.

Momenan, R., Steckler, L. E., Saad, Z. S., van Rafelghem, S., Kerich, M. J., & Hommer, D. W. (2012). Effects of alcohol dependence on cortical thickness as determined by magnetic resonance imaging. Psychiatry Research: Neuroimaging, 204(2-3), 101–111.

Monnig, M. A., Tonigan, J. S., Yeo, R. A., & Thoma, R. J. (2013). McCrady B. White matter volume in alcohol use disorders: a meta-analysis. Addiction Biology, 18(3), 581-592.

Moos, R. H., & Moos, B. S. (2006). Participation in treatment and Alcoholics Anonymous: A 16-year follow-up of initially untreated individuals. Journal of Clinical Psychology, 62(6), 735–750.

Morcuende, A., Navarrete, F., Nieto, E., Manzanares, J., & Femenía, T. (2021). Inflammatory Biomarkers in Addictive Disorders. Biomolecules, 11(12), 1824.

Moussawi, K., & Kalivas, P. W. (2010). Group II metabotropic glutamate receptors (mGlu2/3) in drug addiction. European Journal of Pharmacology, 639(1-3), 115–122.

Mueser, K. T., Noordsy, D. L., Drake, R. E., & Fox, L. (2003). Integrated Treatment for Dual Disorders: A Guide to Effective Practice. Guilford Press.

Muller CP, Homberg JR. (2015). The role of serotonin in drug use and addiction. Behavioural Brain Research, 277, 146-192.

Müller, C. P., & Homberg, J. R. (2015). The role of serotonin in drug use and addiction. Behavioural Brain Research, 277, 146–192.

Müller, C. P., Carey, R. J., Huston, J. P., & De Souza Silva, M. A. (2007). Serotonin and psychostimulant addiction: Focus on 5-HT1A-receptors. Progress in Neurobiology, 81(3), 133–178.

Munafo, M. R., Clark, T. G., & Johnstone, E. C. (2004). Association of the serotonin transporter gene polymorphism with nicotine dependence: A systematic review and meta-analysis. Molecular Psychiatry, 9(4), 356–366.

Murnane, K. S., Edinoff, A. N., Cornett, E. M., & Kaye, A. D. (2023). Updated Perspectives on the Neurobiology of Substance Use Disorders Using Neuroimaging. Substance abuse and rehabilitation, 14, 99–111.

Myrick, H., Brady, K. T., & Malcolm, R. (2001). Divalproex in the Treatment of Alcohol Withdrawal. American Journal on Addictions, 10(3), 232–237.

Naqvi, N. H., & Bechara, A. (2009). The hidden island of addiction: the insula. Trends in Neurosciences, 32(1), 56–67.

National Institute of Mental Health. (2021). Depression. https://www.nimh.nih.gov/health/topics/depression/

National Institute on Drug Abuse (NIDA). (2020). Opioid Overdose Crisis. Retrieved from https://www.drugabuse.gov/drug-topics/opioids/opioid-overdose-crisis

National Institute on Drug Abuse (NIDA). (2021). Monitoring the Future Survey: High School and Youth Trends. Retrieved from https://www.drugabuse.gov/drug-topics/trends-statistics/monitoring-future

Nazari, S., Pourmand, S. M., Makki, S. M., Brand, S., & Vousooghi, N. (2022). Potential biomarkers of addiction identified by real-time PCR in human peripheral blood lymphocytes: a narrative review. Biomarkers in medicine, 16(9), 739–758.

Neisewander, J. L., & Cheung, T. H. C. (2019). Pentz award lecture: Toward a neurobiology of addiction: commentary on Koob (2019). Experimental and Clinical Psychopharmacology, 27(3), 225–228.

Nelson, E. C., Agrawal, A., & Heath, A. C. (2009). Evidence for a gene–environment interaction in predicting behavioral disinhibition in children. Psychological Science, 20(9), 1145–1152.

Nelson, E. C., Agrawal, A., & Pergadia, M. L. (2009). Association of childhood trauma exposure and GABRA2 polymorphisms with risk of posttraumatic stress disorder in adults. Molecular Psychiatry, 14(3), 234–235.

Nerella, S. G., Michaelides, M., Minamimoto, T., Innis, R. B., Pike, V. W., & Eldridge, M. A. G. (2023). PET reporter systems for the brain. Trends in neurosciences, 46(11), 941–952.

Nessa, A., Latif, S. A., Siddiqui, N. I., Hussain, M. A., & Hossain, M. A. (2008). Drug abuse and addiction. Mymensingh medical journal. MMJ, 17(2), 227–235.

Nestler E. J. (2001). Molecular basis of long-term plasticity underlying addiction. Nature reviews. Neuroscience, 2(2), 119–128.

Nestler EJ. (2005). Is there a common molecular pathway for addiction? Nature Neuroscience, 8(11), 1445-1449.

Nestler, E. J. (2004). Molecular mechanisms of drug addiction. Neuropharmacology, 47 (1): 24-32.

Nestler, E. J. (2005). Is there a common molecular pathway for addiction? Nature Neuroscience, 8(11), 1445–1449.

Nestler, E. J. (2014). Transcriptional mechanisms of drug addiction. Clinical Psychopharmacology and Neuroscience, 12(3), 169–177.

Nestler, E. J. (2015). ΔFosB: A transcriptional regulator of stress and antidepressant responses. European Journal of Pharmacology, 753, 66–72.

Nestler, E. J., Barrot, M., DiLeone, R. J., Eisch, A. J., Gold, S. J., & Monteggia, L. M. (2002). Neurobiology of depression. Neuron, 34(1), 13–25.

Newman, A. H., Xi, Z. X., & Heidbreder, C. (2023). Current Perspectives on Selective Dopamine D3 Receptor Antagonists/Partial Agonists as Pharmacotherapeutics for Opioid and Psychostimulant Use Disorders. Current topics in behavioral neurosciences, 60, 157–201.

Nguemeni Tiako, M. J., Shofer, F., Dolan, A., Goldberg, E. B., Rhodes, K. V., Hess, E. P., Bellamkonda, V. R., Perrone, J., Cannuscio, C. C., Becker, L., Rodgers, M. A., Zyla, M. M., Bell, J. J., McCollum, S., Engel-Rebitzer, E., Schapira, M. M., & Meisel, Z. F. (2023). Personalized risk communication and opioid prescribing in association with nonprescribed opioid use: A secondary analysis of a randomized controlled trial. Academic emergency medicine: official journal of the Society for Academic Emergency Medicine, 30(8), 851–858.

Nichols, C. D., & Sanders-Bush, E. (2002). A single dose of lysergic acid diethylamide influences gene expression patterns within the mammalian brain. Neuropsychopharmacology, 26(5), 634–642.

Nichols, D. E. (2004). Hallucinogens. Pharmacology & Therapeutics, 101(2), 131–181.

Nichols, D. E. (2016). Psychedelics. Pharmacological Reviews, 68(2), 264–355.

Nilsson, K. W., Sjöberg, R. L., & Wargelius, H. L. (2011). The monoamine oxidase A (MAO-A) gene, family function and maltreatment as predictors of destructive behaviour during male adolescent alcohol consumption. Addiction Biology, 16(2), 325–332.

Nock, N. L., Minnes, S., & Alberts, J. L. (2017). Neurobiology of substance use in adolescents and potential therapeutic effects of exercise for prevention and treatment of substance use disorders. Birth defects research, 109(20), 1711–1729.

Noonan, M. A., Bulin, S. E., Fuller, D. C., Eisch, A. J., & Reduction, M. (2010). Adult Neurogenesis in the Mammalian Hippocampus: Why the Dentate Gyrus? Learning & Memory, 14(5), 364–377.

Nunes, E. V., Levin, F. R., & Donovan, S. J. (2008). Treatment of depression in patients with alcohol or other drug dependence: A meta-analysis. JAMA, 299(9), 1025–1034.

Nutt, D. J., Lingford-Hughes, A., Erritzoe, D., & Stokes, P. R. (2015). The dopamine theory of addiction: 40 years of highs and lows. Nature Reviews Neuroscience, 16(5), 305–312.

Obara, M., Kwon, J., Yoneyama, M., Ueda, Y., & Cauteren, M. V. (2023). Technical Advancements in Abdominal Diffusion-weighted Imaging. Magnetic resonance in medical sciences: MRMS: an official journal of Japan Society of Magnetic Resonance in Medicine, 22(2), 191–208.

Olasore, H. S., Osuntoki, A. A., Magbagbeola, O. A., Awesu, A. B., & Olashore, A. A. (2023). Association of Dopamine Transporter Gene (DAT1) 40 bp 3' UTR VNTR Polymorphism (rs28363170) and Cannabis Use Disorder. Substance abuse: research and treatment, 17, 11782218231163696.

Olsen, R. W., & Liang, J. (2017). Role of GABAA receptors in alcohol use disorders suggested by chronic intermittent ethanol (CIE) rodent model. Molecular Brain, 10(1), 45.

Oscar-Berman, M., & Marinković, K. (2007). Alcohol: Effects on neurobehavioral functions and the brain. Neuropsychology Review, 17(3), 239-257.

Ossipov, M. H., Morimura, K., & Porreca, F. (2014). Descending pain modulation and chronification of pain. Current opinion in supportive and palliative care, 8(2), 143–151.

Pacula, R. L., Kilmer, B., Wagenaar, A. C., Chaloupka, F. J., & Caulkins, J. P. (2014). Developing Public Health Regulations for Marijuana: Lessons from Alcohol and Tobacco. American Journal of Public Health, 104(6), 1021–1028.

Pacula, R. L., Powell, D., Heaton, P., & Sevigny, E. L. (2015). Assessing the effects of medical marijuana laws on marijuana use: the devil is in the details. Journal of Policy Analysis and Management, 34(1), 7-31

Padwa, H., Guerrero, E. G., Braslow, J. T., & Fenwick, K. M. (2015). Barriers to serving clients with co-occurring disorders in a transformed mental health system. Psychiatric services (Washington, D.C.), 66(5), 547–550.

Pantoja-Urbán, A. H., Richer, S., Mittermaier, A., Giroux, M., Nouel, D., Hernandez, G., & Flores, C. (2024). Gains and Losses: Resilience to Social Defeat Stress in Adolescent Female Mice. Biological psychiatry, 95(1), 37–47.

Pariante, C. M., & Lightman, S. L. (2008). The HPA axis in major depression: classical theories and new developments. Trends in Neurosciences, 31(9), 464-468.

Pattanaik, B., Hammarlund, M., Mjörnstedt, F., Ulleryd, M. A., Zhong, W., Uhlén, M., Gummesson, A., Bergström, G., & Johansson, M. E. (2022). Polymorphisms in alpha 7 nicotinic acetylcholine receptor gene, CHRNA7, and its partially duplicated gene, CHRFAM7A, associate with increased inflammatory response in human peripheral mononuclear cells. FASEB journal: official publication of the Federation of American Societies for Experimental Biology, 36(5), e22271.

Pautrat, M., Le Guen, A., Barrault, S., Ribadier, A., Ballon, N., Lebeau, J. P., & Brunault, P. (2022). Impulsivity as a Risk Factor for Addictive Disorder Severity during the COVID-19 Lockdown: Results from a Mixed Quantitative and Qualitative Study. International journal of environmental research and public health, 20(1), 705.

Pavlov P. I. (2010). Conditioned reflexes: An investigation of the physiological activity of the cerebral cortex. Annals of neurosciences, 17(3), 136–141.

Perry, J. L., & Carroll, M. E. (2008). The role of impulsive behavior in drug abuse. Psychopharmacology, 200(1), 1–26.

Peters, J., & Kalivas, P. W. (2006). The group II metabotropic glutamate receptor agonist, LY379268, inhibits both cocaine- and food-seeking behavior in rats. Psychopharmacology, 186(2), 143–149.

Petry, N. M., Peirce, J. M., Stitzer, M. L., Blaine, J., Roll, J. M., Cohen, A., Obert, J., Killeen, T., Saladin, M. E., Cowell, M., Kirby, K. C., Sterling, R., Royer-Malvestuto, C., Hamilton, J., Booth, R. E., Macdonald, M., Liebert, M., Rader, L., Burns, R., DiMaria, J., … Li, R. (2005). Effect of prize-based incentives on outcomes in stimulant abusers in outpatient psychosocial treatment programs: a national drug abuse treatment clinical trials network study. Archives of general psychiatry, 62(10), 1148–1156.

Piazza, P. V., Deroche-Gamonent, V., Rouge-Pont, F., & Le Moal, M. (2000). Vertical shifts in self-administration dose-response functions predict a drug-vulnerable phenotype predisposed to addiction. The Journal of neuroscience: the official journal of the Society for Neuroscience, 20(11), 4226–4232.

Picci, G., Fishbein, D. H., VanMeter, J. W., & Rose, E. J. (2022). Effects of OPRM1 and DRD2 on brain structure in drug-naïve adolescents: Genetic and neural vulnerabilities to substance use. Psychopharmacology, 239(1), 141–152.

Picciotto, M. R., & Kenny, P. J. (2013). Molecular mechanisms underlying behaviors related to nicotine addiction. Cold Spring Harbor Perspectives in Medicine, 3(1), a012112.

Pinto, F. J., Piepoli, M. F., Ferrari, R., Tsioufis, K., Rosano, G. M. C., Nedoshivin, A., & Kaski, J. C. (2023). Single-pill combination in the management of chronic coronary syndromes: A strategy to improve treatment adherence and patient outcomes? International journal of cardiology, 384, 10–17.

Piper, M. E., Cook, J. W., Schlam, T. R., Jorenby, D. E., & Baker, T. B. (2011). Anxiety diagnoses in smokers seeking cessation treatment: relations with tobacco dependence, withdrawal, outcome and response to treatment. Addiction (Abingdon, England), 106(2), 418–427.

Poian, L. R., & Chiavegatto, S. (2023). Serotonin Syndrome: The Role of Pharmacology in Understanding Its Occurrence. Cureus, 15(5), e38897.

Poisel, E., Zillich, L., Streit, F., Frank, J., Friske, M. M., Foo, J. C., Mechawar, N., Turecki, G., Hansson, A. C., Nöthen, M. M., Rietschel, M., Spanagel, R., & Witt, S. H. (2023). DNA methylation in cocaine use disorder-An epigenome-wide approach in the human prefrontal cortex. Frontiers in psychiatry, 14, 1075250.

Poling, J., Oliveto, A., Petry, N., Sofuoglu, M., Gonsai, K., Gonzalez, G., Martell, B., Kosten, T. R., & Desai, P. (2006). Six-month trial of bupropion with contingency management for cocaine dependence in a methadone-maintained population. Archives of General Psychiatry, 63(2), 219–228.

Pollard, A. A., Hauson, A. O., Lackey, N. S., Zhang, E., Khayat, S., Carson, B., Fortea, L., Radua, J., & Grant, I. (2023). Functional neuroanatomy of craving in heroin use disorder: voxel-based meta-analysis of functional magnetic resonance imaging (fMRI) drug cue reactivity studies. The American journal of drug and alcohol abuse, 49(4), 418–430.

Popoli, M., Yan, Z., McEwen, B. S., & Sanacora, G. (2012). The stressed synapse: the impact of stress and glucocorticoids on glutamate transmission. Nature Reviews Neuroscience, 13(1), 22–37.

Powell, S. B., & Swerdlow, N. R. (2023). The Relevance of Animal Models of Social Isolation and Social Motivation for Understanding Schizophrenia: Review and Future Directions. Schizophrenia bulletin, 49(5), 1112–1126.

Prendergast, M., Podus, D., Finney, J., Greenwell, L., & Roll, J. (2006). Contingency management for treatment of substance use disorders: a meta-analysis. Addiction (Abingdon, England), 101(11), 1546–1560.

Prendergast, M., Podus, D., Finney, J., Greenwell, L., & Roll, J. (2006). Contingency management for treatment of substance use disorders: A meta-analysis. Addiction, 101(11), 1546–1560.

Price, J. L., & Drevets, W. C. (2010). Neurocircuitry of mood disorders. Neuropsychopharmacology: official publication of the American College of Neuropsychopharmacology, 35(1), 192–216.

Price, J. L., & Drevets, W. C. (2012). Neural circuits underlying the pathophysiology of mood disorders. Trends in Cognitive Sciences, 16(1), 61–71.

Primack, B.A., Colditz, J. B., Pang, K. C., Jackson, K.M. (2014). Portrayal of Alcohol Intoxication on YouTube. Alcoholism: Clinical and Experimental Research, 38(11), 3061-3066.

Prosser, J. M., & Nelson, L. S. (2012). The toxicology of bath salts: A review of synthetic cathinones. Journal of Medical Toxicology, 8(1), 33–42.

Pugsley, M. K. (2008). Assessing the cardiovascular safety of new drugs: the importance of integrating knowledge across the pharmaceutical development spectrum. Pharmacology & Therapeutics, 119(3), 213–222.

Puig, M. V., & Gulledge, A. T. (2011). Serotonin and prefrontal cortex function: neurons, networks, and circuits. Molecular Neurobiology, 44(3), 449–464.

Rabinak, C. A., Angstadt, M., Lyons, M., Mori, S., Milad, M. R., Liberzon, I., & Phan, K. L. (2014). Cannabinoid modulation of prefrontal-limbic activation during fear extinction learning and recall in humans. Neurobiology of learning and memory, 113, 125–134.

Radhakrishnan, R., Pries, L. K., Erzin, G., Ten Have, M., de Graaf, R., van Dorsselaer, S., Gunther, N., Bak, M., Rutten, B. P. F., van Os, J., & Guloksuz, S. (2023). Bidirectional relationships between cannabis use, anxiety and depressive symptoms in the mediation of the association with psychotic experience: further support for an affective pathway to psychosis. Psychological medicine, 53(12), 5551–5557.

Rawson, R. A., Huber, A., McCann, M., Shoptaw, S., Farabee, D., Reiber, C., & Ling, W. (2002). A comparison of contingency management and cognitive-behavioral approaches during methadone maintenance treatment for cocaine dependence. Archives of general psychiatry, 59(9), 817–824.

Ray, B., Chen, J., Fu, Z., Suresh, P., Thapaliya, B., Farahdel, B., Calhoun, V. D., & Liu, J. (2023). Replication and Refinement of Brain Age Model for adolescent development. bioRxiv: the preprint server for biology, 2023.08.16.553472.

Ray, L. A., & Hutchison, K. E. (2004). A polymorphism of the mu-opioid receptor gene (OPRM1) and sensitivity to the effects of alcohol in humans. Alcoholism: Clinical and Experimental Research, 28(12), 1789–1795.

Razaghi, E., Farhoudian, A., Pilevari, A., Noroozi, A., Hooshyari, Z., Radfar, R., & Malekinejad, M. (2023). Identification of the socio-cultural barriers of drug addiction treatment in Iran. Heliyon, 9(5), e15566.

Rehm, J., Mathers, C., Popova, S., Thavorncharoensap, M., Teerawattananon, Y., & Patra, J. (2009). Global burden of disease and injury and economic cost attributable to alcohol use and alcohol-use disorders. The Lancet, 373(9682), 2223-2233.

Reich, J., & Schatzberg, A. (2023). Childhood maladaptive coping mechanisms and the subsequent development of depression. Clinical psychology & psychotherapy, 30(3), 528–535.

Reissner, K. J., & Kalivas, P. W. (2010). Using glutamate homeostasis as a target for treating addictive disorders. Behavioural Pharmacology, 21(5-6), 514–522.

Renner HM, Rowland B, Hutchinson D, Toumbourou JW. Modeling Adolescent Social Inclusion to Improve School Completion. J Youth Adolesc. 2023 Aug;52(8):1662-1673.

Richards, M., Iijima, Y., Kondo, H., Shizuno, T., Hori, H., Arima, K., Saitoh, O., & Kunugi, H. (2006). Association study of the vesicular monoamine transporter 1 (VMAT1) gene with schizophrenia in a Japanese population. Behavioral and brain functions: BBF, 2, 39.

Ringwalt, C., Ennett, S., Johnson, R., Rohrbach, L. A., Simons-Rudolph, A., & Vincus, A. (2003). Factors associated with fidelity to substance use prevention curriculum guides in the nation's middle schools. Health Education & Behavior, 30(3), 375–391.

Roberto, M., Gilpin, N. W., & Siggins, G. R. (2012). The central amygdala and alcohol: role of γ-aminobutyric acid, glutamate, and neuropeptides. Cold Spring Harbor Perspectives in Medicine, 2(12), a012195.

Robinson TE, Berridge KC. (2008). The incentive sensitization theory of addiction: some current issues. Philosophical Transactions of the Royal Society B: Biological Sciences, 363(1507), 3137-3146.

Robinson TE, Berridge KC. (2008). The incentive sensitization theory of addiction: some current issues. Philosophical Transactions of the Royal Society B: Biological Sciences, 363(1507), 3137-3146.

Robinson TE, Kolb B. Structural plasticity associated with exposure to drugs of abuse. Neuropharmacology. 2004;47 Suppl 1(Suppl 1):33-46.

Robinson, M. J., & Berridge, K. C. (2003). Addiction. Annual Review of Psychology, 54, 25–53.

Robinson, T. E., & Berridge, K. C. (2008). Review. The incentive sensitization theory of addiction: some current issues. Philosophical Transactions of the Royal Society B: Biological Sciences, 363(1507), 3137–3146.

Robison, A. J., & Nestler, E. J. (2011). Transcriptional and epigenetic mechanisms of addiction. Nature Reviews Neuroscience, 12(11), 623–637.

Rocha, A., Kalivas, P. W., & Role of the prefrontal cortex and nucleus accumbens in reinstating methamphetamine seeking. (2010). European Journal of Neuroscience, 31(5), 903–909.

Romer Thomsen, K., Thylstrup, B., Kenyon, E. A., Lees, R., Baandrup, L., Feldstein Ewing, S. W., & Freeman, T. P. (2022). Cannabinoids for the treatment of cannabis use disorder: New avenues for reaching and helping youth? Neuroscience and biobehavioral reviews, 132, 169–180.

Rong, J., Haider, A., Jeppesen, T. E., Josephson, L., & Liang, S. H. (2023). Radiochemistry for positron emission tomography. Nature communications,

14(1), 3257.

Room R. (2005). Stigma, social inequality and alcohol and drug use. Drug and alcohol review, 24(2), 143–155.

Rotermann M. (2023). Using the Severity of Dependence Scale to examine cannabis consumers with impaired control in Canada. Health reports, 34(6), 3–16.

Rothman, R. B., Baumann, M. H., Dersch, C. M., Romero, D. V., Rice, K. C., & Carroll, F. I. (2001). Amphetamine-type central nervous system stimulants release norepinephrine more potently than they release dopamine and serotonin. Synapse, 39(1), 32–41.

Roy, T. A., Bubier, J. A., Dickson, P. E., Wilcox, T. D., Ndukum, J., Clark, J. W., Rizzo, S. J. S., Crabbe, J. C., Denegre, J. M., Svenson, K. L., Braun, R. E., Kumar, V., Murray, S. A., White, J. K., Philip, V. M., & Chesler, E. J. (2023). Discovery and validation of genes driving drug-intake and related behavioral traits in mice. bioRxiv: the preprint server for biology, 2023.07.09.548280.

Rudd, R. A., Aleshire, N., Zibbell, J. E., & Gladden, R. M. (2016). Increases in Drug and Opioid Overdose Deaths—United States, 2000–2014. Morbidity and Mortality Weekly Report, 64(50-51), 1378–1382.

Rudolph, U., & Möhler, H. (2006). GABA-based therapeutic approaches: GABAA receptor subtype functions. Current opinion in pharmacology, 6(1), 18–23

Ruiz M. E. (2010). Risks of self-medication practices. Current drug safety, 5(4), 315–323.

Rush, B., & Koegl, C. J. (2008). Prevalence and profile of people with co-occurring mental and substance use disorders within a comprehensive mental health system. Canadian Journal of Psychiatry, 53(12), 810-21.

Russo, S. J., & Nestler, E. J. (2013). The brain reward circuitry in mood disorders. Nature Reviews Neuroscience, 14(9), 609–625.

Sáiz, P. A., García-Portilla, M. P., Arango, C., Morales, B., Martínez-Barrondo, S., Alvarez, C., San Narciso, G., Carreño, E., Alvarez, V., Coto, E., & Bobes, J. (2008). Association between heroin dependence and 5-HT2A receptor gene polymorphisms. European addiction research, 14(1), 47–52.

Salamone, J. D., Correa, M., Farrar, A. M., Nunes, E. J., & Pardo, M. (2009). Dopamine, behavioral economics, and effort. Frontiers in behavioral neuroscience, 3, 13.

Salo, R., & Nordahl, T. E. (2015). Neurocognitive features and behavioral characteristics of methamphetamine users. Journal of Psychiatric Research, 60, 10–15.

Saloner, B., & Karthikeyan, S. (2015). Changes in Substance Abuse Treatment Use Among Individuals With Opioid Use Disorders in the United States, 2004–2013. JAMA, 314(14), 1515–1517.

Sanacora, G., & Banasr, M. (2013). From pathophysiology to novel antidepressant drugs: glial contributions to the pathology and treatment of mood disorders. Biological Psychiatry, 73(12), 1172–1179.

Sanacora, G., Zarate Jr, C. A., Krystal, J. H., & Manji, H. K. (2008). Targeting the glutamatergic system to develop novel, improved therapeutics for mood disorders. Nature Reviews Drug Discovery, 7(5), 426–437.

Sandi, C. (2011). Glucocorticoids act on glutamatergic pathways to affect memory processes. Trends in Neurosciences, 34(4), 165–176.

Sansone, R. A., & Sansone, L. A. (2010). SSRI withdrawal: a review of the literature. Current Psychiatry, 9(7), 25–31.

Sarkar, S., & Balhara, Y. P. S. (2023). Telemedicine in addiction treatment: Ethical considerations. Indian Journal of Medical Ethics, VIII(2), 162-163.

Scarpulla, R. C. (2011). Metabolic control of mitochondrial biogenesis through the PGC-1 family regulatory network. Biochimica et Biophysica Acta (BBA)-Molecular Cell Research, 1813(7), 1269–1278.

Schenk, S. (2000). Effects of the serotonin 5-HT(2) antagonist, ritanserin, and the serotonin 5-HT(1A) antagonist, WAY 100635, on cocaine-seeking in rats. Pharmacology Biochemistry and Behavior.67(2), 363-369.

Schultz, W. (2015). Neuronal reward and decision signals: From theories to data. Physiological Reviews, 95(3), 853–951.

Schultz, W. (2016). Dopamine reward prediction error coding. Dialogues in Clinical Neuroscience, 18(1), 23-32.

Schultz, W. (2016). Dopamine reward prediction error coding. Dialogues in Clinical Neuroscience, 18(1), 23–32.

Seymour, B., Daw, N., Dayan, P., Singer, T., & Dolan, R. (2012). Differential Encoding of Losses and Gains in the Human Striatum. Journal of Neuroscience, 32(50), 17762–17768.

Shaham, Y., Shalev, U., Lu, L., De Wit, H., & Stewart, J. (2003). The reinstatement model of drug relapse: history, methodology and major findings. Psychopharmacology, 168(1–2), 3–20.

Shaheen, N., Shaheen, A., Sarica, C., Singh, A., Zanaty, M., Johari, K., Yang, A., Zesiewicz, T., Dalm, B., Bezchlibnyk, Y., Lozano, A. M., & Flouty, O. (2023). Deep brain stimulation for substance use disorder: a systematic review and meta-analysis. Frontiers in psychiatry, 14, 1231760.

Shalaeva, E. V., Bano, A., Kasimov, U., Janabaev, B., Laimer, M., & Saner, H. (2023). Impact of Persistent Medication Adherence and Compliance with Lifestyle Recommendations on Major Cardiovascular Events and One-Year Mortality in Patients with Type 2 Diabetes and Advanced Stages of Atherosclerosis: Results From a Prospective Cohort Study. Global heart, 18(1), 61.

Sharma, R., Batchelor, R., & Sin, J. (2023). Psychedelic Treatments for Substance Use Disorder and Substance Misuse: A Mixed Methods Systematic Review. Journal of psychoactive drugs, 55(5), 612–630.

Shreya, S., Annamalai, M., Jirge, V. L., & Sethi, S. (2023). Utility of salivary biomarkers for diagnosis and monitoring the prognosis of nicotine addiction - A systematic review. Journal of oral biology and craniofacial research, 13(6), 740–750.

Siegle, G. J., Thompson, W., Carter, C. S., Steinhauer, S. R., & Thase, M. E. (2007). Increased amygdala and decreased dorsolateral prefrontal BOLD responses in unipolar depression: related and independent features. Biological Psychiatry, 61(2), 198–209.

Simons, J. S., Wills, T. A., & Neal, D. J. (2014). The many faces of affect: a multilevel model of drinking frequency/quantity and alcohol dependence symptoms among young adults. Journal of abnormal psychology, 123(3), 676–694.

Simons-Morton, B., & Farhat, T. (2010). Recent findings on peer group influences on adolescent substance use. Journal of Primary Prevention, 31(4), 191–208.

Sinha R. (2008). Chronic stress, drug use, and vulnerability to addiction. Annals of the New York Academy of Sciences, 1141, 105-130.

Sinha R. (2011). New findings on biological factors predicting addiction relapse vulnerability. Current psychiatry reports, 13(5), 398–405.

Sinha, R. (2001). How does stress increase risk of drug abuse and relapse? Psychopharmacology, 158(4), 343–359.

Sinha, R., & Li, C. S. (2007). Imaging stress- and cue-induced drug and alcohol craving: association with relapse and clinical implications. Drug and Alcohol Review, 26(1), 25–31.

Sinha, R., Fox, H. C., Hong, K. I., Hansen, J., Tuit, K., & Kreek, M. J. (2011). Effects of adrenal sensitivity, stress- and cue-induced craving, and anxiety on subsequent alcohol relapse and treatment outcomes. Archives of general psychiatry, 68(9), 942–952.

Skinner, M. D., & Lahmek, P. (2016). Disulfiram Efficacy in the Treatment of Alcohol Dependence: A Meta-Analysis. PLOS ONE, 11(9), e0161725.

Skowronek, M. H., Laucht, M., Hohm, E., Becker, K., & Schmidt, M. H. (2006). Interaction between the dopamine D4 receptor and the serotonin transporter promoter polymorphisms in alcohol and tobacco use among 15-year-olds. Neurogenetics, 7(4), 239–246.

Smith, D. A., & Beaumont, K. (2007). Perspective: Animal models of disease: preclinical animal models of safety and efficacy testing. Current Opinion in Pharmacology, 7(5), 469–474.

Sørensen A, Jørgensen KJ, Munkholm K. Description of antidepressant withdrawal symptoms in clinical practice guidelines on depression: A systematic review. J Affect Disord. 2022 Nov 1; 316: 177-186.

Soyka, M. (2017). Treatment of Benzodiazepine Dependence. New England Journal of Medicine, 376(12), 1147–1157.

Spencer, L., Alderson, H., Scott, S., Kaner, E., & Ling, J. (2023). 'The Addiction Was Making Things Harder for My Mental Health': A Qualitative Exploration of the Views of Adults and Adolescents Accessing a Substance Misuse Treatment Service. International journal of environmental research and public health, 20(11), 5967.

Spencer, T. J., Biederman, J., & Mick, E. (2007). Attention-deficit/hyperactivity disorder: Diagnosis, lifespan, comorbidities, and neurobiology. Journal of Pediatric Psychology, 32(6), 631–642.

Spijker, J., & Bijl, R. V. (2001). Predictors of suicidality in depressive spectrum disorders in the general population: results of the Netherlands Mental Health Survey and Incidence Study. Social Psychiatry and Psychiatric Epidemiology, 36(7), 338–345.

Spoth, R., & Greenberg, M. (2011). Impact challenges in community science-with-practice: Lessons from PROSPER on transformative practitioner–scientist partnerships and prevention infrastructure development. American Journal of Community Psychology, 48(1-2), 106–119.

Stahl, S. M. (2013). Stahl's Essential Psychopharmacology: Neuroscientific Basis and Practical Applications. Cambridge University Press.

Staley, J. K., & Krishnan-Sarin, S. (2015). Zoghbi SS. Sex differences in [123I]beta-CIT SPECT measures of dopamine and serotonin transporter availability in healthy smokers and nonsmokers. Synapse, 54(1), 20–32.

Stead, L. F., & Lancaster, T. (2012). Clonidine for smoking cessation. Cochrane Database of Systematic Reviews, (5), CD000058.

Stead, L. F., Hartmann-Boyce, J., Perera, R., & Lancaster, T. (2013). Telephone counselling for smoking cessation. Cochrane Database of Systematic Reviews, (8), CD002850.

Stead, L. F., Perera, R., Bullen, C., Mant, D., & Lancaster, T. (2008). Nicotine replacement therapy for smoking cessation. Cochrane Database of Systematic Reviews, (1), CD000146.

Stead, L. F., Perera, R., Bullen, C., Mant, D., & Lancaster, T. (2012). Nicotine replacement therapy for smoking cessation. Cochrane Database of Systematic Reviews, (11), CD000146.

Stephens, D. N., & King, S. L. (2009). Reflections on the discovery of drug withdrawal. Addiction Biology, 14(1), 1–5.

Stewart, P., Adams, J., & White, D. (2023). Shifting Social Norms and Substance Abuse: An Empirical Analysis. Social Science Research, 65(2), 102391. DOI: 10.1016/j.ssresearch.2023.102391

Stitzer, M. L., & Petry, N. M. (2006). Contingency management for treatment of substance abuse. Annual Review of Clinical Psychology, 2, 411–434.

Strang, J., McDonald, R., Alqurshi, A., Royall, P., Taylor, D., Forbes, B., & Lintzeris, N. (2019). Naloxone without the needle — Systematic review of candidate routes for non-injectable naloxone for opioid overdose reversal. Drug and Alcohol Dependence, 194, 1–7.

Strickland, J. C., Acuff, S. F. (2023). Role of social context in addiction etiology and recovery. Pharmacology Biochemistry and Behavior, 229, 173603.

Stuber, G. D., Sparta, D. R., Stamatakis, A. M., van Leeuwen, W. A., Hardjoprajitno, J. E., Cho, S., Tye, K. M., Kempadoo, K. A., Zhang, F., Deisseroth, K., & Bonci, A. (2011). Excitatory transmission from the amygdala to nucleus accumbens facilitates reward seeking. Nature, 475(7356), 377–380.

Substance Abuse and Mental Health Services Administration (SAMHSA). (2021). Key substance use and mental health indicators in the United States: Results from the 2020 National Survey on Drug Use and Health. Retrieved from https://www.samhsa.gov/data/sites/default/files/reports/rpt29393/2020NSDUHFFRPDFWHTML/2020NSDUHFFR09092022.pdf

Sulzer, D. (2011). How addictive drugs disrupt presynaptic dopamine neurotransmission. Neuron, 69(4), 628–649.

Swendsen, J., Conway, K. P., Degenhardt, L., Glantz, M., Jin, R., Merikangas, K. R., Sampson, N., & Kessler, R. C. (2010). Mental disorders as risk factors for substance use, abuse and dependence: results from the 10-year follow-up of the National Comorbidity Survey. Addiction (Abingdon, England), 105(6), 1117–1128.

Swimmer, K. R., & Sandelich, S. (2024). Substance Use Disorder. Emergency medicine clinics of North America, 42(1), 53–67.

Tammimäki, A. E., & Männistö, P. T. (2010). Are genetic variants of COMT associated with addiction? Pharmacogenetics and genomics, 20(12), 717–741.

Tan, K. R., Brown, M., Labouèbe, G., Yvon, C., Creton, C., Fritschy, J. M., Rudolph, U., & Lüscher, C. (2010). Neural bases for addictive properties of benzodiazepines. Nature, 463(7282), 769–774.

Tan, K. R., Rudolph, U., & Lüscher, C. (2011). Hooked on benzodiazepines: GABAA receptor subtypes and addiction. Trends in neurosciences, 34(4), 188–197.

Tang, Y. Y., Holzel, B. K., & Posner, M. I. (2015). The neuroscience of mindfulness meditation. Nature Reviews Neuroscience, 16(4), 213–225.

Tanti, A., & Belzung, C. (2013). Neurogenesis along the septo-temporal axis of the hippocampus: are depression and the action of antidepressants region-specific? Neuroscience, 252, 234–252.

Tanum, L., Solli, K. K., Latif, Z. E., Benth, J. Š., Opheim, A., Sharma-Haase, K., ... & Kunøe, N. (2017). Effectiveness of injectable extended-release naltrexone vs daily buprenorphine–naloxone for opioid dependence: A randomized clinical noninferiority trial. JAMA Psychiatry, 74(12), 1197–1205.

Teal, L. B., Ingram, S. M., Bubser, M., McClure, E., & Jones, C. K. (2023). The Evolving Role of Animal Models in the Discovery and Development of Novel Treatments for Psychiatric Disorders. Advances in neurobiology, 30, 37–99.

Teasdale, J. D., Segal, Z. V., Williams, J. M., Ridgeway, V. A., Soulsby, J. M., & Lau, M. A. (2000). Prevention of relapse/recurrence in major depression by mindfulness-based cognitive therapy. Journal of Consulting and Clinical Psychology, 68(4), 615–623.

Tetrault, J. M., Crothers, K., Moore, B. A., Mehra, R., Concato, J., & Fiellin, D. A. (2007). Effects of marijuana smoking on pulmonary function and respiratory complications: a systematic review. Archives of Internal Medicine, 167(3), 221–228.

Thanos, P. K., Volkow, N. D., & Freimuth, P. (2001). Overexpression of dopamine D2 receptors reduces alcohol self-administration. The Journal of Neuroscience, 21(12), RC222.

Thompson, A. J., & Lummis, S. C. (2007). 5-HT3 receptors. Current Pharmaceutical Design, 13(28), 28.

Thorsell, A., Michalkiewicz, M., Dumont, Y., Quirion, R., Caberlotto, L., Rimondini, R., Mathé, A. A., & Heilig, M. (2000). Behavioral insensitivity to restraint stress, absent fear suppression of behavior and impaired spatial learning in transgenic rats with hippocampal neuropeptide Y overexpression. Proceedings of the National Academy of Sciences of the United States of America, 97(23), 12852–12857.

Treadway, M. T., & Zald, D. H. (2011). Reconsidering anhedonia in depression: lessons from translational neuroscience. Neuroscience & Biobehavioral Reviews, 35(3), 537–555.

Trivedi, M. H., & Greer, T. L. (2014). Cognitive dysfunction in unipolar depression: Implications for treatment. Journal of Affective Disorders, 152–154, 19–27.

Trivedi, M. H., Fava, M., Wisniewski, S. R., Thase, M. E., Quitkin, F., Warden, D., Ritz, L., Nierenberg, A. A., Lebowitz, B. D., Biggs, M. M., Luther, J. F., Shores-Wilson, K., Rush, A. J., & STAR*D Study Team (2006). Medication augmentation after the failure of SSRIs for depression. The New England journal of medicine, 354(12), 1243–1252.

Trujillo, K. A. (2000). Are NMDA receptors involved in opiate-induced neural and behavioral plasticity? A review of preclinical studies. Psychopharmacology (Berl). 2000;151(2-3):121-141.

Tzschentke, T. M. (2007). Measuring reward with the conditioned place preference paradigm: a comprehensive review of drug effects, recent progress and new issues. Progress in Neurobiology, 81(3), 263–307.

Uhart, M., & Wand, G. S. (2009). Stress, alcohol and drug interaction: an update of human research. Addiction Biology, 14(1), 43–64.

Uhl, G. R., & Grow, R. W. (2004). The burden of complex genetics in brain disorders. Archives of General Psychiatry, 61(3), 223–229.

Uhl, G. R., Koob, G. F., & Cable, J. (2019). The neurobiology of addiction. Annals of the New York Academy of Sciences, 1451(1), 5–28.

Ungless, M. A., & Grace, A. A. (2012). Are you or aren't you? Challenges associated with physiologically identifying dopamine neurons. Trends in Neurosciences, 35(7), 422–430.

United Nations Office on Drugs and Crime (UNODC). (2021). World Drug Report 2021. Retrieved from https://www.unodc.org/unodc/en/data-and-analysis/wdr2021.html

Urban, M. M., Stingl, M. R., &Meinhardt, M. W. (2023). Mini-review: The neurobiology of treating substance use disorders with classical psychedelics. Frontiers in Neuroscience, 17, 1156319.

Ursini, G., Bollati, V., & Fazio, L. (2011). Tobacco smoking is associated with DNA methylation of diabetes susceptibility genes. PLoS ONE, 6(6), e20871.

Valentino, R. J., & Van Bockstaele, E. (2008). Convergence of corticotropin-releasing factor and norepinephrine and the co-ordination of stress and arousal: Focus on the locus coeruleus. Brain Research Reviews, 58(1), 160–172.

van den Brink, W., Sørensen, P., Torup, L., Mann, K., & Gual, A. (2013). Long-term efficacy, tolerability and safety of nalmefene as-needed in patients with alcohol dependence: A 1-year, randomised controlled study. Journal of Psychopharmacology, 27(8), 694–704.

van Draanen, J., & Aneshensel, C. S. (2022). Parental and own substance use disorder: The intersection of gender and early adversity. Drug and alcohol dependence, 234, 109393.

van Namen, D. M., Knapen, V., van Staa, A., de Vries, H., Hilberink, S. R., & Nagelhout, G. E. (2023). Stress and strain: a qualitative study into the impact of having relatives with addiction problems on students' health and daily lives. International journal of qualitative studies on health and well-being, 18(1), 2223864.

Vanderbilt, D., Smith, J., & Carter, M. (2022). Family Dynamics and Substance Abuse: A Longitudinal Analysis. Journal of Family Psychology, 43(2), 189-204.

Vanderschuren, L. J., & Kalivas, P. W. (2000). Alterations in dopaminergic and glutamatergic transmission in the induction and expression of behavioral sensitization: a critical review of preclinical studies. Psychopharmacology, 151(2-3), 99–120.

Vanderschuren, L. J., & Pierce, R. C. (2010). Sensitization processes in drug addiction. Current Topics in Behavioral Neurosciences, 3, 179–195.

Vargas, G., Araya, D., Sepulveda, P., Rodriguez-Fernandez, M., Friston, K. J., Sitaram, R., & El-Deredy, W. (2023). Self-regulation learning as active inference: dynamic causal modeling of an fMRI neurofeedback task. Frontiers in neuroscience, 17, 1212549.

Venniro, M., Caprioli, D., & Shaham, Y. (2016). Animal models of drug relapse and craving: From drug priming-induced reinstatement to incubation of craving after voluntary abstinence. Progress in Brain Research, 224, 25–52.

Ventura, R., & Alcaro, A. (2016). Punding as a Complication of Stimulant Use: A Review of the Literature. Clinical Neuropharmacology, 39(3), 151–161.

Verdejo-García, A., & Bechara, A. (2009). A somatic marker theory of addiction. Neuropharmacology, 56 Suppl 1(Suppl 1), 48–62.

Verdejo-García, A., Lawrence, A. J., & Clark, L. (2008). Impulsivity as a vulnerability marker for substance-use disorders: review of findings from high-risk research, problem gamblers and genetic association studies. Neuroscience and biobehavioral reviews, 32(4), 777–810.

Verdejo-García, A., Pérez-García, M., & Bechara, A. (2006). Emotion, decision-making and substance dependence: A somatic-marker model of addiction. Current Neuropharmacology, 4(1), 17–31.

Vermeulen, I., Isin, E. M., Barton, P., Cillero-Pastor, B., & Heeren, R. M. A. (2022). Multimodal molecular imaging in drug discovery and development. Drug discovery today, 27(8), 2086–2099.

Verovnik, B., Khachatryan, E., Šuput, D., & Van Hulle, M. M. (2023). Effects of risk factors on longitudinal changes in brain structure and function in the progression of AD. Alzheimer's & dementia: the journal of the Alzheimer's Association, 19(6), 2666–2676.

Vezina, P., & Leyton, M. (2009). Conditioning and sensitization to psychostimulants in humans. Current Opinion in Neurobiology, 19(4), 281–286.

Volkow, N. D., & Blanco, C. (2020). The changing opioid crisis: development, challenges and opportunities. Molecular Psychiatry, 25(2), 268-279.

Volkow, N. D., & Fowler, J. S. (2000). Addiction, a disease of compulsion and drive: Involvement of the orbitofrontal cortex. Cerebral Cortex, 10(3), 318–325.

Volkow, N. D., & Morales, M. (2015). The Brain on Drugs: From Reward to Addiction. Cell,162(4): 712-725.

Volkow, N. D., & Muenke, M. (2012). The Genetics of Addiction. Human Genetics, 131(6): 773–777.

Volkow, N. D., Fowler, J. S., Wang, G. J., & Swanson, J. M. (2004). Dopamine in drug abuse and addiction: results from imaging studies and treatment implications. Molecular Psychiatry, 9(6), 557–569.

Volkow, N. D., Fowler, J. S., Wang, G. J., Swanson, J. M., & Telang, F. (2007). Dopamine in drug abuse and addiction: results of imaging studies and treatment implications. Archives of neurology, 64(11), 1575–1579.

Volkow, N. D., Jones, E. B., Einstein, E. B., Wargo, E. M., & Liedtke, W. (2019). Addiction: Beyond dopamine reward circuitry. Proceedings of the National Academy of Sciences, 116(8), 2815-2822.

Volkow, N. D., Koob, G. F., & McLellan, A. T. (2016). Neurobiologic Advances from the Brain Disease Model of Addiction. New England Journal of Medicine, 374(4), 363-371.

Volkow, N. D., Koob, G. F., & McLellan, A. T. (2016). Neurobiologic Advances from the Brain Disease Model of Addiction. New England Journal of Medicine, 374(4), 363–371.

Volkow, N. D., Michaelides, M., & Baler, R. (2019). The Neuroscience of Drug Reward and Addiction. Physiological reviews, 99(4), 2115–2140.

Volkow, N. D., Swanson, J. M., & Baler, R. D. (2015). Understanding the Effects of Stimulant Medications on Cognition in Individuals with Attention-Deficit Hyperactivity Disorder: A Decade of Progress. Neuropsychopharmacology, 40(1), 211–221.

Volkow, N. D., Wang, G. J., Fowler, J. S., & Telang, F. (2008). Overlapping neuronal circuits in addiction and obesity: evidence of systems pathology. Philosophical Transactions of the Royal Society B: Biological Sciences, 363(1507), 3191–3200

Vollenweider, F. X., & Kometer, M. (2010). The neurobiology of psychedelic drugs: implications for the treatment of mood disorders. Nature Reviews Neuroscience, 11(9), 642–651.

Vrieze, E., Demyttenaere, K., Bruffaerts, R., Hermans, D., Pizzagalli, D. A., Sienaert, P., Hompes, T., de Boer, P., Schmidt, M., & Claes, S. (2014). Dimensions in major depressive disorder and their relevance for treatment outcome. Journal of affective disorders, 155, 35–41.

Vyas, A., Mitra, R., Shankaranarayana Rao, B. S., & Chattarji, S. (2002). Chronic stress induces contrasting patterns of dendritic remodeling in hippocampal and amygdaloid neurons. Journal of Neuroscience, 22(15), 6810–6818.

Wade, N. E., Sullivan, R. M., Tapert, S. F., Pelham, W. E., 3rd, Huestis, M. A., Lisdahl, K. M., & Haist, F. (2023). Concordance between substance use self-report and hair analysis in community-based adolescents. The American journal of drug and alcohol abuse, 49(1), 76–84.

Wadsley, M., & Ihssen, N. (2023). A Systematic Review of Structural and Functional MRI Studies Investigating Social Networking Site Use. Brain Science, 13(5), 787.

Walker, B. M., & Koob, G. F. (2008). Pharmacological evidence for a motivational role of κ-opioid systems in ethanol dependence. Neuropsychopharmacology, 33(3), 643–652.

Walter, H., Ramskogler, K., Semler, B., Lesch, O. M., & Platz, W. (2001). Dopamine and alcohol relapse: D1 and D2 antagonists increase relapse rates in animal studies and in clinical trials. Journal of biomedical science, 8(1), 83–88.

Wang, J. C., Hinrichs, A. L., & Stock, H. (2004). Evidence of common and specific genetic effects: Association of the muscarinic acetylcholine receptor M2 (CHRM2) gene with alcohol dependence and major depressive syndrome. Human Molecular Genetics, 13(17), 1903–1911.

Wang, J., Carnicella, S., Phamluong, K., Jeanblanc, J., Ronesi, J. A., Chaudhri, N., Janak, P. H., Lovinger, D. M., & Ron, D. (2007). Ethanol induces long-term facilitation of NR2B-NMDA receptor activity in the dorsal striatum: implications for alcohol drinking behavior. The Journal of neuroscience: the official journal of the Society for Neuroscience, 27(13), 3593–3602.

Wang, L., Gao, M., Wang, Q., Sun, L., Younus, M., Ma, S., Liu, C., Shi, L., Lu, Y., Zhou, B., Sun, S., Chen, G., Li, J., Zhang, Q., Zhu, F., Wang, C., & Zhou, Z. (2023). Cocaine induces locomotor sensitization through a dopamine-dependent VTA-mPFC-FrA cortico-cortical pathway in male mice. Nature Communications, 14(1), 1568.

Wang, Q., Zhao, S., He, Z., Zhang, S., Jiang, X., Zhang, T., Liu, T., Liu, C., & Han, J. (2023). Modeling functional difference between gyri and sulci within intrinsic connectivity networks. Cerebral cortex (New York, N.Y.: 1991), 33(4), 933–947.

Wang, T. Y., Lu, R. B., Lee, S. Y., Chang, Y. H., Chen, S. L., Tsai, T. Y., Tseng, H. H., Chen, P. S., Chen, K. C., Yang, Y. K., & Hong, J. S. (2023). Association Between Inflammatory Cytokines, Executive Function, and Substance Use in Patients With Opioid Use Disorder and Amphetamine-Type Stimulants Use Disorder. The international journal of neuropsychopharmacology, 26(1), 42–51.

Wang, Y., Li, Q., & Zhang, H. (2023). Urban-Rural Disparities in Substance Abuse: A Comprehensive Analysis. Drug and Alcohol Dependence, 231(2), 12-24.

Watts, A. L., Latzman, R. D., Boness, C. L., Kotov, R., Keyser-Marcus, L., DeYoung, C. G., Krueger, R. F., Zald, D. H., Moeller, F. G., & Ramey, T. (2023). New approaches to deep phenotyping in addictions. Psychology of addictive behaviors: journal of the Society of Psychologists in Addictive Behaviors, 37(3), 361–375.

Wee, S., Mandyam, C. D., Lekic, D. M., & Koob, G. F. (2008). Alpha 1-noradrenergic system role in increased motivation for cocaine intake in rats with prolonged access. European neuropsychopharmacology: the journal of the European College of Neuropsychopharmacology, 18(4), 303–311.

Wei, Z. X., Wu, Q., Liu, Q. S., & Cheng, Y. (2020). Neurotransmitter system aberrations in patients with drug addiction. Journal of neural transmission (Vienna, Austria: 1996), 127(12), 1641–1650.

Weinshenker, D., & Schroeder, J. P. (2007). There and back again: a tale of norepinephrine and drug addiction. Neuropsychopharmacology, 32(7), 1433–1451.

Whittaker, R., McRobbie, H., Bullen, C., Rodgers, A., & Gu, Y. (2016). Mobile phone-based interventions for smoking cessation. Cochrane Database of Systematic Reviews, (4), CD006611.

Wilens, T. E., Biederman, J., Spencer, T. J., & Prince, J. (2006). Pharmacotherapy of adult ADHD: Nonstimulant medications. The Primary Care Companion to the Journal of Clinical Psychiatry, 8(6), 366–376.

Williams, J. T., Ingram, S. L., Henderson, G., Chavkin, C., von Zastrow, M., Schulz, S., Koch, T., Evans, C. J., & Christie, M. J. (2013). Regulation of μ-opioid receptors: desensitization, phosphorylation, internalization, and tolerance. Pharmacological reviews, 65(1), 223–254.

Wilson JB, Epstein M, Lopez B, Brown AK, Lutfy K, Friedman TC. The role of Neurochemicals, Stress Hormones and Immune System in the Positive Feedback Loops between Diabetes, Obesity and Depression. Front Endocrinol (Lausanne). 2023 Aug 17; 14: 1224612.

Wise, R. A. (2004). Dopamine, learning and motivation. Nature Reviews Neuroscience, 5(6), 483-494.

Wise, R. A., & Koob, G. F. (2014). The development and maintenance of drug addiction. Neuropsychopharmacology, 39(2), 254–262.

Wise, R. A., & Robble, M. A. (2020). Dopamine and Addiction. Annual review of psychology, 71, 79–106.

Witkiewitz, K., Lustyk, M. K. B., & Bowen, S. (2013). Retraining the addicted brain: a review of hypothesized neurobiological mechanisms of mindfulness-based relapse prevention. Psychology of addictive behaviors: journal of the Society of Psychologists in Addictive Behaviors, 27(2), 351–365.

Witkiewitz, K., Marlatt, G. A., & Walker, D. (2005). Mindfulness-based relapse prevention for alcohol and substance use disorders. Journal of Cognitive Psychotherapy, 19(3), 211–228.

Wolf, M. E. (2016). Synaptic mechanisms underlying persistent cocaine craving. Nature Reviews Neuroscience, 17(6), 351-365.

Wolitzky-Taylor K. (2023). Integrated behavioral treatments for comorbid anxiety and substance use disorders: A model for understanding integrated treatment approaches and meta-analysis to evaluate their efficacy. Drug and alcohol dependence, 253, 110990.

Woodward, D., Wilens, T. E., Glantz, M., Rao, V., Burke, C., & Yule, A. M. (2023). A systematic review of substance use screening in outpatient behavioral health settings. Addiction Science & Clinical Practice, 18(1), 18.

World Health Organization. (2021). Tobacco. Retrieved from https://www.who.int/news-room/fact-sheets/detail/tobacco

Xuan, J., Zhao, X., He, G., Yu, L., Wang, L., Tang, W., Li, X., Gu, N., Feng, G., Xing, Q., & He, L. (2008). Effects of the dopamine D3 receptor (DRD3) gene polymorphisms on risperidone response: a pharmacogenetic study. Neuropsychopharmacology: official publication of the American College of Neuropsychopharmacology, 33(2), 305–311.

Yang, S., Wang, K., Gregory, B., Berrettini, W., Wang, L. S., Hakonarson, H., & Bucan, M. (2009). Genomic landscape of a three-generation pedigree segregating affective disorder. PloS one, 4(2), e4474.

You, I. J., Wright, S. R., Garcia-Garcia, A. L., Tapper, A. R., Gardner, P. D., Koob, G. F., David Leonardo, E., Bohn, L. M., & Wee, S. (2016). 5-HT1A Autoreceptors in the Dorsal Raphe Nucleus Convey Vulnerability to Compulsive Cocaine Seeking. Neuropsychopharmacology: official publication of the American College of Neuropsychopharmacology, 41(5), 1210–1222. https://doi.org/10.1038/npp.2015.268

Zepf, F. D., & Wöckel, L. (2016). Serotonergic modulation of ADHD: Effects of l - 5-HTP and fluoxetine. Human Psychopharmacology: Clinical and Experimental, 31(2), 127–134.

Zhang, W., Liu, Y., Dong, Y., He, W., Yao, S., Xu, Z., & Mu, Y. (2023). How we learn social norms: a three-stage model for social norm learning. Frontiers in psychology, 14, 1153809.

Zhu, Y., Wang, K., Ma, T., Ji, Y., Lou, Y., Fu, X., Lu, Y., Liu, Y., Dang, W., Zhang, Q., Yin, F., Wang, K., Yu, B., Zhang, H., Lai, J., Wang, Y. (2023). Nucleus accumbens D1/D2 circuits control opioid withdrawal symptoms in mice. Journal of Clinical Investigations, 133(18), e163266.

Zhuo, L. Y., Huang, P., Fan, H. Z., Wu, J. J., Wang, Y., Ye, X. Y., & Yu, R. B. (2019). Study on thyroid hormone levels and influence factors in drug users in a drug rehabilitation center in Jiangsu province. Zhonghua liuxingbingxue zazhi, 40(9), 1134–1138.

Zill, P., Büttner, A., & Eisenmenger, W. (2007). Analysis of tryptophan hydroxylase I and II mRNA expression in the human brain: A post-mortem study. PLoS ONE, 2(12), e573.

Zschucke, E., Gaudlitz, K., & Ströhle, A. (2013). Exercise and physical activity in mental disorders: clinical and experimental evidence. Journal of preventive medicine and public health = Yebang Uihakhoe chi, 46 Suppl 1(Suppl 1), S12–S21.

Zubieta, J. K., Smith, Y. R., Bueller, J. A., Xu, Y., Kilbourn, M. R., Jewett, D. M., Meyer, C. R., Koeppe, R. A., & Stohler, C. S. (2001). Regional mu opioid receptor regulation of sensory and affective dimensions of pain. Science (New York, N.Y.), 293(5528), 311–315.